K

61

PRODUCTIVE AGING

PRODUCTIVE

AGING

Concepts and Challenges

Edited by

Nancy Morrow-Howell, James Hinterlong,

and Michael Sherraden

THE JOHNS HOPKINS UNIVERSITY PRESS
Baltimore & London

© 2001 The Johns Hopkins University Press
All rights reserved. Published 2001
Printed in the United States of America on acid-free paper
2 4 6 8 9 7 5 3 1

The Johns Hopkins University Press
2715 North Charles Street
Baltimore, Maryland 21218-4363
www.press.jhu.edu

Library of Congress Cataloging-in-Publication Data

Productive aging : concepts and challenges / edited by Nancy Morrow-Howell,
James Hinterlong, and Michael Sherraden.
p.   cm.
Includes bibliographical references and index.
ISBN 0-8018-6557-3 (hard : alk. paper)
1. Aged. 2. Life span, Productive. I. Morrow-Howell, Nancy, 1952–
II. Hinterlong, James, 1970–   III. Sherraden, Michael W. (Michael Wayne), 1948–
HQ1061 .P777 2001
305.26—dc21   00-010213

A catalog record for this book is available from the British Library.

CONTENTS

III

EMERGENT THEORIES IN GERONTOLOGY

IV

FUTURE DIRECTIONS IN PRACTICE, THEORY, AND RESEARCH

FOREWORD

Will 69 million baby boomers suddenly drop out of the workforce when they turn 65? It is difficult to imagine this generation, with its talent, education, and experience, idling away the last 30 years of life.

In the 1950s, sociologist Ernest Burgess wrote that older people's lives were notably "roleless." Little progress has been made since then. Today, the issue takes on new urgency as the average life expectancy rises to 76.6 and evidence suggests a cause-and-effect relationship among health, productivity, and longevity. Studies begun in 1955 by the National Institutes of Health have demonstrated that older people who have goals and structure have a better chance of living longer. Thus, health supports productivity and productivity encourages health. Productive aging would appear to be in the best interests of both society and the individual.

In 1982, the concept of productive aging was developed at a seminar in Salzburg. Herbert Gleason, James Birren, Alvar Svanborg, Betty Friedan, and I, among others, explored the variety of ways in which older people can continue to contribute to society. That same year, I was asked to give testimony before the National Commission for Social Security Reform, in my capacity as director of the National Institute on Aging. Chairperson Alan Greenspan asked me to comment on the practicality of Americans retiring at age 65, given that our life expectancy has risen substantially since the passage of Social Security in 1935. His point was well taken: there is no logical reason why people must automatically retire at 65. However, unless jobs exist, older Americans cannot be productively employed. Unless the Age Discrimination in Employment law is strictly enforced, they will not be hired. Finally, unless they remain in reasonably good health, older persons will not be able to work.

Extending the productive work life requires extensive education, research, and policy initiatives. Investments must be made today in biomedical and behavioral research, particularly research on aging and studies that help people compensate for disabilities. Programs of health promotion and disease prevention must be undertaken and affordable geriatric care developed.

Employers must be educated in the importance of continuing worker education and sabbaticals so the workforce can retool and upgrade skills throughout life. Accommodations will have to be made to reflect the specific ergonomic requirements and changing physical capabilities of older workers. Flexible and phased retirement options need to be examined.

Imaginative social solutions will be necessary, and we can learn from the experiences of other societies. For example, Japan has provided employer subsidies to retain or hire older workers. In the United States, Medicare might become the first payer of health care costs after 55 years of age, which would lower the costs of hiring older employees.

In the latter part of the twentieth century, we saw a range of efforts to secure human rights. However, we have yet to establish strong legislative and institutional efforts against ageism, nor have we fully implemented human rights as they relate to old age itself. Perhaps future historians will view the past century as an incubator that helped the longevity revolution reach fruition in the century that followed.

Before the twenty-first century is over, we will begin to celebrate the remarkable human achievement of longevity, enhanced by biological and societal advancement. People will enjoy the blessings of gene-based and regenerative medicine. They will gain control over the consequences of gene-related pathology and receive replacement parts for impaired organs, cells, and tissues. New work patterns will emerge that include significant roles for older Americans, in both the paid and the voluntary sectors.

The twenty-first century will become the century of productive old age, but clearly we must be prepared. *Productive Aging* explores the subject in depth, and as such, I find it to be an extremely valuable addition to the literature. Nancy Morrow-Howell, James Hinterlong, and Michael Sherraden have drawn together an impressive array of distinguished scholars, whose keen insights on a variety of important issues illuminate and challenge the reader. The serious analysis of productive aging in our society is very well served by this excellent volume.

Robert N. Butler, M.D.
Professor of Geriatrics and Adult Development,
The Mount Sinai Medical Center
President and CEO, International Longevity Center-US

PREFACE AND ACKNOWLEDGMENTS

The concept of productive aging is of great importance worldwide because of the confluence of three large trends, one demographic, one economic, and one social/cultural. The demographic trend is that more people are living longer, healthier lives. Many people now live into their 70s, 80s, and 90s fit in mind and body, and a large portion of this older population would prefer to be engaged in society and making useful contributions. The economic trend is that information age technologies are changing the way we think about productivity. No longer is it necessary to bend one's back or work in an industrial setting to be productive. Indeed, the most economically productive work is now related to the creation and application of human capital rather than to the operations of plants and machinery. There are multiple implications of this transition, and one is that older people can participate in information age economy as easily as younger people. The social/cultural trend is that older people may be less inclined to retire into near-total leisure in their later years. For example, a 1998 survey by the AARP found that 80 percent of baby boomers in the United States plan to keep working at least part-time after retirement age; this would be a marked change from the current pattern. These trends require that, as a society, we think and act differently about being "old." Yet we have only barely begun to do so. Productive aging is an effort to come to a better understanding of involvement in the society and/or economy as one option during the later years.

Although the concept of productive aging has been with us for close to 20 years, most of the writing on the topic has been to advance an advocacy agenda, challenging the prevailing myth that later life is a period of frailty, disengagement, and consumption of resources. As questions arose about the process and outcomes of various forms of productivity in later life, the advocacy agenda has begun to shift to a research agenda. However, rigorous scholarship on the topic has to date been limited, advanced by only a handful of researchers. A body of literature has begun to take shape, but its boundaries are still diffuse and it is developing without the advantages of commonly accepted definitions and guiding theoretical frameworks.

Symposium

In an effort to improve and coalesce scholarship on productive aging, we assembled a group of prominent gerontologists to offer their best thinking about the concept of productive aging. These contributors were chosen because of their eminence in the psychology of aging, the sociology of aging, the economics of aging, the biomedicine of aging, and the history of gerontology as well as their leadership in gerontological theory development. We asked them to discuss the promises and pitfalls of the concept of productive aging and to offer disciplinary and interdisciplinary theoretical perspectives to guide scholarship.

In his opening remarks at the symposium on "Perspectives on Productive Aging," Harry Moody said that the meeting was like a family reunion. Indeed, many of the leading scholars in gerontology in the United States were in the room. Together, the "family" of authors in this book has done so much to shape academic gerontology, and several of the family members have quite literally defined productive aging.

The symposium was sometimes marked by intense discussions, but our overall sense was that differences were often exaggerated. It is inherent in academic life to debate opposing concepts and ideas, but in the effort to make a particular point, this can sometimes be overly simplistic. For example, we found exaggerated differences in discussions of individual versus collective, market versus state, and freedom versus coercion. It is inevitable and indeed essential to go through this dichotomizing and debating process, but at the end of the day, if this work is to move forward, we will have to develop more complex mental frames and live with greater ambiguities. Regarding the dichotomies listed above, they are in fact more complementary than they are trade-offs. For example, individual choices are in large part defined and regulated by collective public policies. In fact, we found at the symposium a rather surprising degree of agreement on fundamental matters, including the multidimensionality of productive aging, the importance of multiple and diverse opportunities, and the value of choice.

Symposium papers were excellent and discussions were fruitful. It is always a challenge to present ideas and theories and discuss across disciplines, and we knew this at the outset, but we decided to take the risk because the potential benefits, should the meeting be successful, would be great. In a new area of scholarship and practice, where little is established, interdisciplinary exchange and cross-fertilization hold great potential.

The Center for Social Development (CSD) at the George Warren Brown School of Social Work, Washington University, sponsored the meeting. Productive aging is consistent with the center's mission, which is to look for ways in which social research and policy can build capacities of individuals, families, and communities to lead richer lives and, insofar as possible, solve their own problems. At CSD, we intend to use this symposium as a beginning point for a program of research and policy innovation in productive aging.

Organization of the Book

We begin the book with an introductory chapter that summarizes the history of the scholarship of productive aging, highlights the underlying tensions and value issues, and reviews the specific research efforts that have contributed to the literature. In Chapter 2, Andrew Achenbaum places productive aging within the American historical context. He points out that, from its earliest days, society has attended to the productive capacities and engagement of its older members. The changes in social welfare policy following the Great Depression and World War II significantly dampened public and scholarly interest in the productivity of those in later life and formed the now-normative link between old age and leisure—one that no longer serves the purpose for which it was engineered. Achenbaum concludes that we should aim to renew positive images of later life and the productive potential and contributions of older adults.

In Chapter 3, Scott Bass and Francis Caro provide a thorough review of the current state of knowledge on productive aging and an overview of a selection of theories that have relevance for understanding various forms of productive aging. They also offer a revision of their conceptual framework, which was first published in 1996 (Theoretical perspectives on productive aging, in W. H. Crown [Ed.], *Handbook on employment and the elderly.* [pp. 262–275]. Westport, CT: Greenwood). Their conceptual mapping identifies factors influencing individual participation in productive activities in five sectors: environmental, individual, social policy, situational, and outcomes. After defining the scope and nature of each sector, Bass and Caro turn their attention to the effects of public policy on participation in productive activities. They conclude by identifying directions for policy that could increase productive involvement by older adults.

Disciplinary Perspectives on Productive Aging. In each of the next four chapters (4–7), scholars from core social science fields advance a disciplinary review of and directions for scholarship on productive aging. Physician and medical researcher Alvar Svanborg authors the initial chapter in this series, which looks at productive aging from a biomedical perspective. He uses life expectancy data and what is known of age-related physiological changes in the human body as a backdrop for the concept of reactivation. While distinguishing between the effects of exogenous factors, such as lifestyle, and those of aging itself, Svanborg shows how appropriate, timely intervention can enable individuals to maintain or recover functioning and postpone the onset of age-related dysfunction well into later life. He also suggests that productive behavior may in fact contribute to the postponement of age-related physiological decline.

Psychologist James Birren opens his chapter by exploring the motivations of those who call for greater attention to be paid to productive aging. He then presents a constructive critique of current definitions of productive aging, and advances a provocative reformulation of the term to include the creation and dissemination of ideas. These alterations coincide under the concept of the life portfolio, which reflects an individual's chosen distribution of time, energy, and concerns. Noting the difficulty of assigning economic value to these concepts, Birren suggests that it may be necessary to view the consequences of an individual's portfolio investment in terms of the physical and mental health of society in addition to the traditionally measured monetized effects. Thus, in Birren's framework, an individual's net use of resources is an important consideration, but equally important are the extended consequences of that person's actions. Included in these extended consequences are the intergenerational effects of current actions on the productivity of current and future generations, as is seen in the impact of parents' education on their children. Birren concludes with a call for greater interdisciplinary collaboration in research on productive aging.

Contributing from the discipline of sociology, Brent Taylor and Vern Bengtson present an extensive overview of theories and paradigms that have been applied to the study of aging. From these, they identify those most likely to inform and improve research on productive aging. They cite the pressing need for research that uses theoretical perspectives to predict relationships and explain findings, and call for greater attention to cumulative theory development in this work. Emphasizing the importance of the societal context in shaping productivity in later life, Taylor and Bengtson challenge researchers to acknowledge the different realities experienced by various segments of the older adult population. They conclude that careful consideration of the sociological significance of productive aging will ensure that the concept has greater application in addressing the needs of an increasingly heterogeneous aging population.

In Chapter 7, James Schulz opens with an interpretation of the changing political face of aging in the United States, which has led in part to the call for attention to productive aging. He then extends a more traditional economic treatment of productivity by older adults by employing four frames to understand the issues associated with this changing politicized image of later life: age as buffer, the importance of national savings, reallocation of responsibilities and leisure across the life course, and the semantic challenges presented by focusing on productivity. Following an elaboration of these perspectives, he concludes that the economic roles for older adults and the policies associated with those roles are and are likely to remain ambiguous. Moreover, he asserts, the national economy simply does not need older adults to be employed in greater numbers. Therefore, we must look beyond simple economic assessments of what population aging will mean for the nation and begin to recognize the potential for later life to be a period of reflection and pursuit of personally meaningful activity.

Emergent Theories in Gerontology. The third section of the volume highlights provocative assessments of productive aging by proponents of three emergent perspectives on aging. Each chapter in this series identifies promises and pitfalls of the concept. In doing so, these authors raise important questions related to the assumptions and values underlying the concept.

Harry Moody explores the potential of productive aging by placing it alongside three other emergent perspectives: successful aging, radical aging, and conscious aging. Successful aging focuses our attention on the health of the individual. Radical aging is an attempt to place social justice and equality at the fore of society's social welfare agenda. Conscious aging encourages individuals to engage in personal growth and consciousness expansion to achieve meaning as they age. Along with successful aging, he proposes that the productive aging perspective is likely to help shape future, positive images of aging. Moody states that productive aging emphasizes generativity, market efficiency, and achievement through personal growth and social contribution. He finds promise in extending opportunities for productive engagement to older adults, but then cautions that greater attention to late-life productivity could lead society to obligate older adults to productive activities to the exclusion of other fulfilling, meaningful, and self-directed pursuits.

In the next chapter, Carroll Estes and Jane Mahakian evaluate productive aging from a political economy perspective. They assert that an emphasis on productivity, with roots in capitalist principles, will further marginalize and devalue historically disadvantaged segments of the older adult population, such as women and minorities. Estes and Mahakian charge that productive aging must not neglect the central importance of social and economic class in shaping the possibilities of later life. They also see significant political, economic, and social barriers to the efforts of productive aging proponents to reframe the activities and contributions of older adults in order to "redeem old age itself." They ask for whom productive aging, a seemingly individualistic concept, is relevant, and how the answer to that question will change with increasing social and economic inequality. In the light of these concerns, they conclude that community and social institutional responsibility are necessary components of any effort to promote that productive aging.

James Jackson concludes this section by using longitudinal data taken from the Americans' Changing Lives Study to present empirical evidence that highlights the differential influence of race, gender, age, and education on productive engagement within three economic networks: regular, irregular, and social. Proceeding from a life course perspective and a set of theoretical propositions concerning the influence of these factors on productive behavior, Jackson shows that blacks and whites, and men and women vary significantly over time on their level, pattern, and type of engagement. Moreover, education and age appear to have interactive effects on these relationships. His findings offer a valuable conceptual and methodological framework for investigating the influence of race, gender, age, and education on individual patterns of activity.

Future Directions in Practice, Theory, and Research. The final section of the volume comprises three chapters. The first, by Marc Freedman, highlights the manner in which community-based programs across the country provide opportunities for productive aging. Freedman demonstrates how older adults are actively seeking out and creating opportunities for productive engagement. Through these efforts, they alter the structures of opportunity available to those in later life. He concludes that greater public-private partnerships can enhance and expand these efforts to include a larger number of older adults.

In Chapter 12, we evaluate the current state of conceptual and theoretical development on productive aging, as evidenced in the preceding chapters. We offer suggestions for future theory building. We then present a model of productivity in later life in which individuals with varying sociodemographic characteristics, capacities, and resources link to productive roles. Institutions are seen to encourage or inhibit this linking process by providing or restricting information, incentives, and access for these roles, or by facilitating participation. Public policy is presented as the key exogenous factor influencing these institution capacities. When an individual expends resources in the performance of a market-based activity, nonmarket activity with economic value, informal social assistance (caregiving), or formal social and civic activity, the behavior is productive. The model includes the effects of this productive behavior on individuals, families, and society. This model may be useful for identifying areas of applied research and guiding the formation of specific hypotheses.

The volume concludes with a proposed research agenda. We suggest that a multidimensional research agenda is achievable and necessary, if work on productivity in later life is to advance. We include a discussion of the implicit values and assumptions behind the traditional conceptualizations of productive aging, and offer a preliminary research agenda on late-life productivity.

Looking Ahead

This volume represents a collective effort to critically evaluate, clarify, and construct ways of thinking about productive opportunity and action during later life. Our aim is to provide direction for theory building and research on productive aging via the identification of useful concepts, articulation of cautions, and presentation of research questions that might guide future scholarship. We hope that the volume will serve as a catalyst for scholarship and application that extends the biology of successful aging into the social policy of productive aging (Butler, R. N., Oberlink, M. R., & Schechter, M. [Eds.]. [1990]. *The promise of productive aging: From biology to public policy.* New York: Springer). The intellectual challenges ahead can be boiled down to making theoretical choices for undertaking this work, specifying theories so they are testable, formulating and carrying out research agendas, and translating knowledge into policy and practice. This is a lot to do, and note that both theories and research agendas are stated in the plural. Like most applied social science, there is unlikely to be a Holy Grail or a singular idea that will guide productive aging scholarship and practice in the years ahead.

Acknowledgments

We are grateful for the support of the funders of the symposium, "Perspectives on Productive Aging," which led to this volume. They are the National Institute on Aging; the George Warren Brown School of Social Work at Washington University; the Center for Social Development, with funds from the Ford Foundation; and Mrs. John F. (Mary) Roatch.

Special thanks go to Sid Stahl of the National Institute on Aging and Dean Shanti Khinduka of the George Warren Brown School of Social Work for their guidance and support in planning the meeting.

We are grateful to faculty members from Washington University who provided thoughtful responses to the papers and contributed to the rich discussion. They are Martha Storandt, Professor of Psychology; David Carr, Associate Professor of Geriatric Medicine; Letha Chadiha, Associate Professor of Social Work; and Martha Ozawa, Betty Boefinger Brown Professor of Social Policy.

We thank Philip Rozario, a doctoral student at the George Warren Brown School of Social Work, for his considerable assistance with the symposium and this volume. Also, a team of masters' students helped organize and carry out the symposium; they are Kathy McDougall, Melanie Morris, Stacy Rousch, and Di Warner. Thanks also to Hong Li for her assistance. Karen Edwards at the Center for Social Development assisted with travel and other arrangements.

We appreciated the guidance and support of Bob Binstock, consulting editor for the Johns Hopkins University Press. Wendy Harris, senior acquisitions editor, and reviewers at the Johns Hopkins University Press greatly improved the quality of the volume with their comments and suggestions.

CONTRIBUTORS

W. Andrew Achenbaum, Ph.D., is Dean of the College of Liberal Arts and Social Sciences as well as Professor of History at the University of Houston. Previously, he was associated with the Institute of Gerontology at the University of Michigan. Dr. Achenbaum currently chairs the National Council on the Aging.

Scott A. Bass, Ph.D., is Dean of the Graduate School and Vice Provost for Research at the University of Maryland, Baltimore County. He founded the Gerontology Institute at the University of Massachusetts Boston. He organized a major conference on productive aging in 1990 and edited the volume resulting from that conference, *Achieving a Productive Aging Society* (1993).

Vern L. Bengtson, Ph.D., is Professor of Sociology and AARP/University Professor of Gerontology at the University of Southern California. He is past President of the Gerontological Society of America and has been granted a MERIT award for research from the National Institute of Aging. Recently he published *The Handbook on the Theories of Aging* (1999) with K. Warner Schaie.

James E. Birren, Ph.D., is Founding Dean of the Andrus Gerontology Center at the University of Southern California and the first Director of the Borun Center for Gerontological Research at UCLA. Currently he is Associate Director, UCLA Center on Aging. He has served as the Chief of the Section on Aging of the National Institute of Mental Health, as President of the Gerontological Society of America, and as President of the Division on Adult Development and Aging of the American Psychological Association.

Francis G. Caro, Ph.D., is Director of the Gerontology Institute and Professor of Gerontology at the University of Massachusetts Boston. He coedited *Achieving a Productive Aging Society* (1993) with Scott Bass. More recently, Dr.

Caro coauthored *Personal Assistance: The Future of Home Care* (1998) with Robert Morris and John Hansan.

Carroll L. Estes, Ph.D., is the Founder and first Director of the Institute for Health & Aging (IHA) and Professor of Sociology at the Department of Social and Behavioral Sciences and School of Nursing at the University of California, San Francisco (UCSF). Dr. Estes is past President of the Gerontological Society of America, the American Society on Aging, and the Association for Gerontology in Higher Education.

Marc Freedman, M.B.A., is President of Civic Ventures and Co-Founder of Experience Corps, a program that mobilizes older adults to serve children in school and community organizations. He recently completed the book *Prime Time: How Baby Boomers Will Revolutionize Retirement and Transform America* (2000). His earlier book, *The Kindness of Strangers*, was described by the *Los Angeles Times* as the "definitive book on the mentoring movement."

James Hinterlong, M.S.W., is a Ph.D. student at the George Warren Brown School of Social Work at Washington University in St. Louis. He was awarded an AARP Andrus Fellowship for predoctoral work on productive aging. He currently is a research associate at the Center for Social Development and serves on the public policy committee for the St. Louis Alzheimer's Association as well as the Project Research Team of the national OASIS Health Stages program.

James S. Jackson, Ph.D., is Director and Senior Research Scientist at the Research Center for Group Dynamics, Institute for Social Research, Director of the Center for Afroamerican and African Studies, and Faculty Associate at the Institute of Gerontology, the University of Michigan. He is past Chair of the GSA Section on Behavioral and Social Sciences and the Social Psychology Training Program at the University of Michigan.

Jane L. Mahakian, Ph.D., is Principal of Pacific Senior Services, a geriatric case management service that specializes in older adults with memory loss. She is a Visiting Adjunct Professor at the University of California, San Francisco, Institute for Health and Aging, and is past Director of the UCSF Elder Care Referral Program. She also consults to assisted living facilities and conducts corporate seminars on elder care, work/life issues, and healthy aging.

Harry R. Moody, Ph.D., is National Program Director of the Faith in Action Program with the Robert Wood Johnson Foundation. He is the Co-Founder and past Executive Director of the Brookdale Center on Aging at Hunter College in New York. He is Vice Chairman of the board of Elderhostel.

Nancy Morrow-Howell, Ph.D., is Associate Professor and Chair of the Ph.D. program at the George Warren Brown School of Social Work at Washington University in St. Louis. She is a national mentor for the Hartford Geriatric Scholars Program, the past Practice Concepts Editor for *The Gerontologist*, and the past Vice President of the Association for Gerontology in Social Work Education.

Philip Rozario, M.S.W., is a Ph.D. student at the George Warren Brown School of Social Work at Washington University in St. Louis. He is Project Coordinator for the Post-Hospital Service Use by Depressed Elders Project at the Center of Mental Health Services Research. His academic interest area is family caregiving.

James H. Schulz, Ph.D., is Emeritus Professor of Economics and the former Kirstein Professor of Aging Policy and Associate Dean for Faculty Affairs at the Florence Heller Graduate School, Brandeis University. Dr. Schulz is past President of the Gerontological Society of America and Founding Fellow of the National Academy on Social Insurance.

Michael Sherraden, Ph.D., is Benjamin E. Youngdahl Professor of Social Development and Founding Director of the Center for Social Development at Washington University in St. Louis. He has extensively studied youth services and worked on policy initiatives that contributed to the creation of AmeriCorps in 1993. With this work on productive aging, he is extending his focus to service across the life span.

Alvar Svanborg, M.D., Ph.D., is Emeritus Professor of Medicine and the Beth Fowler Vitoux and George E. Vitoux Distinguished Professor of Geriatric Medicine, Former Chief of the section of Geriatric Medicine, and Clinical Director of Research in Gerontology at the University of Illinois in Chicago. He is Emeritus Professor in Geriatric Medicine, Goteburg University, Sweden. He is credited, along with Robert Butler, with originating the concept of "productive aging."

Brent A. Taylor, Ph.D., is Assistant Professor at San Diego State University, Marital and Family Therapy Program, Department of Counseling and School Psychology. He has a Ph.D. in Sociology with an emphasis in Gerontology from the University of Southern California. His clinical work has focused on low-income inner-city Latino families, and he specializes in working with men and fathers.

THE HISTORY AND

CURRENT STATE

OF PRODUCTIVE AGING

PRODUCTIVE AGING

Principles and Perspectives

James Hinterlong, M.S.W., Nancy Morrow-Howell, Ph.D.,
and Michael Sherraden, Ph.D.

The common human experience of aging has changed dramatically during the past century, particularly in developed areas of the world. We build relationships, contribute to our families and communities, develop skills, and garner experiences over a life course that can extend almost twice as long as that of our ancestors born just 100 years ago. As we enter "old age," we are faced with opportunities, choices, and expectations that differ considerably from those we encountered in our youth and middle age and that are heavily dependent on assumptions about the effects of aging on abilities and desires. Our engagement in roles and behaviors that have traditionally been viewed as productive often declines. We typically lessen our participation in the workforce and reduce the number of hours we spend in formal volunteer roles.

Yet, if the definition of *productive* is broadened to include activities that occur outside the market, we find that many people do remain productively engaged, although their contributions may go unnoticed or be undervalued, overshadowed by their departure from the labor market (Herzog & Morgan, 1992; Bass, 1995). More important, it is clear that older adults perceive significant barriers and disincentives to their continued or renewed participation in formal productive roles (Bass, 1995). While they may wish or even need to participate in these roles, they are unable to do so, or do so only with great difficulty. This observation coincides with that of sociologists, like Ogburn (1957) and Riley (1972), who have long asserted that the institutionalized structure of opportunity has failed to keep pace with increases in the capacity and desire of older adults to fill productive roles. Society is not adequately equipped to provide opportunities for continued productive engagement to older adults.

The productive aging perspective has emerged as a positive response to this lag between rising individual capacity and the availability of institutionalized productive roles. Proponents of productive aging challenge the perception that the majority of older adults are unable to remain active contributors to the commonweal, and must be net consumers of resources. Indeed, the vast majority of older adults today do engage in some form of productive behavior, although research has shown that there is great variability in the amount and form of that behavior within the older adult population, as individuals are able to spread their time and energies across a variety of activities (Bass, 1995). Their contributions as workers, volunteers, caregivers, and active citizens have important and underappreciated benefits for their personal welfare as well as that of their families and communities.

The Case for Productive Aging

As we move through the dawn of a new demographic era, the perspective of productive aging highlights another dimension of later life by recognizing the current and potential contributions of older adults through meaningful action. Through an emphasis on opportunity, advocates of productive aging hope to ensure that older adults are allowed to choose the forms of engagement that best fit their needs, interests, and skills, and that have the potential to produce benefits to others. Older adults currently face a set of very limited choices, despite the marked advances in our ability to preserve and enhance late-life functional ability. Many older adults are pushed toward less meaningful participation or into roles for which there are no market equivalents, no compensation, little recognition, and few institutional supports. Advocates for productive aging argue that society simply cannot afford to continue to overlook the potential of the older population to serve as a resource for social change and economic growth. Moreover, they charge that withholding from older adults opportunities for productive involvement may lend greater credence to the generational equity debate.

In recent decades, many elder advocates and gerontological scholars have proffered hopeful visions of later life, in which opportunities for personal growth and productive contribution are readily available. Nearly 25 years ago, physician Robert Butler identified several myths about aging in his Pulitzer Prize–winning book, *Why Survive? Being Old in America* (1975). He asserted that the "myth of unproductivity" is largely unfounded and leads to "dismal conclusions" about older adults' productive and creative capacities. Butler noted that creative contribution by the older adult is not an uncommon occurrence, but as a matter of course occurs when dysfunction and "social adversity" do not thwart attempts to be productive. Similarly, Betty Friedan, in *The Fountain of Age* (1993), asks why "the aging are kept out of the places where the productive activities of society go on" (p. 26). Thinking differently about what constitutes productivity and recognition of the immense potential of older adults may generate what she called "new visions, new values, new states of personal realization" for later life. Finally, writing in this volume, Harry Moody expresses hope that attention to productive aging and other emerging ideological platforms can open and keep us alive to the possibilities inherent in an extended, functional lifetime and help form a new and positive vision for later life.

Advocacy to Academia

Productive aging developed credence first among advocates as a response to ageism, and has only recently received attention in academia as a useful construct. As an advocacy position, support for productive aging presupposes benefits to both the individual and society. There is evidence to support the general claim that productive involvement is good for self and others, particularly in later life. Research on successful aging led John Rowe and Robert Kahn (1997) to assert the importance of productive engagement to continued health and well-being for older adults. Productive aging generates social improvements as well, leading some scholars to call for explicit recognition of the broad range of contributions through which older adults increase social welfare (Achenbaum, 1996). Moreover, by extending the definitional boundaries of productive aging beyond traditional, narrow market-based activity, we can identify a large and developing body of literature on the extent of older adults' productive engagement.

The most recent review finds that this knowledge base, while substantial, has grown unevenly (O'Reilly & Caro, 1994). However, rising interest in the potential and realized contributions of those in later life has pressed academic work on productive aging to a critical juncture. This work is currently coalescing as distinct bodies of knowledge concerned with discrete forms of productivity: employment, volunteer work, caregiving, and education/training (O'Reilly & Caro, 1994). Thus, this work is not cohesive enough to answer to general questions about productivity or to incorporate cross-disciplinary interests. In addition, research has proceeded without the benefits of solid theoretical specification or a multilevel research agenda.

The contributions in this volume represent a unique, collective effort to critically evaluate, clarify, and construct ways of thinking about productive behavior during later life. Our aim is to provide direction for theory building and future research on productive aging via the identification of useful concepts, the articulation of cautions, and the presentation of research questions that challenge future scholarship. We hope that the volume will serve as a catalyst for research and scholarship that extends the biology of successful aging into the social policy of productive aging (Butler, Oberlink, & Schechter, 1990).

Defining Productive Aging

The term *productive aging* draws our attention away from a narrow biological treatment of aging and toward the contributions made by older adults. Inherent in the concept is the assumption that the skills, expertise, and experience of those in later life are presently inefficiently employed and can be used better. Proponents of productive aging therefore take interest in the actual and potential contributions of older adults. They challenge the persistent "myth of unproductivity" (Hendricks, 1995). As we discuss in Chapter 12 of this volume, productive aging is an applied concept or viewpoint; it suggests lines of inquiry and courses of action to understand and enhance productivity in later life.

Productive aging can be seen as a new formulation of old questions about later life. Historian W. Andrew Achenbaum reminds us (Chapter 2) that individuals have long contemplated the meanings and experiences of growing older. Exploration of our patterns of engagement in later life led to some of the earliest social theories on aging, such as disengagement theory and activity theory. However, scientific inquiry into the causes, nature, and effects of productivity in later life is a newly emerging area in gerontology.

To date, work on productive aging has proceeded without the benefit of a commonly accepted definition of what constitutes "productive" activity or behavior, and without a multidisciplinary research agenda. From its roots as an advocacy position, the term *productive aging* has been adopted by a small but growing number of scholars to label and draw attention to a selection of activities performed by older adults as productive—that is, having social and economic value. Several scholars have offered definitions of *productive aging* to guide research, policy, and program development. These differ in the breadth of activity considered productive, and sometimes include capacity-building and self-care as forms of productivity.

The Salzburg Conference of 1982 resulted in an edited volume by Drs. Robert Butler and Herbert Gleason entitled *Productive Aging: Enhancing Vitality in Later Life* (1985). In this work, a collection of scholars focused on productive aging as "the notion that we can, and must, express and facilitate our personal and social productivity as we grow older." The following year, James Morgan (1986) offered a definition more in keeping with the traditional economic conceptualization of productivity, stating that it includes "anything that produces goods and services. . . . It should reduce demand on goods and services produced by others." Herzog and colleagues extended the scope of the concept in 1989 by suggesting that "any activity that produces goods or services, whether paid or not, including activities such as housework, childcare, volunteer work, and help to family and friends" should be considered productive.

Four years later, Scott Bass and Francis Caro offered a definition that explicitly labeled capacity-building a productive behavior. In *Achieving a Productive Aging Society,* they contend that the concept should include any activity that "produces goods or services, whether paid or not, or develops the capacity to produce goods or services" (Bass, Caro, & Chen, 1993). Most recently, Robert Butler and Mal Schechter (1995), in a contribution to the *Encyclopedia of Aging,* proposed that *productive aging* refers to "the capacity of an individual or a population to serve in the paid workforce, to serve in volunteer activities, to assist in the family, and to maintain himself or herself as independently as possible."

There are significant differences among these definitions. Some scholars would have us consider capacity-building or self-directed action as productive; others make an explicit attempt to include those activities traditionally performed outside the formal market and often performed by members of marginalized groups such as women and minorities. Still, some activities are not labeled "productive" under any of the definitions. Critics such as Harry Moody, Martha Holstein, Carroll Estes, and Jane Mahakian have expressed concern over the concept's emphasis on production, whether inside or outside of the market, because it leads to monetization of activity and individuals. Moody (see Chapter 8) argues that we should spread our attention across the broad range of activities that infuse our lives with meaning, not simply those for which an external reward system exists. Holstein (1992, 1993) and Estes and Mahakian (see Chapter 9) raise more fundamental disagreements with the concept, fearing that the emphasis on productivity, particularly paid work, could serve to further marginalize historically disadvantaged segments of the older population (namely, women and minorities) and lead to commensurate changes in public policy that endanger the already precarious welfare of these individuals. These criticisms and cautions expose several important tensions, which merit further discussion.

Challenges for Productive Aging

It is useful to conceive of these tensions along several dimensions: natural versus artificial limits, opportunity versus obligation, and meaningful engagement versus exploitation.

Natural versus Artificial Limits

One fundamental question for those interested in productive aging is "Productive aging for whom?" Advancements in biomedicine and cognitive science throughout the twentieth century shed considerable light on how human functioning is influenced by the physiological aging process. We are now able to predict more accurately and assess a person's physical, cognitive, and emotional capacity throughout later life. This is important because engagement in productive behavior requires a basic level of physical, cognitive, and emotional functioning. Robert Butler calls this connection between health and productivity a "basic premise" of the productive aging concept (Butler, Oberlink, & Schechter, 1990).

Research has revealed that most older adults have the physiological and cognitive capacity to engage in some form of productive activity late into life (Sterns, Sterns, & Hollis, 1996) and can retain that capacity or regain functioning with assistance (Svanborg, Chapter 4 in this volume). Even among the oldest-old, productive engagement remains a potentiality.

We cannot, however, predict on the basis of age alone when an individual will no longer be capable of productive contribution. Dysfunction—and ultimately death—can and will apply real natural limits to our engagement.

Changing physiological status represents only one facet of aging. The social dimensions of growing old are equally powerful in establishing limits for productive behavior. It is crucial that we recognize the role social institutions play in shaping the choices we face in later life, individual capacity for productivity notwithstanding. The institutionalization of the life course has had a profound impact on our personal expectations for how we will age (Mayer, 1986; Settersten & Hägestad, 1996a, 1996b). Unfortunately for older adults in the United States, society raises significant artificial limits to late-life productive engagement through public policy and social institutions (Mayer & Schoepflin, 1989), which serve to reify incomplete visions of later life. We experience these limits as reduced opportunities to participate in and encouragement to move out of productive roles. For example, institutionalized ageism within the private sector, born from the "myth of unproductivity," results in buyouts for older workers to make way for younger counterparts. Although we might express interest in continued or renewed involvement in contributory roles, these barriers prevent us from pursuing that interest (Bass, 1995). As Betty Friedan asserts, new public policies and reformed social institutions are required to make use of the new dimensions of human vitality (Friedan, 1993, p. 31).

The perspective of productive aging accentuates the importance of the individual-societal interaction. Enhancing productive aging requires mitigation of the natural and artificial limits we face as we age. Improved understanding of the physiological processes of aging and changes in lifestyle can further enable us to postpone age-related functional decline. Proactive social policy can secure access to productive roles and spark the formation of innovative public-private programs that provide opportunities for meaningful productive activity.

Opportunity versus Obligation

Estes and Mahakian (Chapter 9) caution us that values such as social adequacy and individual equity heavily influence our expectations and perceptions of older adults. Changes in U.S. social welfare policy in the early twentieth century created the institution of retirement. Thus, the idea that leisure in later life is the appropriate counterpoint to a lifetime of productive contribution is relatively new. It also has been a privilege of only certain segments of society. Critics of productive aging assert that older adults may find themselves obliged to be productive for two reasons. First, they may have significant economic needs that require them to work, or social commitments that demand their time be spent in a particular form of productive behavior (i.e., caregiving). Second, added attention to the capacity of older adults to be productive could cause society to conclude that their participation in the labor market or volunteer roles is necessary, leading to changes in social policy that eliminate the choice of leisure as an acceptable form of late-life activity. Each of these points now is discussed in greater detail.

Those on the margins, women and members of minority groups, are particularly affected by structural biases throughout their lives and tend to have restricted choices as they enter old age. For example, among those in the current generation of older adults, it is not uncommon to identify women who have never worked in the formal labor market or who did so only to a limited extent; as a consequence, these women have no pension income. Their contributions were made within the household: childrearing, homemaking, and caring for a frail spouse, activities that are viewed as marginally productive and that are seen as keeping individuals out of the labor market. Minority elders, who may have worked their entire adult lives, find that their history of low earnings—the product of discrimination and restricted opportunity—leaves them insufficient income from public and private pensions and financial assets. The only real option for many older adults, therefore, is to continue (or begin) working or, when social and economic inequalities prevent access to paid work, to remain in unpaid positions, such as that of caregiver (Estes, 1998). For these individuals, productive behavior is not an opportunity but an obligation. Moreover, they often are unable to select the form of their productive behavior. As a result, the real contributions they make during their lives go unrecognized and unrewarded.

A second cause for concern is that increases in longevity have significantly extended the period in which older adults are repaid for past productivity. Yet, concurrent improvements in late-life functioning, possibly the result of a compression of morbidity, have made it possible for individuals to sustain or undertake productive behaviors well into their later years. The question now is: Should society continue to reward individuals for years of contribution, when they may collect these benefits for an equal or greater period of time? Emphasis on productive aging, the critics contend, could lead to the conclusion that equity demands an extended period of contribution to offset the costs of providing benefits over such a potentially long period of repayment. Moreover, can the standard of adequate support for those in later life be maintained when some of these individuals have made limited contributions through labor market participation?

Estes and Mahakian, along with critics such as Martha Holstein (1992, 1993), argue that the freedom of older adults to choose the extent and forms of their engagement in both productive and nonproductive activities could be jeopardized further by an emphasis on productivity. In large part, their concern stems from the connection of productivity to activity in the marketplace—the traditional, narrow, money-for-time concept of production. If society replaces the current normative vision of later life as a period of earned leisure with an equally strong expectation or mandate that older adults remain productively engaged, later life will become filled with continued obligation rather than expanded opportunity. Perhaps worse, we could come to press older adults into paid work, rather than support them in other forms of productive behavior.

As economics and demography combine to bring more challenging public policy questions to the fore, it is likely that the current vision of late-life leisure will give way to more balanced and sustainable expectations of what we can and should do as we age. Indeed, aging adults are themselves redefining the possibilities for that period. They are balancing contribution with leisure, and actively responding to the lag in opportunities for productive engagement by creating new options for themselves (Freedman, Chapter 11, this volume). The productive aging perspective can serve as a theme around which society can form public policies, programs, and social institutions that support and enhance older adults' participation in many forms of productive behavior.

Meaningful Engagement versus Exploitation

A third tension in the discussion of productive aging concerns the meaning we attach to the activities we perform. In his classic article, "The Busy Ethic," David Ekerdt (1986) contends that we hold a normative belief that an active, engaged lifestyle is morally and ethically preferable. Even our leisure is consumed with activity. Ekerdt contends this is especially true of the retirement period. Older adults, generally no longer obligated to remain in the labor force full-time, are expected to pursue other activities. Consequently, it may be that efforts to enhance productive aging could lead to the creation of roles or opportunities for the older adult that emphasize busyness over meaning—which Marc Freedman metaphorically refers to as "jogging in place" (Chapter 11, this volume). Instead of asking older adults to contribute in essential ways, we might further limit their value as a social and economic resource by expecting them to underemploy their skills and expertise in menial work. This problem has already been noted in the areas of employment (Crown & Leavitt, 1996) and voluntarism (Morris & Caro, 1994). Moreover, while the concept of "productive" may assign positive value to age (Moody, 1988), it also could lead older adults to feel they can seek meaning only through contribution to others (Mahakian & Estes, this volume).

The creation of meaning in one's life can be achieved in many ways. For some, productive behavior may be the key. However, the definitional differences discussed earlier make clear the difficulties in distinguishing what constitutes productive behavior. The inclusion of activities that occur outside the formal market raises problems in measurement and valuation (see Chapter 13), but acknowledges that enabling older adults to choose among a variety of meaningful and fulfilling activities, whether productive or not, could help restore their status as "full people, not just objects of our compassionate or contemptuous care" (Friedan, 1993, p. 199).

As stewards of civic society, older adults can bring to bear the wisdom born of a lifetime's experiences to shaping individual lives, communities, and social institutions. The gifts of age should be seen as important societal resources that are too easily overlooked and underused. Crafting meaningful and productive roles that can address the aspirations and fully employ the generative capacity of the older population is a necessary but difficult task (Morris & Bass, 1988). If these efforts are guided by the developing knowledge base on productive aging, they are more likely to be successful.

Research on Productive Aging

Research has progressed sporadically and unevenly, as scholars have explored productive aging in its various manifestations rather than general patterns of productive behavior regardless of form. Readers will note that a significant amount of research has focused on older adults' participation in work, voluntarism, caregiving, self-care, education, social networks, and other types of activity that fit under various definitions of productive aging. (See O'Reilly & Caro, 1994, for an excellent overview of this research.) It is difficult to make generalizations about older adults' willingness and capacity to assume productive roles, since this research has been conducted on widely divergent samples. As a result, we can identify lines of research on specific forms (sectors) of late-life productivity, but there has been no effort to create a unified agenda that can guide future work across these areas. The concluding chapter in this volume marks our attempt at crafting this agenda.

Some data on productive engagement have been collected and are currently available for analysis. Although several large studies include significant content pertaining to the productivity of older and have made substantial contributions to our understanding of later life, these research initiatives were not developed to explore specifically productive aging. However, the Productive Aging Study and the Americans' Changing Lives Study were specifically developed to explore productivity in later life and across the life course, respectively.

The Productive Aging Study

The Productive Aging Study is the only large-scale survey study to date designed specifically to assess the extent of older adults' involvement in multiple forms of productive activity and to ascertain their desire to engage more heavily in these activities. The study attempted to explore the extent, timing, and potential of late-life productive activity.

Conducted by The Commonwealth Fund, ICF Incorporated, Louis Harris and Associates, and the University of Massachusetts at Boston in 1991, the Productive Aging Study examined the incidence of activity across five areas: working, volunteering for organizations, helping children and grandchildren, helping the sick and disabled, and education and retraining. The sample was comprised of 2,999 noninstitutionalized adults over the age of 55. In addition to determining the incidence of productivity within these five areas, the study assessed respondents' interest in initiating or increasing their engagement in productive activity. The study also asked respondents to identify barriers that influenced their decision to become or remain productively engaged. The findings from this survey, as well as an overview of the findings, were published in 1995 as the volume *Older and Active* (Bass, 1995) and referred to by Bass and Caro in this volume (Chapter 3).

Americans' Changing Lives Study

The Americans' Changing Lives Study (ACL) was initiated in 1986, with waves II and III conducted in 1989 and 1994, respectively. The ACL aims to document the broad array of productive activities in which people engage and the consequences of that behavior. The initial multistage stratified area probability sample contained 3,617 adults between the ages of 25 and 96, with an oversampling of blacks and those over age 60. In wave I, 1,183 older adults were included in the sample. Attrition reduced the total sample to 2,562 proxy and nonproxy respondents by wave III.

Data from the ACL have been used to investigate age difference in productive activity (Herzog et al., 1989), the relationships among age, economic status, and health (House et al., 1990), and by James Jackson in this volume (Chapter 10) to explore race differences in engagement across three economic and quasi-economic networks.

Other National Studies Relevant to Productive Aging

Several other important survey research initiatives have explored respondents' involvement in productive activity. John Rowe and Robert Kahn (1987, 1997), through their contributions to the MacArthur Foundation Study of Aging, have drawn attention to the concept of successful aging. This work has recently attracted much attention in the field of gerontology and beyond. Evidence from this study suggests that continued productive activity (paid or unpaid) in later life is desirable and can lead to greater well-being. The book *Successful Aging* summarizes many of the findings from this study (Rowe & Kahn, 1998). Readers are also directed to the related work of Glass, Seeman, and colleagues, which uses the MacArthur study data to explore productivity in later life (Glass et al., 1995; Seeman et al., 1994, 1995).

The Health and Retirement Survey (HRS) and Asset and Health Dynamics among the Oldest-Old (AHEAD) surveys are both conducted through the University of Michigan's Institute for Social Research–Survey Research Center (ISR-SRC). Each longitudinal study contains questions pertaining to the time use and labor force participation of its participants. The information gathered in these studies does not address the reasons why particular patterns of activity are undertaken, nor does it offer a sense of whether greater or lesser degrees of productive engagement are desired. To date, over 50 of the nearly 300 publications using the data from these two studies have related to late-life productive behavior. Those interested in reviewing the entire list of publications should refer to the ISR-SRC Internet site (http://www.umich.edu/~hrswww).

It would be desirable for more researchers to use publicly available data, such as that from HRS, AHEAD, and the ACL, to explore the nature of older adults' involvement in productive roles. Secondary data from these studies are longitudinal and thus afford the opportunity to pursue many interesting lines of inquiry related to productive aging. In particular, we should strive to test analytic models that capture the dynamics of productive behavior, its antecedents, and its effects.

Concluding Thoughts

The contributors to this volume offer a variety of recommendations and cautions for those interested in or investigating productive aging. A broad range of viewpoints are presented that can inform the choices we make in all areas of our work related to productive engagement in later life. Readers are encouraged to consider these viewpoints when asking questions, selecting research methods, interpreting findings, evaluating programs, or proposing new policy initiatives that aim to understand or influence productive behavior by older adults.

Efforts to improve our understanding of the nature, causes, and consequences of productive aging will face three key challenges. First, scholars must specify productive aging as an applied concept, with utility in developing programs and policies. To do this, work on productive aging must establish a firmer foothold in academia and, specifically, a more prominent place in gerontology. Second, this scholarship should aim to illuminate the factors, both individual and societal, that lead to or inhibit productive engagement. This requires interdisciplinary research collaboration, which addresses questions at a variety of levels and employs micro, midrange, and macro theories. Finally, research on productive aging must look beyond participation levels and toward the outcomes of engagement for the individual, family, community, and society. Of particular interest is how older adults' increased productive involvement can and does alter the terms under which society seeks their engagement.

Scholars, educators, and policy makers interested in late-life productivity will find useful the concepts and cautions raised in this volume. These perspectives clearly outline the challenges of calling for expanded opportunities in later life. We believe attention to productive will serve to promote a positive discussion rather than simply present a normative vision of later life. The promise of productive aging lies in its ability to inspire new and fuller visions of old age, which stimulate the formation of innovative policies and programs that broaden the possibilities for older adults.

References

Achenbaum, W. A. (1996). View from academe. *Aging Network News, 14* (3), 2, 7.

Bass, S. A. (Ed.). (1995). *Older and active: How Americans over age fifty-five are contributing to society.* New Haven: Yale University Press.

Bass, S. A., & Caro, F. G. (1996). Theoretical perspectives on productive aging. In W. H. Crown (Ed.), *Handbook on employment and the elderly* (pp. 262–275). Westport, CT: Greenwood.

Bass, S. A., Caro, F. G., & Chen, Y.-P. (Eds.). (1993). *Achieving a productive aging society.* Westport, CT: Auburn House.

Butler, R. N. (1975). *Why survive? Being old in America.* New York: Harper & Row.

Butler, R. N., & Gleason, H. P. (Eds.). (1985). *Productive aging: Enhancing vitality in later life.* New York: Springer.

Butler, R. N., Oberlink, M. R., & Schechter, M. (Eds.). (1990). *The promise of productive aging: From biology to public policy.* New York: Springer.

Butler, R. N., & Schechter, M. (1995). Productive aging. In G. L. Maddox (Ed.), *The encyclopedia of aging* (pp. 763–764). New York: Springer.

Crown, W. H., & Leavitt, T. D. (1996). *Underemployment and the older worker: How big a problem?* Washington, DC: AARP.

Ekerdt, D. (1986). The busy ethic: Moral continuity between work and retirement. *The Gerontologist, 26* (3), 239–244.

Estes, C. (1998, November). *Crisis, the welfare state and aging.* Paper presented at the meeting of the American Gerontological Association, San Francisco, CA.

Friedan, B. (1993). *The fountain of age.* New York: Simon & Schuster.

Glass, T. A., Seeman, T. E., Herzog, A. R., Kahn, R., & Berkman, L. F. (1995). Change in productive activity in late adulthood: MacArthur Studies of Successful Aging. *Journal of Gerontology: Social Sciences, 50B* (2), S65–S76.

Hendricks, J. (1995). Productivity. In G. L. Maddox (Ed.), *Encyclopedia of aging* (pp. 764–765). New York: Springer.

Herzog, A. R., Kahn, R., Morgan, J. N., Jackson, J., & Antonucci, T. (1989). Age differences in productive activity. *Journal of Gerontology: Social Sciences, 44,* 129–138.

Herzog, A. R., & Morgan, J. N. (1992). Age and gender differences in the value of productive activities. *Research on Aging, 14* (2), 169–198.

Holstein, M. (1992). Productive aging: A feminist critique. *Journal of Aging and Social Policy, 4* (3–4), 17–33.

Holstein, M. (1993). Women's lives, women's work: Productivity, gender, and aging. In S. A. Bass, F. G. Caro, & Y.-P. Chen (Eds.), *Achieving a productive aging society* (pp. 235–249). New Haven: Yale University Press.

House, J. S., Kessler, R. C., Herzog, A. R., Mero, R. P., Kinney, A. M., & Breslow, M. (1990). Age, socioeconomic status, and health. *Milbank Quarterly, 68,* 383–411.

Mayer, K. U. (1986). Structural constraints on the life course. *Human Development, 29,* 163–170.

Mayer, K. U., & Schoepflin, U. (1989). The state and the life course. *Annual Review of Sociology, 15,* 187–209.

Moody, H. R. (1988). *Abundance of life: Human development policies for an aging society.* New York: Columbia University Press.

Morgan, J. N. (1986). Unpaid productive activity over the life course. In Committee on an Aging Society et al., *Productive roles in an older society* (pp. 250–280). Washington, DC: National Academy Press.

Morris, R., & Bass, S. A. (1988). *Retirement reconsidered: Economic and social roles for older people.* New York: Springer.

Morris, R., & Caro, F. G. (1994). *Productive retirement: Stimulating greater volunteer efforts to meet national needs.* Boston: Gerontology Institute, University of Massachusetts Boston.

Ogburn, W. F. (1957, January–February). Cultural lag as theory. *Sociology and Social Research, 41,* 167–174.

O'Reilly, P., & Caro, F. G. (1994). Productive aging: An overview of the literature. *Journal of Aging and Social Policy, 6* (3), 39–71.

Riley, M. W. (1972). *Aging and society.* Vol. 3, *A sociology of age stratification.* New York: Russell Sage Foundation.

Rowe, J. W., & Kahn, R. L. (1987, July). Human aging: Usual and successful. *Science, 233,* 143–149.

Rowe, J. W., & Kahn, R. L. (1997). Successful aging. *The Gerontologist, 37* (4), 433–440.

Rowe, J. W., & Kahn, R. L. (1998). *Successful aging.* New York: Pantheon.

Seeman, T., Berkman, L. F. Charpentier, P. A., Blazer, D. G., Albert, M. S., &

Tinetti, M. E. (1995). Behavioral and psychosocial predictors of physical performance: MacArthur Studies of Successful Aging. *Journals of Gerontology, 50A* (4), M177–M183.

Seeman, T., Charpentier, P. A., & Berkman, L. F. (1994). Predicting changes in the physical functioning in a high-functioning elderly cohort: MacArthur Studies of Successful Aging. *Journals of Gerontology, 49,* M97.

Settersten, R. A., & Hägestad, G. O. (1996a). What's the latest? Cultural age deadlines for family transitions. *The Gerontologist, 36* (2), 178–188.

Settersten, R. A., & Hägestad, G. O. (1996b). What's the latest? II. Cultural age deadlines for educational and work transitions. *The Gerontologist, 36* (5), 602–613.

Sterns, A. A., Sterns, H. L., & Hollis, L. A. (1996). The productivity and functional limitations of older workers. In W. H. Crown (Ed.), *Handbook on employment and the elderly* (pp. 276–303). Westport, CT: Greenwood.

2

PRODUCTIVE AGING
IN HISTORICAL PERSPECTIVE

W. Andrew Achenbaum, Ph.D.

Physicians, philosophers, and social commentators as well as ordinary men and women from ancient times have contemplated the meanings and experiences of growing older (Cole, 1992; Achenbaum, 1995). Nonetheless, most of the features of senescence that grab headlines are unprecedented, making gerontology a "modern" field of scientific and humanistic inquiry. Roughly two-thirds of all increases in human longevity, claim demographers, occurred during the twentieth century (Riley & Riley, 1986). Population aging has affected political economies everywhere. The rising costs of old-age entitlements have attracted attention worldwide since the 1970s. So has the mounting price of medical and financial aid for the very old (Myles, 1984; Light, 1988).

Not all the news about aging is grim. Scientific and technological advances have demonstrably improved older people's capacity to maintain their healthfulness. Those who survive to advanced years prove remarkably adaptable, quite capable of staying independent (Vaupel, 1997). Such "great modifications in the course of the last period of life" (Metchnikoff, 1903/1908, p. 208) were only dreamt about in the early twentieth century. Now, we are poised to capitalize on the vitality manifest in old age. Researchers and practitioners are fulfilling the hope of Elie Metchnikoff, who coined the term *gerontology*.

Given gerontologists' penchant for accentuating novelty, it is not surprising that the contributors to this volume tell us repeatedly that "productive aging" is a recent addition to the lexicon. Robert N. Butler, the first director of the National Institute of Aging and Pulitzer Prize–winning author who added *ageism* to our vocabulary, is credited with introducing the phrase. He wanted to counterbalance images that cast old people as burdens to their families and society. Most elderly men and women, Butler asserted, made invaluable contributions as volunteers, caregivers, and advisors. Other scholars and journalists in the United States, Japan, and Western Europe soon adopted the phrase *productive aging*. They offered quantitative proof to show that senior citizens could and did remain useful until advanced ages. Emphasizing the present and projected value of late life undercut those who charged that the aged's rapacious consumption of resources was jeopardizing younger people's futures.

My colleagues' interpretation of productive aging is good as far as it goes. Asking whether (old) age is relevant in allocating finite resources has fueled anxieties since the 1980s. If trade-offs between rich and poor, male and female, and young and old amount to the "paradigm zero-sum game" (Thurow, 1981, p. 189), then caring for youth is problematic. Public policies, many Americans fear, disproportionately reward past performance rather than investing in the future. Invoking productive aging has been a useful rhetorical tack because it highlights the elderly's current and anticipated contributions. Rather than scapegoating the old as greedy geezers, as drains on resources, the concept debunks stereotypes that are bound to polarize age groups.

Paradoxically, focusing on the recent history of productive aging ignores the broader sweep of developments. The major point of this essay can be simply stated: by choice and by necessity older people have had to be productive during most of recorded history. In the United States, virtually everyone was expected to contribute to the common good. Only those deemed too young, too decrepit, or too incapacitated were exempt. The Protestant work ethic and market efficiencies demanded that Americans remain active over the life course. Productive aging has been the norm here. There have been turning points in descriptions of elderly workers, to be sure. Sometimes their assets and experience were extolled; at other times veterans of productivity have been marginalized. This is hardly surprising, given the fluidity and diversity of ideas dominant in various segments of American culture. To this must be added the volatility of U.S. capitalism, which has never been impartial in rewarding effort. Rookies generally receive less pay than those who can coast on their seniority. Women and minorities on average have faced greater barriers than older people in getting jobs and keeping positions wherein they might truly have been productive.

In Praise of Productive Aging in the Early American Republic

One of the earliest descriptions of America, a play entitled *Eastward Hoe* (1605) by George Chapman, Ben Jonson, and John Marston, portrayed Virginia as a place where "gold is more plentiful than copper is with us . . . and for rubies and diamonds they go forth on holidays and gather 'em by the seashore to hang on their children's coats" (quoted in Potter, 1954, p. 78). Wave after wave of immigrants came to the New World expecting to find streets paved with gold. They quickly discovered that extracting America's rich natural resources required hard work and persistence. Still, the effort paid off in most instances. *The Autobiography of Benjamin Franklin* (1771/1965) dangled rewards before apprentices willing to improve their skills. Franklin cited the opportunities enjoyed by the mature man, who was "sensible and sagacious in himself, and attentive to good advice from others, capable of forming judicious plans, and quick and active in carrying them into execution" (p. 155). In his *Letters from an American Farmer* (1782), Hector St. John de Crevecoeur claimed that workers could prosper in the New World:

There is room for every body in America: has he any particular talent, or industry? He exerts it in order to procure a livelihood, and it succeeds. Is he a merchant? The avenues of trade are infinite; is he eminent in any respect? He will be employed and respected. Does he love a country life? Pleasant farms present themselves; he may purchase what he wants, and thereby become an American farmer. Is he labourer, sober and industrious? He need not go many miles, nor receive many informations before he will be hired, well fed at the table of his employer, and paid four or five times more than he can get in Europe. Does he want uncultivated lands? Thousands of acres present themselves, which he may purchase cheap. Whatever be his talents or inclinations, if they are moderate, he may satisfy them. I do not mean, that every one who comes will grow rich in a little time; no, but he may procure an easy, decent maintenance, by his industry. Instead of starving, he will be fed; instead of being idle, he will have employment; and these are riches enough for such men as come over here. (Quoted in Potter, 1954, p. 79)

Few paupers grew rich in the New World, yet those willing and able to work rarely ended up losing everything. Most Americans in the early Republic could satisfy their wants if they refined their skills and adopted a moderate lifestyle. Success was possible to Franklin's urban workers and Crevecoeur's farmers who aged productively.

Farmers were especially likely to remain productive throughout their lives. "We have an immensity of land courting the industry of the husbandman," Thomas Jefferson pronounced in *Notes on the State of Virginia* (1785/1954, pp. 164–165), adding that "those who labour in the earth are the chosen people of God, if ever he had a chosen people, whose breasts he has made his peculiar deposit for substantial and genuine virtue." In the Jeffersonian political economy, virtuous men and women cultivated natural resources so as to assure national prosperity. The commonweal's health was sustained by ordinary citizens' creativity and sweat: "The rights of the whole can be no more than the rights of individuals" (quoted in Appleby, 1984, p. 97). Nature afforded space for individuals to grow and, in the process, to add the fruits of their labor to the products created by others. Social comity fostered economic productivity, and vice versa.

There were, the Founding Fathers believed, indirect benefits to the new nation's underdeveloped vistas. Not only was there plenty for everybody to do, but the very act of being productive promoted societal well-being. "The virtues of hospitality, temperance, industry, and oeconomy [sic] delight to dwell" in "the present state of society in America," observed Samuel Whiting in 1796, "and which, from its characteristic spirit of enterprise, exertion and vigour, is most favourable to the cultivation of the useful arts and sciences" (quoted in McCoy, 1980, p. 170). Laborers embraced knowledge-building with good reason: to them, pragmatism, usefulness, and productivity were intertwined.

Nor were such paeans to agrarian virtues simply ideological dross. According to the first federal Census, 95 percent of all Americans were rural dwellers in 1790. The percentage was slightly less 30 years later, but Census takers reported that roughly three-quarters of all workers were farmers (Shover, 1976, p. 3). Almanacs and other writings from the period indicate that most aged workers were farmers. When no longer able to clear land or plow fields, the old did other tasks—shoeing horses, caring for tools, and minding the books. Seasons of experience gave the elderly insights worth respecting. Hence their children and younger friends heeded their advice concerning where to plant crops or when to sell property (Achenbaum, 1978).

Older farmers were not the only workers who remained active in their chosen occupations until late in life. George Washington, John Adams, and Thomas Jefferson were about 65 when they retired from the presidency. John Quincy Adams left the White House at 61; elected to Congress in 1832, he served until suffering a fatal stroke at the age of 81. State and municipal officials stayed in their posts past 70; few jurisdictions forced magistrates to quit the bench. Army and navy officers grew old in rank. The elderly remained active in the clergy, business, and medicine (Achenbaum, 1978). Senior citizens did not need to possess wealth or special gifts to be perceived as productive. An orator dedicating a canal in Ohio on July 4, 1825, extolled the community's ability to mobilize "all the vigor and firmness of youth, the strength and firmness of manhood, and the wisdom of age. Great as is the undertaking, your powers are equal to its completion; be but united, firm and persevering, and if heaven smile on your labors, success is sure" (quoted in Achenbaum, 1978, p. 9). Achieving a "novus ordo seclorum"—a new order of the ages—hinged on the ability of all age groups to remain productive, committed to working together for the benefit of all.

Alexis de Tocqueville underscored the connection between individual productivity and societal progress in *Democracy in America* (1835–1840/1956), arguably the most insightful commentary about the United States ever written. The French aristocrat saw that Americans desired the best of all possible worlds: "We find them seeking with nearly equal zeal for material wealth and moral good,—for well-being and freedom on earth, and salvation in heaven . . . a career without bounds, a field without a horizon was opened before them" (p. 48). Americans' ambitions and productivity assured the advancement of democratic ideals. Democracy in turn "swells the number of working-men," de Tocqueville postulated (p. 214).

In the United States, the greatest undertakings and speculations are executed without difficulty, because the whole population are engaged in productive industry, and because the poorest as well as the most opulent members of the commonwealth are ready to combine their efforts for these purposes. The consequence is that a stranger is constantly amazed by the immense public works executed by a nation which contains, so to speak, no rich men. . . . What astonishes me in the United States is not so much the marvelous grandeur of some undertakings, as the innumerable multitude of small ones. . . . The Americans make immense progress in productive industry, because they all devote themselves to it at once. (pp. 215–216)

Alexis de Tocqueville predicted that the genius of U.S. democracy was its ability to capitalize on the productivity of ordinary people. Americans were willing to pool their resources to accomplish tasks both great and small.

The preceding quotation illustrated how class differences theoretically were overcome. Other passages in *Democracy in America* attested to ways of bridging age disparities. Tocqueville's emphasis on the solidarity of all productive members of society jibed with the impressions of his contemporaries. Advanced age mitigated neither the right nor the responsibility to be productive. All age groups had to contribute to the progress of *Democracy in America*. Should disabilities diminish the capacity to work, then younger members of society were expected to make the necessary provisions, to treat their elders as "worthy poor" (Trattner & Achenbaum, 1983, pp. 259–261). Old age per se was not considered license for desuetude.

Questioning the Elderly's Capacity for Productive Aging (ca. 1880–1950)

Ideas about older people's capacity for productive aging did not suddenly change. Many attitudes expressed by the Founding Fathers remained in vogue. Foreign visitors reiterated the prevailing sentiment that everybody should work for their own benefit and for the common good. Thus *The American Commonwealth* (1888/1959), written by Oxford law professor James Bryce, echoed themes enunciated in *Democracy in America*. Like Tocqueville, the Englishman was struck by the great value Americans placed on self-reliance over the life course: "Everything tends to make the individual independent and self-reliant. He goes early into the world; he is left to make his way alone; he tries one occupation after another, if the first or second venture does not prosper; he gets to think that each man is his own best helper and adviser" (p. 308). Americans, observed Bryce, were "a busy people . . . accustomed to reckon profit and loss" (pp. 309–311). Viewed as no less pragmatic, rootless, or energetic than earlier cohorts, a new wave of citizens sought niches that would provide them material well-being for life.

Gradually, however, forms of superannuation (not related to health conditions) came into vogue. Railroads and steel companies—enterprises that relied on economies of scale and maximizing worker efficiency to generate profits—developed ideas and instituted practices that tended to devalue older workers' contributions. American Express in 1875 granted retirement packages calculated on the basis of employees' ages and years of experience. Only seven other companies followed suit during the next quarter-century, but 151 corporations implemented age-based policies between 1900 and 1915 alone (Latimer, 1932, p. 50). To make way for younger employees, a small but growing number of municipal, state, and federal agencies also offered retirement to certain categories of workers.

New images of older workers took shape, ones that seemed to justify private- and public-sector initiatives to discharge older workers:

> In the search for increased efficiency, begotten in modern time by the practical universal worship of the dollar . . . gray hair has come to be recognized as an unforgivable witness of industrial imbecility, and experience the invariable companion of advancing years, instead of being valued as common sense would require it to be, has become a handicap so great as to make the employment of its possessor, in the performance of tasks and duties for which his life work has filled him, practically impossible. (Anonymous, 1913, p. 504)

Employers wished to recruit young blood and retain employees in full flower. To get the right mix of workers, companies wanted rid of older workers who no longer offered much. This strategy seemed reasonable insofar as productivity was measured in terms of speed and efficiency. But there was a price. Managers overlooked some hidden assets of age. They discounted the time veteran employees spent teaching novices. They did not appreciate the quality of work seniors performed under artificial time constraints.

What impact, if any, did this rhetorical shift have on the elderly's ability to get gainful employment? Historians disagree. In *Old Age in the New Land* (1978), I argued that white men's workforce participation declined modestly, even in heavily industrialized states like Massachusetts. I estimated that roughly two-thirds of all men over 65 worked in 1900. Twenty years later, the percentage dropped to 56 percent; only 42 percent of all older males were working in 1940. Employment statistics, I found, vary historically by race and gender. Throughout the period most African Americans, concentrating in the agrarian sector, worked until they became chronically disabled or died. Few white women of any age were employed outside of the home. Opportunities were greatest for single young females and for widows who took in boarders or worked in sales. This is not to say that most elderly women were unproductive, however. Grandparents helped with caregiving. Well-to-do native-born women spearheaded many voluntary agencies and social service initiatives. Immigrant women, particularly older widows, tended to be active in their neighborhood parishes.

Other social and economic historians (such as Brian Gratton, Carole Haber, Roger Ransom, and Richard Sutch) interpret labor force participation trends differently. Imaginatively adjusting Census data, they contend that there was considerable movement in and out of the labor force. "Older men with sufficient wealth and other sources of income from the household could reduce the amount of work they did or leave the work force for a time, especially if they were sick or less physically able. . . . The family economy allowed these work choices" (Haber & Gratton, 1993, p. 105). These historians further stipulate that the ranks of older workers increased as a result of new employment opportunities in the late nineteenth century in department stores, railroads, and financial services. Disabled and superannuated workers found a niche serving as guards or advisors, or performing other ancillary tasks.

More work must be done to reconstruct the history of retirement. But let us assume that the revisionists' estimates about older people's employment histories are more valid than mine. If this were so, then note their relevance to the history of productivity. Although corporate structures were becoming inimical to the elderly, the aged managed to remain active. That said, we must not discount the long-term effects of the ageism that arose during the take-off phase of America's industrial revolution. Cumulatively, negative images constrained older workers' ability to be productive. Historians agree that employment practices became honeycombed with age-based barriers during the first three decades of the twentieth century. Few firms recruited workers over 40. Personnel departments reported that elderly employees were sicker and slower than young people. Mid-sized companies and new businesses joined the pacesetters in establishing pension plans to foster loyalty and to eliminate redundancy among blue- and white-collar workers. At every turn the press took swipes at the inefficiencies and foibles of those who were "over the hill."

Taking to the defensive, some writers questioned derogatory assumptions about the aged's productivity. Consider the efforts of the distinguished psychologist G. Stanley Hall, who wrote *Senescence: The Last Half of Life* (1922) upon his retirement from the presidency of Clark University. Among other things, Hall piled example upon example of late-life creativity in *Senescence*. He reported the results of a survey he sent to older friends and distinguished citizens. Hall received mixed opinions about how greatly the aged wished to stay involved in business or the professions. Some were happy to retire. Other correspondents wanted to bring their life's work to completion. Still others, such as the retired men in the Borrowed-Time Club or the women over 60 who belonged to the Sunset Club, intended to pursue new activities. Schools for Maturates, a precursor of Elderhostel, were started. Stanford's professor emerita Lillien J. Martin (1944) proposed practical strategies for members of her generation to "salvage old age."

Despite attempts to refurbish the aged's image as productive workers, few analysts of the United States prior to the Great Depression actually devoted much attention to the elderly's role in increasing the nation's wealth. Their silence speaks loudly. For instance, economists in *Recent Social Trends* (Mitchell, 1933, vol. I, pp. 332–334; vol. II, 805), an ambitious if ill-timed survey of American society, attributed the 34 percent rise in agricultural output and industrial productivity during the 1920s to scientific inventions and advances in mechanization. Human resources— including the increasing employment of women outside of the home and new roles played by various racial and ethnic groups—were also cited as factors. Experts noted that the proportion of the population over 16 who were "customarily employed" had risen 5 percent between 1870 and 1920; this age group, they claimed, now "shouldered the load of the nation's gainful work" (Mitchell, 1933, vol. I, p. 274). Absent from *Recent Social Trends* was any documentation of older workers' contributions. Comments about elderly Americans in the two-volume analysis dealt with their need for pensions and housing.

The images of productive aging that animated thinking about Social Security were even more Janus-faced than those appearing in *Recent Social Trends*. Legislators and other public officials, corporate executives, and labor leaders as well as representatives from the voluntary sector and from the ranks of the elders themselves all agreed that the federal government had to do something to help workers who had lost their jobs, savings, and pensions during the Great Depression. Some planners felt that the aged should retire, in order to create positions for younger workers. A careful reading of the documents that culminated in the 1935 Social Security Act, however, suggests that New Dealers did not intend to foment a mass senior citizen exodus from the labor force. *The Report of the Committee on Economic Security,* which provided the intellectual rationale for the landmark legislation, reiterated that prosperity depended on productivity. Honoring this premise led to a distinctively "American" approach to crafting social insurance measures.

Social Security in the United States departed from European precedents. "In placing primary emphasis on employment, rather than unemployment compensation, we differ fundamentally from those who see social insurance as an all-sufficient program for economic security" (Committee on Economic Security, 1935/1985, p. 70). Americans focused on replacing lost wages because they assumed that most adults would be productive: "We deem provision of work the best measure of security for able-bodied workers" (p. 30). Guaranteed employment, declared Social Security's architects (p. 42), was preferable to unemployment benefits. Social insurance had to be broad enough in scope to provide an adequate income to every citizen, young and old, but not so generous as to reward shiftlessness. Workers, not sycophants, deserved protection from modernity's hazards.

Individuals surely would gain once Social Security were enacted, but the nation would be the true beneficiary: "The program will promote social and industrial stability and will operate to enlarge and make steady a widely diffused purchasing power upon which depends the high American standard of living and the internal market for our mass production, industry, and agriculture" (Committee on Economic Security, 1935/1985, p. 70). Policy makers, respecting "the deep essentials of [the U.S.] Republican form of government," used language reminiscent of Jefferson and de Tocqueville. Social Security's architects thought in broad terms. They claimed that this legislation complemented other New Deal bills designed to promote Reconstruction, Recovery, and Relief. The omnibus bill was transgenerational: the aged got special attention because attending to their needs helped everybody else.

Program designers were disturbed by the fact that "four times as many old people over 65 [were] on relief lists as are in receipt of old-age pensions" (Committee on Economic Security, 1935, p. 47). Older people unable to find suitable work or no longer healthy enough to stay active, stressed New Dealers, deserved financial subsidies. Yet Social Security was not envisaged simply as a human resource tool. It took cues from the Townsend Movement, which wanted people over 60 to get monthly pensions worth $200 to stimulate the economy. Franklin Delano Roosevelt, like the Townsendites, saw old-age pensions as more than a retirement tool: "We have so far failed to create a national policy for the development of our land and water resources and for their better use by those people who cannot make a living in their present positions" (Committee on Economic Security, 1935, p. 137). Definitions of "productive aging" by the 1930s had become elastic enough to embrace the aged's vital role as consumers.*

The actual Social Security measures defined the aged's place in society with ambivalence. Title I of the 1935 Act created a federal-state program for providing assistance to the elderly poor. Because states set eligibility criteria, the federal government ceded its right to establish "minimal standards of decency and health." To prevent welfare rolls from growing too great, Title II established a mechanism whereby employers and employees collected funds for future retirements. (The 1939 amendments, which went into effect before the original legislation, extended coverage to workers' families.) Aged workers were not required to retire, but a ceiling was placed on how much they could earn and still collect pensions (Achenbaum, 1986). Coverage was uneven. Not all states provided Title I benefits; older agricultural workers initially did not contribute to Title II. But Social Security became a benchmark for all subsequent policies concerning the elderly's work and retirement behavior. The 1935 Act was the cornerstone of FDR's 1944 Economic Bill of Rights: "America must remain the land of high wages and efficient production. Every full-time job in America must provide enough for a decent living" (Achenbaum, 1986, pp. 153–154). By allaying workers' fears of old-age dependency, Social Security lay the financial foundations for well-being in late life.

---

*It is worth noting that historians consider the 1930s a critical decade in consolidating the modern American consumer society. Advertisers, academics, and bureaucrats often joined forces to effect "the link between the emergent consumer culture and the ideal of a beautifully orders, methodically managed society" (Fox & Lears, 1983, p. 104).

Postwar Realities Alter the
Meanings of Old-Age Productivity

The United States emerged from World War II as the most powerful nation on earth. For the next 25 years the economy grew. Most U.S. workers earned steadily bigger paychecks. Not everybody benefited. Women and minorities faced barriers and ceilings. Even so, individual successes far outweighed failures during the boom years. "Expert opinion regards the qualities of a people and the techniques and institutions of a society as vital factors in the process of economic growth," declared David M. Potter in his highly influential *People of Plenty* (1954, p. 88). "The qualities which are regarded as important are initiative and capacity for productive work." The nation's vital center, which consisted mainly of its middle- and working-class wage earners, was judged capable of sustaining growth for the foreseeable future. These workers' families, it was said, ought to benefit as well. Ways were developed to enable ordinary Americans to profit from this happy situation—with the government's blessing.

In the spirit of nineteenth-century pioneers who sang that "Uncle Sam is rich enough to give us all a farm," postwar Americans made all sorts of claims on the federal Treasury. Veterans received special housing allowances and tuition benefits under the GI Bill. Defense contracts provided entrepreneurs lucrative incentives to do work for the government. The Supreme Court ruled that public and private pensions, once viewed as a gratuity for a select few, were a right. In the late 1940s pension plans were made subject to collective bargaining by the United Auto Workers, United Steel Workers, and other unions. Congress liberalized Social Security benefits and increased average benefits. Citizens took these entitlements seriously. Retirement became the norm, not just the province of the rich or sick. Between 1945 and 1968, years of affluence when workers' expectations rose, one might have surmised that Americans had a golden opportunity to rethink the possible meanings of productivity in the later years. Instead, they segmented the labor market, generally ignoring what older people could contribute.

Capitalizing on productive aging was not a priority at first; academics claimed that they did not really know how to define "productivity." The term did not even appear in the first two editions of *Cowdry's Problems of Ageing,* the first gerontology handbook published in the United States. The third edition stated that "existing knowledge of the effects of ageing on productivity is perhaps more deficient than in any other phase of the older worker problem" (Lansing, 1952, p. 1004). We should take this observation at face value. The paucity of comments about older workers' productivity, a reticence that first became evident in the 1920s, persisted until the 1980s. Perhaps this is why my colleagues find Dr. Butler's use of the phrase *productive aging* so novel. In their lifetimes few gerontologists thought along these lines.

I should not overstate the case. I spent several days in the University of Michigan libraries tracking down possible references to "productive aging." Anecdotal evidence was reported in scholarly journals during the 1950s; studies such as Harvey Lehman's *Age and Achievement* (1953) received widespread attention. Nevertheless, little information could be found for determining the role of age per se in industrial output, according to researchers at the time. There were surprisingly few occupations in which a substantial number of workers were employed on work of equal difficulty, the speed of which was governed by the worker himself, and for which individual production records, such as piece-rate earnings, were maintained. Experts stated that the transition into retirement needed to be analyzed in far greater detail. On the basis of workers' differential expectations, researchers hypothesized that retirement experiences varied by occupation. But they clearly did not expect to find much by way of productive activities among those who were retired.

In their manner of framing issues, gerontologists probably accorded higher priority to the nature of "work" than the concept of "productivity." And this focus deflected attention away from anything that was not income-producing. University of Chicago researchers Eugene A. Friedman and Robert J. Havighurst, for instance, posited five dimensions to the functions and meanings of work. They asserted that work was a source of income, an expenditure of time and energy, a way to identify one's status, a means of association, and a source of meaningful life experiences. Attitudes toward retirement varied due to work experiences. "Retirement is one of the very few approved forms of unemployment which our society allows its male members. . . . As a reward it may have a varying degree of appeal for the individual, ranging perhaps on one extreme from a form of 'time off for good behavior' to the other extreme as a successful culmination of a lifetime of labor and a chance to make one's fondest dreams come true. The reality of the matter probably lies somewhere in between" (Friedman & Havighurst, 1954, p. 185).

Once retirement became the norm, American workers viewed "the golden years" either as a reward or as a right. Under both scenarios, it is understandable why researchers prior to the 1980s reckoned that late-life productivity no longer mattered much. Retirement meant leisure, even self-indulgent consumption. To the extent that experts pursued the question of how to create meaningful opportunities for older workers, they were likely to start by acknowledging that it was going to be hard to persuade Americans that rehabilitating senior citizens deserved to be a higher national priority. "Vocational rehabilitation services for aging workers have lagged, partly because of the general lack of employment opportunities for older people," observed Wilma Donahue (1953, p. 1) at a conference on aging at the University of Michigan. Rehabilitation of workers over 40 was reduced by this logic to a preventive measure, in case labor shortages among youth dampened economic growth.

At first glance Wilma Donahue's case for rehabilitation does not seem to fit easily with the thrust of her other pioneering efforts in advancing gerontology during the 1950s. Through her radio shows, summer programs, and fieldwork, Donahue extolled the assets of age. She stressed the value of volunteerism, caregiving, and other nonpaying activities. Although Donahue did not at the time link these contributions to any notion of "productive aging," it is not anachronistic to posit that a connection could have been made. In 1955, moreover, Donahue did make a case for productive aging in her edited collection from the sixth annual conference on aging at the University of Michigan. *Earning Opportunities for Older Workers* assessed the feasibility of paid employment (especially for elderly women) and offered methods for adapting jobs to create earnings opportunities for aging workers. What links this volume with the earlier emphasis on rehabilitation? Both focus on ways to eliminate barriers by readjusting the aged. And the emphasis on "human readjustment" was hardly accidental: it was to be the hallmark of gerontological training and service in Ann Arbor under the aegis of Donahue and Tibbitts until the 1970s (Achenbaum, 1995).

Not only did her interest in "rehabilitation" mesh with broader institutional aims, but it also served as a bridge to the policy world. And Donahue was keen to feature speakers who were bright and pragmatic. So it is not surprising that she invited John Thurston, a deputy administrator of the Federal Security Agency, to keynote the University of Michigan conference on rehabilitation. Thurston told participants that "all are needed." His remarks indicated how dramatically public policy initiatives and negative stereotypes undercut the elderly's place in the marketplace. "We are slowly beginning to recognize," Thurston opined (in Donahue,

1953, p. 8), "that the older population and so-called 'disabled' are people—people who, if given a proper chance to seize opportunities, will enjoy more fully the fruits of our economy and be blessings to our nation."

Citizens in the early American Republic would have appreciated the connections that federal officials such as John Thurston made among productivity, fruitfulness, and blessings. But they would have been shocked to see how far twentieth-century generations had gone in discounting the aged's paid and unpaid contributions to the commonweal. And they would have been perplexed by the irony embedded in the failure of the 1967 Age Discrimination in Employment Act to protect workers over 65. The Act defined "older workers" as people over 40 who toiled until they normally retired.

Conclusion

No wonder Robert Butler wrote as if the notion of "productive aging" were novel. He makes no reference to the concept in *Why Survive?* (1975). Nor did the other major work of the decade, Simone de Beauvoir's *Coming of Age* (1972). Scholars did not focus on the topic: there are no references to productive aging in the first (1976) or second (1985) edition of the *Handbook of Aging and the Social Sciences* edited by Robert Binstock and Ethel Shanas.

There is one major exception, and it is an important source. In the first volume of *Aging and Society: Inventory of Research Findings,* Matilda White Riley and Anne Foner devote more than a dozen pages to analyzing productive aging. Relying only on those data that met their stringent criteria for scientific reliability, Riley and Foner stress that workers with greater experience tend to have high productivity. Older workers tend to be steady and stable. Contrary to popular opinion, illness only explained one-third of their absenteeism—which, in any event, was less than existed among the young. Even allowing for variations in labor market conditions and occupations, the aged on average performed as well as the young. Riley and Foner also considered some examples of nonpaid work. Roughly half of all Americans over 80, they noted, did housework (Riley & Foner, 1968, pp. 425–435).

Despite such evidence, which has been reconfirmed by many scholars in subsequent studies, most Americans continued to believe that illness, diminished intellectual capacity, diminished psychomotor skills, and an unwillingness to learn diminished productive aging. "Despite the fact that little or no empirical evidence exists to support such a view," observed Jon Hendricks, "the myth of productive decline has shown remarkable persistence" (1987, p. 540). Yet if we take an even longer view, a different perspective emerges. History teaches us that the elderly have always contributed to our prosperity. There are enough historical examples to warrant re-creating positive images of late-life productivity.

References

Achenbaum, W. A. (1978). *Old age in the new land: The American experience since 1790.* Baltimore: Johns Hopkins University Press.

Achenbaum, W. A. (1986). *Social security: Visions and revisions.* New York: Cambridge University Press.

Achenbaum, W. A. (1995). *Crossing frontiers: Gerontology emerges as a science.* New York: Cambridge University Press.

Anonymous. (1913, August 28). Independent opinions. *Independent,* vol. 75.

Appleby, J. (1984). *Capitalism and a new social order: The republican vision of the 1790s.* New York: New York University Press.

Binstock, R., & Shanas, E. (Eds.). (1976). *Handbook of aging and the social sciences.* New York: Academic.

Binstock, R., & Shanas, E. (Eds.). (1985). *Handbook of aging and the social sciences.* New York: Academic.

Bryce, J. (1959). *The American commonwealth* (Vols. 1–2). New York: G. P. Putnam's Sons. (Originally published 1888)

Butler, R. N. (1975). *Why survive? Being old in America.* New York: Harper & Row.

Chapman, G., Jonson, B., & Martson, J. (1605). *Eastward Hoe.* London: William Aspley.

Cole, T. R. (1992). *Journey of life: A cultural history of aging.* New York: Cambridge University Press.

Committee on Economic Security. (1985). *The report of the Committee on Economic Security of 1935* (50th anniversary ed.). Washington, DC: National Conference on Social Welfare. (Originally published 1935)

de Beauvoir, S. (1972). *Coming of age.* New York: G. P. Putnam's Sons.

de Crevecouer, St. John. (1782). *Letters from an American farmer : describing certain provincial situations, manners, and customs, not generally known; . . . of the British colonies in North America. Written for the information of a friend in England.* London: Thomas Davies & Lockyer Davis.

de Tocqueville, A. (1956). *Democracy in America.* New York: New American Library. (Originally published 1835–1840)

Donahue, W. (Ed.). (1953). *Rehabilitation of the older worker.* Ann Arbor: University of Michigan Press.

Donahue, W. (1955). *Earning opportunities for older workers.* Ann Arbor: University of Michigan Press.

Fox, R., & Lears, T. J. (1983). *Culture of consumption.* New York: Basic Books.

Franklin, B. (1965). *The autobiography of Benjamin Franklin.* New York: Airmont. (Originally published 1771)

Friedman, E. A., & Havighurst, R. J. (1954). *The meaning of work and retirement.* Chicago: University of Chicago Press.

Haber, C., & Gratton, B. (1993). *Old age and the search for security.* Bloomington: Indiana University Press.

Hall, G. S. (1922). *Senescence: The last half of life.* New York: D. Appleton.

Hendricks, J. (1987). Productivity. In G. L. Maddox (Ed.), *Encyclopedia of aging* (1st ed.). New York: Springer.

Jefferson, T. (1954). *Notes on the State of Virginia.* Chapel Hill: University of North Carolina Press. (Originally published 1785)

Lansing, A. I. (Ed.). (1952). *Cowdry's problems of ageing: Biological and medical aspects* (3rd ed.). Baltimore: Williams & Wilkins.

Latimer, M. W. (1932). *Industrial pension systems in the United States and Canada* (Vols. 1 & 2). New York: Industrial Relations Counselors.

Lehman, H. C. (1953). *Age and achievement.* Princeton: Princeton University Press.

Light, P. C. (1988). *Baby boomers.* New York: Norton.

Martin, L. J. (1944). *A handbook for old age counselors.* San Francisco: Geertz.

McCoy, D. R. (1980). *The elusive republic: Political economy in Jeffersonian America.* Chapel Hill: University of North Carolina Press.

Metchnikoff, E. (1908). *The nature of man: Studies in optimistic philosophy* (trans.). New York: G. P. Putnam's. (Original work published 1903)

Mitchell, W. (1933). *Recent social trends in the United States* (Vols. 1 & 2). New York: McGraw-Hill.

Myles, J. (1984). *Old age in the welfare state: The political economy of public pensions.* Boston: Little, Brown.

Potter, D. M. (1954). *People of plenty: Economic abundance and the American character.* Chicago: University of Chicago Press.

Riley, M. W., & Foner, A. (Eds.). (1968). *Aging and society: Inventory of research findings.* New York: Russell Sage Foundation.

Riley, M. W., & Riley, J. W. (1986). Longevity and social structure: The potential of added years. In A. Pifer & L. Bronte (Eds.), *Our aging society: Paradox and promise* (pp. 53–78). New York: Norton.

Shover, J. L. (1976). *First majority—last minority: The transforming of rural life in America.* DeKalb: Northern Illinois University Press.

Thurow, L. C. (1981). *The zero-sum society: Distribution and the possibilities for economic change.* New York: Penguin Books.

Trattner, W. I., & Achenbaum, W. A. (Eds.). (1983). *Social welfare in America: An annotated bibliography.* Westport, CT: Greenwood.

Vaupel, J. W. (1997). The average French baby may live 95 or 100 years. In J. M. Robine (Ed.), *Longevity: To the limits and beyond* (pp. 11–27). New York: Springer.

3

PRODUCTIVE AGING

A Conceptual Framework

Scott A. Bass, Ph.D., and Francis G. Caro, Ph.D.

It has been nearly 15 years since the term *productive aging* first appeared in the literature. When he first introduced the term at the 1982 Salzberg Seminar, Robert Butler addressed the issue of elder productivity as a way of countering the prevailing wisdom at the time (see Butler & Gleason, 1985). Then, it was dominated by an overwhelming concern about elder dependency and the burden posed to society by an aging population. Butler and others at the Salzberg Seminar sought to begin a more objective and balanced discussion about aging and the aged focusing on the productive capacity of older people and their significant contributions to work, family, and community.

Butler writes, "How do we orient our attention toward productivity rather than dependency? For example, we might very well have entitled the three-week seminar in Salzburg, 'Dependency and Aging.' Many people express concern about the costs and dependency of old age. But we wanted to look at aging from a more positive point of view. I wanted to stress the mobilization of the productive potential of the elders of society" (Butler & Gleason, 1985, p. xii).

Over the years, considerable debate and discussion have taken place at conferences and scientific meetings concerning the engagement and participation of older people in the workplace, volunteer agencies, community service, family support, self-management, and education. Several books, articles, and reports have discussed the barriers and opportunities for participation of older people in employment, higher education, and public life (e.g., Moody, 1988). National, state, and local aging-related groups have advocated for programs that support and enrich opportunities for older people. A few foundations, most notably The Commonwealth Fund, have been interested in examining the level of participation of older people in full-time or part-time employment, voluntary activity in formal organizations, assistance in caregiving, and formal preparation for career enhancement. The examination has been informed by the desire to expand the potential of that participation. Further, articulation of the concept of productive aging has not been limited to just the United States or North America. European scholars have expressed interest in the productive aging movement, and in Japan, the term *productive aging* is specifically mentioned in the national long-range plan for aging seniors (Bass, Morris, & Oka, 1996).

Initially, the literature consisted of ideas and qualitative studies, but more recently, a number of large-scale surveys have provided a detailed quantitative examination of the involvement of older people in a variety of productive activities, including work, volunteering, caregiving, and education. A result of this quantitative research has been a clarification of concepts and definitions of the term *productive aging.*

Nevertheless, despite the growing interest among scholars, practitioners, and older people themselves in the area of productive aging, additional theoretical work is needed to better understand the multiple variables associated with the choices people make regarding work, learning, and leisure later in life. Also, for the productive aging movement to become a more respected part of the gerontological lexicon and intellectual framework, additional conceptual work is required. This chapter reflects revision and extension of an earlier chapter on the subject by Scott A. Bass and Francis G. Caro (1996) entitled "Theoretical Perspectives on Productive Aging," which appeared in the *Handbook on Employment and the Elderly,* edited by William H. Crown. Work by other scholars has brought additional insight to the subject and has helped clarify earlier work. The conceptual framework presented in this chapter, building on the earlier conceptual work, reflects current knowledge on the subject and dramatizes the complexity of the multidisciplinary subject. This framework is multifaceted and interactive, representing an identification of salient variables descriptive of phenomena, but it is not yet at the stage of articulated theory. It is the hope of the authors that others may use this discourse in developing a theory of productive aging.

The Meaning of Productive Aging

The term *productive aging* here refers to any activity by an older individual that contributes to producing goods or services, or develops the capacity to produce them (whether or not the individual is paid for this activity). This was the definition developed by Caro, Bass, and Chen in 1993 (p. 6). Productive aging, under this definition, is restricted to activities that can be quantified as to some form of economic value. These activities are socially valued in the sense that, if one individual or group did not perform them, there would be demand for them to be performed by another individual or group. The term excludes activities that are simply enriching to the older person who performs them. Physical exercise and intellectual and spiritual activities, for example, are excluded. More specifically, the term includes paid employment, unpaid volunteer work for service organizations, certain unpaid tasks performed for family members such as care of grandchildren, and unpaid care at home to relatives, friends, or neighbors who are sick or disabled. Education or training that strengthens an older person's ability to be effective in paid work, in volunteering for organizations, or in informal productive family or community activities is also included in this definition of productive aging. Education for personal growth, such as provided through Elderhostel, although of great personal value, is excluded in that it is not expected to enable participants to make contributions that are economically valuable for themselves or society.

Those who have written on the subject of productive aging disagree on some of the specifics of the definition. For example, Caro, Bass, and Chen (1993, pp. 6–7) do not include housework in their definition. Herzog et al. (1989) do include housework in their definition, as do Rowe and Kahn (1998a) in their study supported by the MacArthur Foundation. In this case, there is ambiguity about the extent to which housework left undone by an older person would need to be done by someone else. Butler and Gleason (1985) use an overarching definition of productive aging that includes a wide range of activities. They state that productive aging is "the capacity of an individual or a population to serve in the paid workforce, to serve in volunteer activities, to assist in the family, and to maintain himself or herself as independently as possible." Their definition includes self-care activities performed by elders in spite of impairments, thereby reducing the need for assistance from others.

The fact that the productive aging discussion focuses on "aging" rather than the "aged" further highlights the fact that the age of older people mentioned in the literature varies; it is often loosely defined. In some cases, the lower age limit is set at 40 years of age, since federal legislation on age discrimination in employment specifies that age as a lower boundary. Other discussions use adults 50 or 55 years of age as starting points because this is when age-related departure from the workforce begins to be substantially evident. In research conducted by The Commonwealth Fund, age 55 is frequently used as a starting point. A pervasive theme in the productive aging literature is that chronological age is a weak predictor of capacity for productive performance (Sterns & Sterns, 1995). Significant evidence has accumulated to show that older people have the capacity to perform all but the most physically demanding tasks; further, there is evidence that they have the ability to learn new skills that may be required for work or other productive activities. The popular beliefs that older people are unable or unwilling to take on new training for skills or new intellectual demands associated with work later in life have been found to be myths (e.g., Rowe & Kahn, 1998a).

The use of the term *productive aging* for analytic purposes should not be confused with the terminology used in public discourse. A number of small programs and centers have been established that use *productive aging* in their titles, often to refer to "lifelong engagement," and as a way of distinguishing their commitment to a positive view of aging (an example is the Center for Productive Aging at Towson University in Maryland). Advocates for the productive aging movement emphasize the need for expanded opportunities for older people to engage in productive and meaningful activities (e.g., Morris & Bass, 1988). Critics of this movement have expressed concern that there may be unrealistic expectations for productive activity, with adverse effects for vulnerable older people, notably women and members of minority groups (Holstein, 1993; Jackson, Antonucci, & Gibson, 1993).

"Productive aging" is language used by both conservatives and liberals, with interesting consequences for public policy. With the recognition of the underutilized capability of older people, some have argued for an increase in the Social Security retirement age, perhaps to age 70, thereby creating financial incentives to postpone the retirement date. The concern of liberals is that the concept or endorsement of "productive aging" not be used to obligate older people to more years of work, but to remove barriers and to provide opportunities and incentives for those who want to work. In this chapter, we refer to productive aging in its narrow analytic sense as any activity by an older individual that produces socially valued goods or services, whether paid for or not, or that develops the capacity to produce these goods or services. Our goal is to provide a conceptual framework within which to better understand the individual and societal forces that restrict or encourage such behavior.

Attention to productive aging as defined here does not, by implication, devalue *successful aging, healthy aging, normative aging, meaningful aging, personal enrichment,* or other terms that describe activities older people undertake to promote their own physical and mental health, their appreciation for life, their spirituality, or their satisfaction with their lives. The authors believe that many of the concepts that promote health and happiness among older people are important and should be supported.

The knowledge base for various aspects of productive aging is highly uneven (O'Reilly & Caro, 1994). Extensive research has been conducted on employment among older people, with particular emphasis on circumstances surrounding retirement (e.g., Schulz, 1992; Crown, 1996). A number of studies have also been conducted on volunteering for service organizations among older people; that literature emphasizes the extent of volunteering and personal characteristics associated with volunteering (e.g., Fischer & Schaffer, 1993). The community-based long-term care literature, in spite of its focus on the recipients of care, provides extensive evidence of the role played by older people, particularly spouses, as caregivers (e.g., Doty, 1995). Informal help to the younger generation, including care of grandchildren, is receiving increased research attention. A number of studies have been conducted on grandparenting (Pruchno & Johnson, 1996; Robertson, 1995), and some general research has been conducted on the reciprocal patterns of assistance between older parents and their children (Rossi & Rossi, 1990). Several studies have been conducted that examine the circumstances under which older people enroll in college courses (Lambdin, 1997; Lowy & O'Connor, 1986); however, retraining to strengthen work or volunteering skills has received much less research attention (Peterson & Wendt, 1995).

The 1991 Commonwealth Fund Productive Aging Survey was unique in examining the productive activity of older people across institutional sectors. The study surveyed a representative sample of noninstitutionalized people in the United States 55 years of age and older. Evidence was collected on the extent of employment, volunteering for service organizations, provision of help to the younger generations, and informal caregiving to sick and disabled relatives, friends, and neighbors. In addition, participation in work-related education and training was covered. Analysis of the data focused on four sectors: employment, volunteering for organizations, help to children and grandchildren, and help to the sick and disabled (Taylor, Bass, & Barnett, 1992).

The survey showed evidence of extensive involvement in productive activity (Table 3.1). Among those 65 to 74 years of age, 73.1 percent were engaged in at least one of the four forms of productive activity; even among those 75 years of age and older, 48 percent reported at least one form of productive activity. The extent of productive activity varied enormously, with some people engaged only a few hours a week and others engaged almost around the clock, seven days a week. A substantial percentage was active at least the equivalent of a half-time job (20 hours a week or more). Of those 65 to 74 years of age, 35.7 percent were active at least half-time. Even among those 75 years of age and older, 17.4 percent were active half-time or more.

The relationship between chronological age and participation varied among the four sectors. These relationships are shown in Figure 3.1 through quadratic regression lines. The relationship between age and employment was relatively strong; employment rates of those in the older age groups were much lower only among those 75 years of age and older. The percentage helping the sick and disabled was also relatively stable across ages. The differences among the four sectors are important for two reasons. First, among older people, the rate of employment is highly deceptive as a general indicator of productive activity. The sharply lower rates of employment in older age groups should not be taken as an indicator of general decline in productive activity associated with age. In contrast, volunteering and informal caregiving to the sick and disabled are remarkably stable across older age groups. Second, the data suggest that characteristics of the institutional sectors themselves must be examined to explain how they provide opportunities for productive activity for older people.

TABLE 3.1   The Commonwealth Fund Productive Aging Survey,
Age and Productive Activity (%)

Age	One or More Productive Activities	20 or More Hours per Week of Productive Activity
55–64 years	87.4	64.5
65–74 years	73.1	35.7
75 years and older	48.0	17.4

SOURCE: Bass and Caro (1996), 264. Copyright © 1996 by William H. Crown. Used by permission of Greenwood Publishing Group, Inc., Westport, Conn.

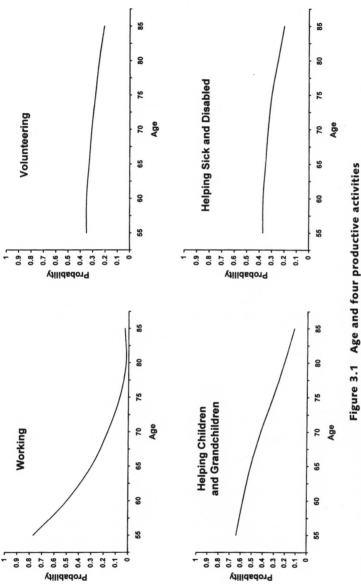

Figure 3.1 Age and four productive activities

SOURCE: Bass, S. (Ed.). (1995). *Older and active: How Americans over 55 are contributing to society.* New Haven: Yale University Press. Copyright © 1995 by Yale University.

Both participation and the extent of participation in any one of the four sectors are, at best, weakly related to participation or the extent of participation in the three other sectors. Rates of volunteering, for example, are not associated with employment status. Rates of volunteering do *not* increase in the period immediately after healthy people stop working. However, among those who volunteer, the number of volunteering hours is slightly greater among those who are not working than it is among those who are employed.

Conceptual Work on Aging and the Aging Society

Early theoretical work in gerontology often focused on the individual as the central unit of study (Achenbaum, 1995). Engagement or disengagement theories were largely social-psychological theories that explored the individual in relation to his or her self or to social forces such as age discrimination. A conceptual framework for productive aging needs to go beyond social forces and examine the interrelationships among policies, norms, cohort effects, the economy, individual personality, and individual behavior.

As John Creighton Campbell points out in his book *How Policies Change,* much of the policy and conceptual work in gerontology within the United States has focused on aging per se, that is, it has centered on older people themselves with the emphasis on the aged and frail (Campbell, 1992). Traditional theoretical work about aging has been driven by the established disciplines of psychology and sociology, and by the allied health professions, and for the most part has centered on work within the disciplinary parameters. Only recently has economic theory been applied extensively to issues in aging. Much of this disciplinary-based inquiry in aging has been criticized as fragmented, contributing too little to the development of a theoretical understanding of individual aging and the implications for society (Thornstam, 1992). The notion of shifting from disciplinary-based study to the study of individual aging in a societal, political, and economic context is particularly appealing to researchers interested in the interaction between individual and social structures. From a societal perspective, long-term care, pensions, social supports, housing, career training, employment, and health care delivery, for example, are primary areas of inquiry that cut across disciplinary boundaries. Productive roles for older people, the subject of this chapter, can be examined from a variety of disciplinary lenses, including individual behavior, societal norms, culture, public policy, and the economy. The challenge herein is to develop a conceptual framework for productive aging that is interdisciplinary, drawing elements from the discrete disciplinary frameworks.

The status and role of older people, for example, is an important consideration in the examination of productive aging. Within the typology of status-role permutations developed by sociologists, there are two relevant groupings: (1) institutional, in which roles and status are defined and institutionalized with clear positions and attributes (most commonly found among defined occupations or obligations such as workers, managers, doctors, etc.); and (2) tenuous, where roles are unclear and status is not defined (e.g., the chronically unemployed and frequently the role of the elderly).

Writing from the sociological perspective, Rosow (1985) argued that the tenuous roles available to many older people in America are the result of a normative process in which older people are removed from highly valued institutional roles (are devalued) and are ascribed less defined and more ambiguous roles. The devaluing process is fairly universal for an entire cohort of people who then must individually seek to adjust to old age, a different phase of their lives.

Alternatively, some psychologists have looked to intrapsychic causes to explain the decline of participation among older people in productive activities. In this view, the decline in participation is viewed individually, based on personality, motivation, interest, and drive. Certainly how older people adjust to changes in later life varies from person to person. People cope and respond differently to changing circumstances. For example, an individual's interest in being engaged in productive activity following the loss of a loved one, or after withdrawing from a lifelong career, or while experiencing economic hardship, or after undergoing surgery, or after aging with a series of painful chronic ailments will vary substantially from one person to another. Nevertheless, the authors believe that a description of an individual's participation in productive activities later in life cannot be fully explained without an understanding of the economic and social contexts that confront the individual older person.

Economists have also contributed to the examination of certain aspects of productive aging. They have been particularly interested in the changing patterns of employment of older adults, and have found that pension policies act as incentives or disincentives to the retirement decisions of individuals (Mutschler, 1996; Schulz, 1992; Turner & Doescher, 1996). The finding that workers respond to economic incentives in the timing of retirement is consistent with the microeconomic theory that people seek to maximize their economic advantage. Although, for the most part, economists have not been identified with productive aging theory, their contributions to the understanding of the linkage of economic incentives and disincentives to individual behavior provide important theoretical groundwork for the multidisciplinary study of productive aging.

Thus far, research about productive aging contributed by social scientists from their disciplinary perspectives has documented the current activity of older people and explored their interest in expanded societal roles. Researchers and policy makers have just begun to examine the established policies and practices that can be altered through litigation, education, programmatic change, and policy reformulation to expand the opportunities for enhanced roles and status in later life. A conceptual framework for productive aging needs to draw on this earlier disciplinary work in psychology, sociology, economics, policy sciences, and anthropology, and to link it together in a more integrative approach.

A Conceptual Framework for Productive Aging

In our effort to develop a conceptual framework from which to view productive aging, we have sought from the outset to develop one that examines the variety of influences that enhance or reduce individual participation in productive activities. Our desire through such conceptual mapping is to find those points in the system at which interventions can be designed to influence behavioral outcomes. We begin with the observation that older people are in large measure underrepresented in the roles of employee, volunteer, and student. By understanding and explaining this phenomenon, we seek to identify those avenues that will increase opportunities for engagement and result in a higher level of participation. Our framework is designed to be informative for the scholar as well as illuminating for those seeking to change participatory outcomes.

Figure 3.2 illustrates the conceptual scheme we have developed from which to view productive aging. It involves five sectors: situational, individual, environmental, social policy, and outcomes. The description is dynamic and interactive, with the variables from one sector affecting another. As factors in the first four sectors change, the participation of older people in productive activities, the fifth sector (Sector E), can change. The framework is sufficiently comprehensive so that if large numbers of older people become much more engaged in productive aging, or alternatively,

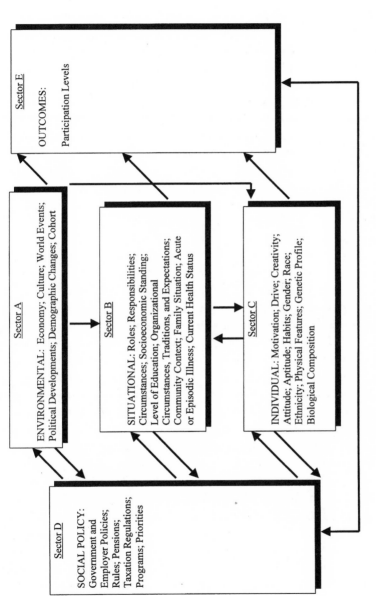

Figure 3.2 A conceptual model of productive aging

Sector E

OUTCOMES:

Participation Levels

Sector A

ENVIRONMENTAL: Economy; Culture; World Events; Political Developments; Demographic Changes; Cohort

Sector B

SITUATIONAL: Roles; Responsibilities; Circumstances; Socioeconomic Standing; Level of Education; Organizational Circumstances, Traditions, and Expectations; Community Context; Family Situation; Acute or Episodic Illness; Current Health Status

Sector C

INDIVIDUAL: Motivation; Drive; Creativity; Attitude; Aptitude; Habits; Gender; Race; Ethnicity; Physical Features; Genetic Profile; Biological Composition

Sector D

SOCIAL POLICY: Government and Employer Policies; Rules; Pensions; Taxation Regulations; Programs; Priorities much less engaged, public policy can be influenced, which can eventually affect other sectors and, ultimately, participation levels.

The framework operates as a comprehensive system, but without a predetermined or defined sequence of events. At any point in time, the interaction of sectors can occur, influencing an individual's choice of participation levels. Unlike in a mechanical system, however, any one of the sectors at any time can trigger an event. Some sectors are less influenced by other sectors. For example, the environmental sector is not influenced by individual, situational, or outcome variables; it is set by much larger world events. Nevertheless, the larger external environment can influence an individual's situational or personal profile. Finally, the outcomes sector has little effect on the larger environment, or individual or situational variables.

Sector A, shown in Figure 3.2, consists of major forces in the political, economic, and social environment, including war, famine, political revolution, worldwide economic conditions, substantial demographic shifts, unique historical events, particular influences of a culture, and major world events. The individual has no control over the forces in Sector A; yet active participation in later life can be influenced by these forces. Historical influences that are unique to a generation are referred to as cohort effects. They can be based on contemporary events or they can be the consequence of a legacy of past events. These larger external forces and historical events all influence decisions made by policy makers, the particular situation or circumstance individuals find themselves encountering, and the degree of productive participation of an individual. In each instance, the environment can affect other variables. Certainly, larger environmental experiences affect the way public policy is developed or the way policies within private institutions are considered, discussed, and acted on.

The environment and cohort in which a person grew up can have a profound influence on his or her choices in later life. Individuals facing retirement from a generation that lived through a deep economic depression might approach retirement quite differently than those who grew up in a time of economic prosperity and job growth. Current and historical environmental circumstances could influence an individual's attitude toward working. They could affect the specific situational context older persons find themselves in, for example, the lack of availability of an antibiotic to fight an infection in one's youth might have lingering effects later in life. Further, the environmental context, both past and present, could influence the decisions of policy makers. Policy makers facing budget surpluses and a growing economy may consider policy options differently than if they were operating in a time of budget deficits and recession. But the environment is not just something that acts on other variables; it also can be acted on—the decisions of policy makers can influence the environment. Taxation, interest rates, and public spending can influence the course of the nation's economy, which in turn influences individual and situational variables.

Sector B in Figure 3.2 consists of the situational variables, including formal institutional roles and more tenuous roles that are assigned through both opportunity and circumstance. Included are family obligations to spouse, children, relatives, grandchildren, and so forth; personal financial resources; educational level; traditions; social expectations; acute or episodic illness; and health. In addition, an individual may encounter specific organizational situations, for example, within a church or synagogue, company, agency, or club that prescribe certain expectations or traditions inhibiting or enhancing productive contributions. The same is true for a community or neighborhood context; the living situation may bring expectations, either defined or not, that may weigh heavily in restricting or expanding individual options. For example, those living in close proximity to other older people, such as in a trailer park or senior housing, may encounter specific circumstances that are different from those living in a suburban, age-integrated, single-family, residential neighborhood. The influence of situation can affect individual performance outcomes. The power of the situation an individual finds his or her self in certainly has the most profound effect on outcomes for those living in prisons, mental health facilities, and nursing homes, for example.

For the most part, an older person has limited immediate flexibility in altering these situational variables; they are a result of circumstance, and frequently change over time, for example, in the situation of an older person needing heavy caregiving because of chronic illness. The responsibility for providing care may be undertaken willingly or unwillingly by the spouse, who then has a new role as a caregiver. Another example is the loss of an elderly family patriarch. As a result, family members may lean on the eldest son to assist in social and economic support for the rest of the family. This pressure may cause this individual to indefinitely delay his retirement decision. Such a situation reflects the sort of real circumstances that confront people in their late 50s and 60s. Challenges are posed or, alternatively, new opportunities for subsequent activity are created.

Sector B also includes those situational variables that are affected as a consequence of nutrition, diet, exercise, lifestyle, and preventive care. Geriatricians are primarily concerned with intervening and mitigating those health hazards that may negatively influence productive aging. John Rowe and Robert Kahn, in their book *Successful Aging* (1998a), focus heavily on preventive care designed to foster a successful and productive aging experience. In each case in Sector B, the circumstances of the older person that are largely unforeseen and outside his or her control have been altered in ways that influence the assumption of new responsibilities.

Sector C in Figure 3.2 consists of individual psychological variables such as motivation, drive, creativity, attitude, and aptitude. Also, it includes the factors that were determined at birth: gender, race, ethnicity, physical features, genetic profile, and biological composition. Individuals draw on the personal resources included in Sector C to interpret and adjust to environmental and situational forces or are limited by them. For example, individuals with limited peripheral vision may need to find accommodation in the workplace as they age and have increased difficulty with visual acuity. If the employer is unwilling or unable to make necessary adjustments, the older worker may be forced to retire. Individuals are saddled or blessed with specific psychobiological characteristics that help them find unique accommodations to the realities of aging. Some of the psychobiological traits found in Sector C such as motivation, drive, attitude, aptitude, and habits, within a range, are amenable to change over time. They are influenced by circumstances, therapeutic treatment, and self-adjustment. But genetic diseases, inherited ailments, and disabilities, as well as personal attributes, may prevent or restrict individuals as they seek productive engagement later in life.

In addition, older individuals may encounter discrimination and unfair treatment based on their individual characteristics; how they mediate these circumstances will vary from individual to individual. Indeed, there are remarkable individuals who may be able to navigate a course and overcome barriers that lead to high levels of societal participation in later life. These individuals—"super elders" as they are sometimes called—are individuals who have overcome major obstacles to achieve significant productive roles in later life. Although we can point to individuals who obtain a college degree in their late 70s, people who find new jobs after retirement, and older adults who are providing extraordinary community service, these super elders are the exception rather than the rule. The evidence indicates widespread productivity among older people, but survey findings also indicate significant untapped potential (Caro & Bass, 1995). And earlier research on older people has provided a substantial body of knowledge on the cognitive ability, physical ability, motivation, and personality attributes of older people that indicates the capacity for sustained productive activity well beyond the traditional retirement age of 62 (Sterns & Sterns, 1995).

Perhaps it is individual differences in interest and motivation that are most frequently noted when productive outcomes for older people are discussed. Many interventions at the policy level are aimed at influencing individual behavior. If, for example, most older people are leaving work and want to retire early, and policy makers think that older people should work longer, what they might seek to do is alter the age of Social Security eligibility. Although such a policy change would indeed influence decisions for many older people, eligibility for Social Security is not the only factor used in determining the point of retirement.

The authors have sought in this conceptual chapter to point out that a fully productive society is more complex, and involves a wide array of interactive variables that affect policy and participation levels. It is Sector D, primarily concerned with the policies and practices in institutional settings such as government and business, which historically has received the least scholarly attention. These include government and employer policies, rules, pensions, taxation, and the norms and priorities set by established institutions outside the family. Despite the limited academic discourse, elder advocates and elected officials have sought to develop legislative programs and policies to protect older people from employment discrimination and provide resources for career retraining. As the prevailing rules and regulations change, older people may experience changes in both the circumstances and the incentives available, ultimately influencing their productive participation in society. Social policy interacts with each of the other sector variables and they in turn with social policy.

For example, under the 1992 Americans with Disabilities Act (ADA), all workers with disabilities are given new protections in the workplace. Among these protections is the requirement that employers adapt and modify working environments for disabled adults (Gelfand, 1993). Although this does little to influence the situational variable of the disability itself, the requirement opens doors for those with disabilities. The Act has implications for older people who develop disabling conditions later in life and seek to continue to work. Prior to passage of the ADA, these older people might have been forced to retire or leave work; now there is a possibility of paid employment being sustained.

Sector D is not simply limited to existing governmental policies, but also includes those areas where policy has not been formulated. In addition, Sector D includes the many different rules and regulations developed by the private sector, be they in the area of work or voluntary services. For example, an agency seeking volunteers may, on occasion, want the volunteer to drive a vehicle. Those interested in volunteering but unable to drive would be excluded. Or, an employer may support a defined-benefit pension program, which has distinct incentives for early retirement. Or, as a result of declining membership, a church may ask its parishioners, many of whom are older, to take on additional responsibilities. The work obligations may exceed an individual elder's physical stamina and rather than ask for a special dispensation, the elder stops going to church. In each case social policy interacts with individual, situational, and environmental variables in synergistic ways that ultimately influence productive participation levels.

Based on the conceptual framework, the outcomes—specifically, the participation levels of older people in productive activities (Sector E)—can be influenced at the margins by changes or modifications to the environmental, individual, situational, and social policy factors. Should participation levels change significantly, one direction or another, to the point that they are of concern to policy makers, elders' participation in turn will influence the policy process and policy decision making.

Sector E is not just limited to individual participation in productive activities, but includes the consequences of an elder's work or service for an employer or care recipient. In addition, when many older people productively participate, benefits accrue to the larger community in terms of social and economic well-being. This collective outcome to the civic good of society is an important contribution of the productive aging society.

In sum, the framework works as a system, with relationships across the different sectors and a degree of connectivity and interaction that influences subsequent participation levels and their impact. For example, a recently retired 65-year-old man lives through a deep economic recession, reducing his income derived from retirement savings (Sector A). He is physically healthy and is unhappy about changing his lifestyle at this point in time. As a consequence of the economic circumstances, he considers returning to work (Sector C). His spouse also desires to maintain her standard of living and as a result he feels pressure to bring in more money. The retiree does not have social or caregiving obligations but does have the time and good health to work (Sector B). As a consequence of the economic downturn, the federal government decides to create a new employment program for retirees, providing part-time work in community service (Sector D). The retiree, in consultation with his wife, decides to interview for the new federal program and return to part-time work. This provides important help to an employer in the town in need of skilled labor. The resulting conditions, circumstance, and public policy result in triggering productive participation of the retiree (Sector E).

The conceptual framework also provides a perspective from which to consider changes in behavioral outcomes. If, for example, we desire to increase or decrease participation levels of older people in career-related higher education, we could examine the individual variables, the environmental circumstances, and the situational context the older person is in, and provide policy incentives or disincentives to alter participation levels.

Theoretical Perspectives on Four Forms of Productive Activity

Employment

Productive aging researchers have sought to explain the obstacles to high levels of participation of older people, particularly in the areas of paid work. Not only is paid work the major source of personal income, but occupation is central to identity for many adults. The decline in labor force participation that has taken place in recent decades (particularly among older men), in spite of major gains in health and longevity among older people, has received extensive research attention. Those studying productive aging have tried to identify ways in which volunteering for organizations might be increased. Their interest is less in the characteristics of individual older people that would explain their patterns of productive activity than it is in the institutional forces that both account for opportunities for productive participation and help to shape public opinion on productive participation among older people.

Caro, Bass, and Chen (1993) hypothesized that the obstacles in this society to the successful employment of older people are so widespread that the term *institutionalized ageism* should be used to describe them. They argued that these obstacles are often so subtle that they are not recognized. They may include not only discrimination against older people in the hiring process, but also a lack of full recognition of the achievements of older workers, lack of consideration of promotions, less-than-equal access to retraining that may be key to job retention or promotion, and exclusion from informal work groups dominated by younger workers. Underlying these discriminatory practices may be unjustified beliefs that older workers are less productive than their younger counterparts, less capable of being retrained, less open to change in organizational practices, more vulnerable to injury and illness, and more costly than younger workers from a fringe benefit perspective. The institutionalized norms that minimize the capabilities of older people in the workplace may be so pervasive that they are internalized even by older people themselves. Through negative images of aging, older people may underestimate their own capabilities and accept the notion that they should leave productive roles at relatively young ages.

A fundamental question about the institutionalized ageism hypothesis concerns the evidence supporting it. The extent to which there are patterns of discriminatory practices toward and prejudicial attitudes about older people in work organizations is an empirical issue. From a scientific perspective, it is not sufficient to invoke institutionalized ageism as a residual explanation of various employment problems of older people. While there is scattered evidence of discriminatory practices and prejudicial beliefs directed toward older workers, pervasive patterns are very difficult to document. Because of the difficulty of obtaining such data, the absence of evidence does not, however, provide a basis for ruling out the possibility of institutionalized ageism in the workplace. To the extent that such ageism can be established, an explanation of the phenomenon is needed.

A basic hypothesis designed to explain the relatively low levels of participation of older people in the workforce might be termed the "affluence/leisure preference" hypothesis, reflecting both the relative affluence of many current older Americans (or Europeans) and the preference of many of them for leisure activities. Implicitly, according to this hypothesis, prevailing social norms define old age as a time in which older people are encouraged to pursue leisure activities. Older people are relieved of their obligations to be economically productive. Again, according to the hypothesis, people work largely for economic reasons, that is, because they "need the money." When they can afford to, older people retire. In this context, the decline of the typical retirement age is attributed to societal as well as individual affluence. The economic prosperity of the United

States and Western European countries after World War II has made it possible for many older people, through government pension programs and employer-financed pension programs, to live comfortably without working. Essentially, the hypothesis asserts that prosperity makes it economically possible for many older people to retire; a great many of them not only take advantage of the opportunity for leisure activities but also concentrate on them, rather than on other productive activities such as volunteering for organizations.

Intergenerational conflict is a second potential explanation of both the current low levels of workforce participation of older people and institutional ageism more generally. According to conflict theory, social groups make competing claims on scarce resources. Each group pursues its own interest, attempting to maximize its share of societal rewards without regard for the welfare of other groups. The pursuit of competing claims need not always be overt. On the surface, groups with conflicting interests may maintain civil relationships, but they may be engaged in energetic covert struggles, each to maximize their advantage. Older and younger people sometimes have conflicting economic interests. When jobs are scarce, older people can be seen by younger people as competitors. If older people hold attractive positions within a firm, this is sometimes seen as blocking opportunities for younger people. Thus, the removal of an older person from such a position is interpreted as an opportunity to make the position available to a younger person. Institutional arrangements that encourage older people to leave jobs, such as early retirement incentives, can be instruments of conflict between older and younger people over jobs.

Conflict theory predicts that pressure to exclude the elderly is affected by labor market conditions. During recessions when jobs are scarce, pressure to remove the elderly from the workforce is expected to increase. In periods of economic prosperity when workers are in short supply, conflict theory predicts that older workers will be seen in a much more favorable light, and therefore, the employment of older people is then more likely to be actively encouraged.

Cultural lag is a third potential explanation for the limited participation of older people in attractive, paid work roles, and is also a potential explanation of institutional ageism. Cultural lag theory, which was introduced by Ogburn (1964) to explain slow societal responses to the improved conditions made possible by technological advances, differs from conflict theory in its assumptions about the underpinnings of institutional patterns. The cultural lag hypothesis asserts that as a society, we simply are slow to adjust our institutions in response to changing conditions. The premise is that institutional arrangements are inherently difficult to change because of their complexity and rigidity and our shortsighted satisfaction with them.

According to cultural lag theory, a learning process is required to understand the implications of technical and social change and to make sound adjustments in institutional policies and practices. Our society may not recognize, for example, that contemporary retirement policies that encourage early retirement are premised on an oversupply of labor. As a result, although the labor supply may diminish to a point where greater numbers of older workers are needed, those who control pension policies may be slow to recognize the need to adjust them to reflect the economic value of continuing the employment of older workers. Certain existing pension policies may be formalized in contracts that cannot be modified quickly. Similarly, our society may simply be slow in reorganizing its educational institutions to provide the lifelong training for work necessary in a changed economy characterized by sharper competition and rapid technological advances. Moreover, according to cultural lag theory, we may be slow to recognize that people now have the potential for remaining productive later in life as a result of improved health and reduced physical demands in the workplace.

Perhaps the most prolific writers on cultural lag as an explanation for the underutilization of the elderly are Matilda White Riley and John Riley (see Riley, Kahn, & Foner, 1994). Riley and Riley (1994) argue that the current life course pattern of education, work, and retirement is inconsistent with the demands of contemporary society—a society that requires lifelong learning and retraining. With the rapid change in technology and the speed of innovation, individuals in virtually every profession and occupation are in need of lifelong learning. The current dominant life course pattern that emphasizes education when one is young, and heavy work demands in the early and middle career years (at the same time as family responsibilities are at their zenith), may be incongruous with the pattern necessitated by a life course plan. Such a life course plan might be one where work demands are reduced in middle years and extended into the later years. It might also involve phased retirement, where sustained activity much later in life is a more rational and reasonable response to the current human capacity.

These regimens of education, work, and leisure may be structural, age-based expectations of behavior. In contrast, cohorts of individuals may experience opportunities or pressures to change these normative behaviors. Changing economic, health, and social circumstances may force individuals to question the expected behavior. For example, younger adults take on many roles through necessity while older people often lack sufficient roles for a productive life. The pressures and circumstances of both older and younger people raise the possibility of needed structural changes in the life course patterns.

As they look into the future, Riley and Riley (1994) anticipate greater age integration in education, work, and leisure. They see our society moving from a pattern in which education will be spread more evenly over one's life so that it will be more common for middle-age and older people to participate in educational programs. They also envision increased numbers of older people remaining in the workforce. In exchange for longer careers, adjustments will be made in the middle years (providing for greater flexibility with careers), with more time devoted to family and leisure. In their minds, the prevailing norms, institutions, and structures always lag behind the changing circumstances of individuals in the society, and at some point the pattern of individual circumstances and prevailing societal structures are reconciled.

The conceptual work of Matilda White Riley has been nicely summarized by Schooler, Caplan, and Oates (1998). They point out that Riley has established four basic principles of aging and society which include: (1) the principle of cohort differences in aging—the unique social and economic events of the historical period in which one grows up; (2) the principle of cohort influence on social change—aging cohorts interact and influence the policies and norms of their milieu; (3) the principle of asynchrony—aging and social change are not sequential or orderly; and (4) the dialectic between aging and social change—the interaction among cohort patterns, individual aging, and social change (Schooler et al., 1998). The conceptual model presented herein (Figure 3.2) reflects the dynamics outlined by Riley.

In *Successful Aging,* another highly publicized work, mentioned earlier, Rowe and Kahn (1998a), drawing on The Commonwealth Fund Productive Aging Survey and other sources, point out the understated contributions of older people to society. They indicate the potential and capacity of older people in later life for continued activity and engagement. In their theory of successful aging, Rowe and Kahn point out that the key elements of it are to avoid disease, maintain high cognitive and physical functioning, and stay engaged with life. Riley (1998) responds to Rowe and Kahn's work in a letter in *The Gerontologist* as ignoring the profound effect of changing lives and changing structures. They have largely described ways individuals can mediate aging and do not discuss the opportunities and challenges afforded when major institutions engage older people in meaningful ways. Riley argues that the interaction between individual behaviors and larger societal structures and opportunities are essential ingredients for successful aging. In a rebuttal in the same journal, Rowe and Kahn (1998b) state that they are limited by the lenses of disciplinary study and the difficulty of testing societal interventions. We agree that the disciplinary lens is a barrier to the theoretical formulations. A goal of our work is to push that frontier.

Although three theories have been developed to explain the underutilization of older people in society in a historical context, they also can be used to explain certain present-day variations in productive activity among older people. The affluence/leisure preference theory, for example, predicts that among older workers, the greater the accumulated savings and the stronger the pension benefits, the earlier the likely age of retirement. Further, the more intrinsically satisfying the occupation, the later the likely age of retirement. Conflict theory predicts that policy toward the older worker is a function of an industry's prosperity. More specifically, in expanding industries, employers' policies will tend to encourage the retention of older workers. In contracting industries, employers' policies will tend to discourage it. On the other hand, cultural lag theory predicts that receptivity to older workers is a reflection of industry "enlightenment." To the extent that industry leaders are well informed about the potential contribution of older workers and make efforts to modify industry policies accordingly, opportunities for older workers will be relatively better.

The three theories differ in their implications for change. The affluence/leisure preference theory suggests that older people will seek to remain in the workforce longer if their economic circumstances are less favorable or if their lifestyle preferences shift from less to more productive activities. If the age of eligibility for Social Security benefits is increased, early retirement will seem less attractive from an economic perspective.

Conflict theory suggests that change is most likely to occur when there are shifts in the relative strength of opposing forces. The baby boom generation has the potential to assert itself effectively in the political process because of its extraordinary numerical strength. As time goes on, the baby boom generation will find itself affected by older-worker issues. In the coming decade, the number of young people entering the workforce will be declining. To the extent that votes reflect political strengths, older workers will have the potential to improve their relative position through legislative measures that strengthen their position in the workforce. At the same time, the underlying tension between older and younger workers will remain. In periods of economic recession when jobs are scarce, competition for jobs will be an issue, and age will be one of the factors considered when workers contest for access to jobs.

Cultural lag theory offers a basis for optimism about the potential for improved opportunities for the productive participation of older people. It suggests that the basis for change lies in part in education. Further, it suggests that social engineering can be successful in adapting societal institutions to changing conditions. Through the education of employers and older workers, myths about the liabilities of older people as workers can be replaced by a more accurate understanding of their potential. As a result, employers will make it more attractive for older workers to remain in the workforce and older workers will be more eager to do so.

Volunteering

The environmental and policy sectors in our model provide an important starting point for consideration of the potential for a substantial expansion of volunteering among older people. Although volunteering is deeply embedded in American social organization, it is currently a relatively minor form of social participation. Contemporary volunteering has roots in both religious and secular traditions. To varying degrees, religious groups encourage volunteering both to support their churches and to address broader community needs under either secular or religious auspices. In the period of settlement of the North American continent, volunteering played an important role in the formation of new communities. Contemporary social and health services typically began as entirely volunteer efforts, often with religious sponsorship (Ellis & Noyes, 1990).

Some aspects of that community service volunteering tradition continue to the present. Many villages and small towns, for example, continue to be served by volunteer fire departments (Brudney & Duncombe, 1992). Small towns, in particular, also continue to rely heavily on volunteers to serve on legislative and regulatory bodies, to help staff libraries, and to help in the staffing of recreational programs.

During the twentieth century, professionalization and commercialization of services led to a vast reduction in the importance of volunteers in many aspects of community life. Health and social service agencies that began early in the century with volunteer staffing tended over time to deemphasize volunteers in favor of paid personnel, both because the supply of volunteers was insufficient and because the expertise that could be provided by paid professionals was valued. In the typical transformation of service organizations formed by volunteers, paid personnel were introduced to supplement volunteers. Subsequently, paid personnel almost entirely displaced volunteers.

Commercialization of many services has undermined the rationale for volunteering. Some service sectors once dominated by nonprofit organizations are now dominated by profit-making organizations (Weisbrod, 1988). The nursing home industry is a good example of a service once predominantly nonprofit that is now dominated by for-profit organizations (Kaffenberger, 1998). Citizens can much more readily be persuaded to volunteer on behalf of a nonprofit organization that serves the community than for a profit-making organization that provides identical services.

In spite of the fundamental changes in the organization of community services, the need for volunteer services remains great because of the complexity of community needs, public resistance to the higher levels of taxation required for stronger community services staffed entirely by paid personnel, the large numbers of low-income people who cannot afford to pay for needed services, and the persistence of nonprofit organizations.

Dramatic increases in labor force participation among women have made the "young elderly" increasingly important as volunteer resources. The middle-class women who provided leadership for voluntary organizations in the United States during the first half of the twentieth century are now much less often available for volunteer assignments because they are likely to be employed on a full-time basis. The combination of widespread early retirement from paid employment and increases in health and longevity among older people have made the young elderly increasingly attractive candidates for substantial volunteer roles (Morris & Caro, 1996). The forces that explain individual volunteering are somewhat different from those that explain individual employment. Empirical evidence is available to support continuity theory as an explanation of volunteering among older people. Continuity theory emphasizes consistency in interests and behavior throughout the life course; it provides a basis for hypothesizing that the roles that people perform in old age are similar to those that they performed throughout their adult lives. Volunteering throughout adult life has been found to be predictive of volunteering in old age (Chambre, 1987; Fischer & Schaffer, 1993). Those who early in life internalized volunteering as a value, who have well-developed skills as volunteers, and who have contributed effectively as volunteers are more likely to be volunteers as older people than those who consider volunteering as an option for the first time late in life.

Affluence may facilitate volunteering among older people. Strong financial resources may make it feasible for some older people to devote substantial time to a highly valued volunteer activity. But preference for leisure activities may explain some of the reluctance of older people to volunteer, especially if a volunteer assignment involves a substantial time commitment. Some older people resist volunteer assignments that require long-term, regularly scheduled time commitments because of their interest in travel for pleasure.

Conflict theory is important in understanding the relationship between paid workers and volunteers of all ages. Both paid workers and volunteers can be regarded as sources of labor. In some instances, paid workers may view volunteers as competitors who have the potential to eliminate paid jobs or to depress wages (Brudney, 1990). In some of these cases, the organizations that make use of both paid workers and volunteers take deliberate steps to structure volunteer roles so that they are distinct from those of paid personnel. Typically, this structuring of roles emphasizes the expertise of paid personnel and the supporting roles performed by volunteers. When volunteers are relegated to marginal supporting roles, able people who want to make full use of their abilities when they volunteer are likely to lose interest in their assignments. Some would-be volunteers who are sympathetic with working people are also detracted from doing so because they do not want to take a paid job away from a person who needs it.

To reinforce their dominance, paid personnel may set lower standards for volunteers. When volunteers, then, perform at mediocre level because nothing better is expected of them, the volunteers provide proof of the limited potential of volunteers. Consequently, organizations have further reason to entrust serious work exclusively to paid personnel.

Cultural lag may explain the modest volume of volunteering on the part of the current generation of healthy, younger elders who are out of the labor force. Their approach to retirement may have been affected greatly by an earlier period in which the normative climate encouraged healthy retirees to pursue leisure. In time, the normative climate may change in directions that place more emphasis on community service volunteering on the part of the well elderly. Elder volunteering may also be inhibited by weak institutional arrangements to recruit and place older people as volunteers. Research conducted by the authors shows that although rates of volunteering among the young elderly are not affected by employment status, receptivity to volunteering is greater among recent retirees than it is among either those employed or those out of the workforce on a long-term basis (Caro & Bass, 1997). As the potential for major volunteer contributions on the part of recent retirees gains greater recognition, improved institutionalized arrangements to engage people in new volunteer assignments at the time of retirement may emerge.

Assistance within Families

Many of the productive contributions of older people are made informally, particularly in family settings. The focus here will be on two informal roles within the family: providing long-term care and caring for grandchildren. While older persons are often seen as recipients of long-term care, older people are also important unpaid providers of long-term care. In this role, they may provide assistance at home to a spouse, a very old parent, and perhaps even an adult child or a grandchild with a serious disabling condition. In other cases, they provide informal long-term care to siblings, other relatives, friends, or neighbors. Long-term care roles are wide-ranging. Informal long-term care includes assistance with such varied tasks as bathing, dressing, shopping, meal preparation, house cleaning, management of personal affairs, escort, and transportation. The productive contributions that older people make through the care of grandchildren range from occasional babysitting to long-term substitute parenting.

For purposes of this discussion, informal long-term care and care of grandchildren have important commonalities. In most instances in which older people provide informal long-term care or provide help to grandchildren, their effort measured by hours is modest. However, a minority provides an extensive amount of assistance. In The Commonwealth Fund Productive Aging study, for example, 37 percent of respondents with grandchildren reported providing at least one hour of help in the previous week. Only 8 percent reported helping 20 hours a week or more. Approximately 30 percent of the respondents reported providing help to a sick or disabled person in the previous week. Of them, the typical respondent provided five hours of help. However, of those providing informal care, 19 percent provided 20 hours or more of care and 8 percent provided more than 40 hours of care (Caro & Bass, 1995).

While family members have long been the major providers of long-term care in the United States, a rapid increase in the role of grandparents as substitute parents has been observed in the past decade (Robertson, 1995). In 1997, 5.5 percent of all American children were living in grandparent-headed households (Lugaila, 1998). Although grandparenthood is a status popularly associated with aging, it is as much a status associated with middle age. Half of grandparents in the United States are estimated to be less than 60 years of age (Schwartz & Waldrop, 1992). Grandparents who are substitute parents tend to be younger than grandparents are generally; in 1992, 73 percent of grandparent caregivers were less than 60 years of age (Harden, Clark, & Maguire, 1997).

Hareven (1994) argues that the recent increase in intergenerational interdependency is consistent with long-term patterns. She argues that the welfare state, which had a major impact in Western countries in the middle of the twentieth century, represented a historical aberration. The welfare state emphasized the nuclear family by providing support that had previously been supplied by intergenerational families. The recent weakening of public income supports for poor families through welfare reform is likely to increase the reliance of poor nuclear families on their extended families. Hareven (1994) also observes that new complex and more flexible kinship relationships are developing because of increased diversity within families, remarriage, cohabitation, and the formation of blended families. Eggebeen and Wilhelm (1995) characterized the demographic changes in the families that include weaker marital ties, reduced numbers of children, and stronger intergenerational links as a weakening of horizontal ties and a strengthening of vertical ties. Using more graphic language to describe the same phenomenon, Bengtson, Rosenthal, and Burton (1990) described contemporary families headed by single parents with a small number of children and extensive involvement of grandparents in raising grandchildren as "beanpole" families.

The assistance provided by grandparents to their children and grandchildren takes many forms. Eggebeen and Hogan (1990) categorized these types of assistance as child care, monetary and material resources, household assistance, companionship, and advice. Parents of adult children tend to provide more assistance to their children and grandchildren than they receive in return except in the late stages of life (Rossi & Rossi, 1990).

Many older people welcome opportunities to provide assistance within their families and take initiatives to offer their help. However, their roles as informal long-term care providers and as surrogate parents are largely driven by difficult circumstances experienced by the recipients of help.

Older people are drawn into informal long-term care when a close relative, friend, or neighbor needs assistance. The extent of the recipient's care needs has a strong effect on the extent of the help that they provide. Often their participation has an obligatory quality. Spouses, for example, are expected to care for one another even if they are old and the care provider has some self-care limitations (Morris, Caro, & Hansan, 1998). The strength of their relationship to the care recipient, the availability of other family members, and residential proximity to the care recipient all affect the degree to which participation has an obligatory quality.

Similarly, the involvement of older people in the care of grandchildren is affected by the number of grandchildren they happen to have, the age-based needs of grandchildren for supervision, the residential proximity of grandchildren, the capacity of parents to provide care, and special needs of grandchildren. Frequently older people welcome the opportunity to be of assistance in providing modest and temporary help with grandchildren. Aldous (1987) reports that it is adult children who initiate helping contacts. Further, they tend to do so selectively. Usually they seek episodic assistance, especially in times of special need such as illness in the family. When grandparents are extensively involved in caring for grandchildren on a long-term basis, they are likely to be led to do so by a breakdown in the ability of parents to provide care for their children, such as divorce, drug addiction, or adolescent pregnancy (Pruchno & Johnson, 1996).

Career-Related Education

In addition to work, volunteering, and caregiving activities, older people who are preparing for new career options through further study are also included in the definition of productive aging proposed by Caro, Bass, and Chen (1993). The literature in the area of education for older adults seems to be divided into two forms of learning: that which is expressive and that which is instrumental. Expressive education refers to many popular educational programs that offer older people opportunities for personal enrichment. These programs include the ever-growing listing of activities from Elderhostel, centers for creative retirement, senior center educational programs, "universities for the third age," and adult education experiences. These are often educational experiences involving travel, personal skill development, creative expression, or intellectual reading and reflection. Programs that are instrumental include formal educational experiences that often provide credit or certification. Such instrumental programs are usually found in vocational training centers, community colleges, industry training centers, professional workshop programs, or university settings. Programs that are designed for personal enrichment, although enormously useful for the participant, would not be included in the definition of productive aging because their value is for the personal growth of the individual. Such courses are not designed to be translated into a measurable good or service. The term *productive aging* as discussed by Caro, Bass, and Chen seeks to identify those measurable activities that contribute to the capacity to produce socially valued goods or services. Therefore, learning for the purposes of employment or service would be included in the definition, while learning for personal growth and enhancement would not.

In 1986, the late Louis Lowy and Darlene O'Connor wrote *Why Education in the Later Years?* In this classic work, they ask two fundamental questions: Why should society invest educational resources in older people? Aren't educational resources best invested in the young who will receive a lifetime of benefits from the educational opportunity? The authors argue that as the result of changing technology, extended human capacity to work and learn until very late in life, a need to keep abreast of new developments in a profession or field, the desire among some to enjoy multiple careers, and as a response to economic shifts, learning needs to be a lifelong activity. Learning new skills and acquiring knowledge is a process that is ongoing and a part of remaining current and active. Older people, even those in their advanced years, can benefit from the information acquired through formal learning experiences.

Despite the value of adult learning, the largest numbers of older learners are not found in colleges and universities but in corporate training centers and programs. According to *Training* magazine, in the late 1980s nearly 35.5 million individuals received formal employer-based training (Eurich, 1990). In contrast, according to the U.S. Department of Education, in 1995 there were 14.2 million students enrolled in all of higher education, of which 1.24 million were age 40 or older. Even smaller numbers of students age 50 or older are registered. In 1995, 356,500 students age 50 or older were registered at any college or university in the United States. For those who are 65 or older, an age where most older people have retired, the numbers drop to 85,000; although small, this group has grown from 63,500 just three years earlier (The Chronicle of Higher Education Almanac, 1998).

Despite the need for continued education, older learners are less likely to receive training in traditional higher education settings. Cross (1981) identifies three barriers to the participation of older people in higher education: (1) situational barriers—restrictions on participation as a result of circumstances; (2) dispositional barriers—older people who are unwilling to participate in the educational process as structured; and (3) institutional barriers—inflexible operating procedures at colleges and universities. For these reasons and others, many older people who may have the time, ability, and need to benefit from participating in higher education have shied away.

Experiments at selected universities have demonstrated that colleges can mitigate institutional barriers by offering conveniently scheduled programs, providing support services to older students unfamiliar with collegiate expectations, and adjusting the pedagogical approach to be sensitive and responsive to the prior learning accumulated through lifelong experience (see Morris & Bass, 1986). But, for the most part, colleges and universities have established invisible barriers that discourage older people. The question remains as to whether higher education simply lags behind the potential and capacity of older learners and that circumstances will change the institutional barriers or whether there will be more of a conflict between the needs of older learners and higher education.

As Lamdin notes, lifelong learning remains a "new frontier in an aging society" (Lamdin, 1997). Federal programs for the retraining of older workers (such as the Jobs Training Partnership Act, which maintains a set-aside for older workers, or Title V of the Older Americans Act, which provides job training for older workers) remain important training programs for unemployed or underemployed older workers. Even though public programs are limited, the private sector seems committed to the importance of training its existing workforce. The importance of such retraining, whether publicly or privately supported, will only grow as we look into the future.

Policies to Strengthen Productive Aging

Employment Policy

As a consequence of the dramatic withdrawal from the workforce, the current participation levels among older people as they age in paid work reflects a very different pattern than that of their participation in other productive activities. Interestingly, findings from the 1989 Commonwealth Fund Labor Force 2000 Survey (The Commonwealth Fund, 1993), a nationally representative sample of older people, indicated that a small but sizable percentage of those who had already retired were interested in returning to work. In addition, of those then working, 26 percent of men and 24 percent of women would work longer than they then had planned to if their employer pension contributions were to continue past the age of 64; 31 percent of men and 30 percent of women indicated that they would do so if they were offered fewer hours and responsibilities with the proportionate reduction in pay. Recent secondary analysis of this data set by Quinn and Burkhauser (1994) indicated that respondents surveyed would like to work longer; 59 percent wanted to return to work for economic reasons and 41 percent wanted to return more for social and psychological reasons. In either case, these are powerful reasons to work. Quinn and Burkhauser have noted that this may be an indication of increased interest in later-life paid work. They point to increased longevity, better health, a reduction in corporate pensions, declining interest rates, and the social rewards for work as reasons to expect more older people to remain on the job or to return to work after retirement. Still, powerful disincentives exist in public policy that discourage people from working past the age of 65.

Bass, Quinn, and Burkhauser (1995) identified a series of policy changes that would make it much easier for those older people who want to work to continue working beyond the traditional retirement years. Their suggestions are rather specific; undoubtedly, the significance of each will change over time. They are based on the belief that social outcomes are alterable through macro-level policy changes. New and different work-incentive policies will need to be adopted in the future if we choose to be proactive about encouraging able-bodied individuals to remain in the workforce. Policy changes that could be implemented in the future include the following:

1. Provide part-time employees with pro-rated fringe benefits, depending on the number of hours they work. This would be a significant incentive for older people to return to work.
2. As part of health care reform, reduce private health care costs for the employer employing older workers.
3. Allow the over-65 worker to opt out of Social Security contributions, saving the older worker and the employer money.
4. Allow low-income older workers without children to qualify for the Earned Income Tax Credit.
5. Provide tax credits to employers who provide or pay for older worker retraining.
6. Expand federal employment training programs to older people.
7. Provide a personal tax credit to older workers who pay for work-related educational expenses.
8. Mandate through federal legislation that employer pensions be age-neutral.
9. Develop state plans for older workers to encourage their retraining and hiring.
10. Expand the enforcement of age discrimination laws.

Some of these changes will cost money, but older people who work are taxpayers and generate new revenues for the state and federal governments. Further, if older people work, they are less likely to draw on Social Security resources. There are economic reasons as well as social benefits to consider in expanding the roles of older workers in an aging society that is nonetheless productive.

Quinn has argued that, as a result of earlier adjustments to Social Security, the elimination of mandatory retirement, the enforcement of the Age Discrimination in Employment Act, shifts in pension programs and coverage, the promulgation of Americans with Disabilities Act, and economic growth, the trend toward early retirement "is over and has been so since the mid-1980s" (Quinn, 1998, p. 257). He argues that there is a relationship between macroeconomic forces and specific public policies that influence the retirement choice people make, and we are seeing this in current retirement patterns. We agree with this argument and believe that our conceptual model incorporates this perspective.

Policies regarding Volunteering

The federal government could increase its modest efforts to promote volunteering by older people. Currently, it administers several programs that explicitly encourage older people to volunteer. One is the Retired Senior Volunteer Program (RSVP), administered in conjunction with local organizations. RSVP provides a variety of volunteer opportunities for older people. Federal funds help with the costs of administration and cover insurance for volunteers and limited volunteer expenses. The Senior Companion Program and the Foster Grandparent Program support more targeted community assignments and provide stipends to the low-income elders who are eligible. (These programs can be considered supported employment programs as much as they are senior volunteer programs.) The Senior Executive Corps provides opportunities for retired executives to serve as short-term consultants. People of all ages are eligible to participate in other federal volunteer programs such as the Peace Corps, VISTA, and AmeriCorps.

The federal government can encourage more senior volunteering by expanding and generally strengthening its existing senior programs. It can also encourage more volunteer opportunities within programs that are open to people of all ages like AmeriCorps. Recognizing that federal programs represent only a small minority of senior volunteering, the federal government might engage in other strategies to encourage volunteering by older people. It might support initiatives to strengthen volunteer administration in nonprofit organizations. Many nonprofit organizations would benefit by employing volunteer administrators with skills in creation of roles suitable for volunteers, recruitment of volunteers, matching volunteers with available assignments, training paid employees to work effectively with volunteers, and providing recognition to volunteers. Public funding could also be used to encourage development of innovative models to deploy volunteers. Morris and Caro (1996), for example, have advocated demonstrations of organizational models that would encourage more older people to assume challenging assignments as volunteers and to make major time commitments.

The suitability of public policies that offer financial incentives to shape behavior is uncertain in efforts to expand senior volunteering. As indicated above, some public programs currently make stipends or expense payments available to volunteers. Tax incentives might also be considered. The introduction of significant financial incentives threatens to transform volunteering into a form of supported employment. The greater the financial incentive, the greater are the reasons for concern about the transformation of volunteering into supported employment.

Recognizing the importance of continuity in volunteering, employers may sponsor programs that generally encourage community-service volunteering among their employees. Further, employers can offer programs that provide assistance in finding attractive volunteer assignments for employees as they approach retirement.

Policy Focused on Assistance within Families

In the American political system, the public sector generally intervenes in family matters through regulation or by offering assistance only in exceptional circumstances. The public sector, for example, does not take an explicit interest in the typically modest assistance that older people most often provide as informal caregivers or in helping their grandchildren. One reason may be that when needs are modest and transitory and the help provided is similarly modest and temporary, public-sector intervention is not needed (Doty, 1995). Nor does it seem likely that a public intervention would be effective if it sought to orchestrate modest increases in contributions of older people in these matters.

However, advocates for families argue that the public sector does have a role when extensive needs in families trigger exceptional and burdensome informal care. Public agencies are expected to protect minor children whose parents do not provide adequately for them. The public sector is also expected to assure adequate long-term care arrangements for those who are functionally disabled and poor. For these reasons, the public sector has reason to be interested when older people serve as substitute parents or provide extensive informal assistance to relatives with multiple functional disabilities and modest financial resources. When a public intervention provides assistance to overburdened providers of informal care, its aim may be to permit a *reduction* in this form of productive activity. Public-sector intervention to provide relief to those extensively involved in informal assistance can take a variety of forms, including subsidies for community services that are potential substitutes for family assistance. The options include both services explicitly designed to provide respite and community services for which eligibility is based on the condition of care recipients. Also pertinent are various financial incentives that provide care providers with greater flexibility in managing their responsibilities.

Some social welfare advocates argue that the public sector should reward or explicitly assist those who provide extensive informal assistance in a family context. Others disagree for various reasons, which include skepticism about the ability of the public sector to target assistance efficiently, the high cost of significant but inefficiently targeted assistance to families, and concern about the possibility that public interventions to assist certain families will contribute to a subtle erosion of the expectation that families in normal circumstances assume full responsibility for the care of dependent children and the functionally disabled of all ages.

Even if the public sector is reluctant to provide extensive direct support to older people who give informal assistance to others in a family context, it has reason to be highly appreciative of this informal assistance. A significant reduction in the informal long-term care and child care provided by older people would result in pressure on the public sector for increases in both publicly funded long-term care services and child care (Doty, 1995). Full discussions of the role of the public sector in regulating and supporting families with minor children or in financing and regulating long-term care are far beyond the scope of this essay.

Various private-sector policies also have implications for the assistance that older people provide within the family. Employers' human resource policies that are insensitive to employees with young children result in greater demands by working parents for assistance with child care from retired grandparents. On the other hand, employer policies that enable working parents to take time off to tend to emergency needs of their children reduce the demands made on older people to care for grandchildren in these circumstances. Similarly, employers who allow their personnel to take time off to meet elder care needs indirectly reduce demands on older informal caregivers to provide that assistance. In another domain entirely, employer policies regarding relocation of their employees have implications for informal intergenerational assistance. Employers who ask their personnel to move substantial distances for job purposes indirectly tend to reduce opportunities for grandparents to provide child care for grandchildren. On the other hand, airline companies that offer attractive fares to nonbusiness travelers make it easier for older people to travel to children living at a distance to provide temporary assistance care for grandchildren.

Career-Related Education Policy

Historically, there has been little interest on the part of colleges, government, or employers in enticing the retired or near-retired into career-related training programs. Although there have been a few isolated programs that have been exemplary in attracting students age 60 or older to college and university settings for career training, most institutions of higher education equate young high SAT–achieving students with national stature and prominence. Scholarships and tuition waivers are provided on a merit or need basis to those students who frequently are of traditional college age. In fact, although often unstated, the human capital theory of the economic value of a college education is widely embraced. It holds that the costs associated with a college education are high and older people, as a result of life expectancy and available productive years, will provide a lower return on investment than a younger student. Despite the growing evidence that college education is a lifelong involvement, with many technical fields changing so rapidly that graduates require retraining every five years, most people still subscribe to the belief that education is for the young.

Nevertheless, career-related training is a necessity for older people to remain vital and successful in their work. While credit-bearing programs in colleges and universities provide one avenue for education, other non-credit programs are offered by colleges and universities as well as many specialized training centers supported by companies and agencies. Bass and Barth (1992) argue that the nation's community college system, which has been so responsive to the changing racial and ethnic composition in America, and has provided access to thousands of minority students seeking an opportunity for career training, is an ideal collection of institutions to turn its attention to career needs of older people.

Today's older people are the best-educated cohort in history, and this trend toward increases in level of education among this group should continue well into the future. Nearly 61 percent of those 55 and older in America have studied beyond the high school level, with 13.3 percent earning a college degree. Fifty years earlier, only 17.4 percent of those 55 or older studied beyond high school, with 3.5 percent earning a college degree. With more and more older people having strong basic academic skills, the capacity to provide enhanced job skills remains accessible to most older people. Further, older workers understand the value of career training. In the 1989 Louis Harris survey conducted for The Commonwealth Fund, 37 percent of employees age 50–64 said they would continue to work past the traditional retirement age if their employers would provide training for a new position. Of those who were already retired, 27 percent stated that they would have participated in a retraining program if it had been offered so that they could continue work past their age of retirement (Taylor & Leitman, 1989).

Findings of the 1992 Louis Harris survey reinforce the 1989 results (Taylor, Bass, & Barnett, 1992). Among those who had completed high school, 30 percent had received formal job training past the age of 50. Of those with some college experience, 44 percent received some formal job training past the age of 50. A surprising 54 percent of those older individuals who took training courses did so on their own, with their own funds and without the encouragement of their employers; 44 percent of those who took classes paid for them themselves. What is quite clear is that older people are interested in career-related education. The 1992 Louis Harris survey found that of those who want to return to work, 55 percent would be willing to take classes to assist with retraining. The biggest barrier to taking these courses is cost: 43 percent of those who did not take a course past the age of 50 cited cost as the major obstacle.

With most older people having the ability to successfully engage in retraining programs and some evidence that there is interest among the population in them, what policy changes might convert more of those with interest into participants?

The first and primary issue is cost. Federal, state, employer, and college-based programs that subsidize tuition costs are crucial. Specific legislation, such as tuition waivers for those age 60 or older, could be enacted at minimal cost. Scholarship programs for older learners and employers' tuition reimbursement programs could be considered. Whatever the mechanism used to defray costs, initiatives that provide direct tuition subsidies for older learners need to be enhanced and expanded.

Community colleges are among the most affordable training institutions, and their accessibility in local neighborhoods nationwide makes them ideal for serving older learners and working with local companies in need of a skilled workforce. This target population needs to be explicitly included in community college mission statements and program and recruitment priorities.

With the vast majority of training taking place within companies, employers need to be encouraged to invest in the training of older workers. In a tight job market, employers are more likely to invest in older workers. To avoid cyclical investments, government can provide tax or financial incentives for companies to provide training to older workers or develop tuition reimbursement programs. Also, employers can reward those who participate in training programs with opportunities for advancement or salary enhancements.

In summary, changes in attitudes that bring about changes in policies and practices, along with incentives, are needed among individuals, employers, and government to further assist older people to invest in their own training and career development.

Conclusion

In this chapter, we have attempted to develop a conceptual framework from which to consider the productive engagement of older people in our society and policies that can be designed to influence participation in paid work, increase volunteer activities in formal organizations, support assistance with caregiving, and encourage participation in career-related education. Within this framework is the explicit examination of the interplay among environmental variables, situational variables, individual variables, and social policy regarding the productive involvement and engagement of older people. We hypothesize that changes in prevailing social policies will alter the interactions between situational and individual variables, resulting in different participatory outcomes. Either increasing or decreasing participation among older people can be achieved through various social policies, rules, and regulations.

In addition, we have examined the theories of affluence/leisure preference, intergenerational conflict, and cultural lag as potential explanations for the relatively low levels of participation by older people in the United States in certain productive activities. Finally, we have identified specific policy directions for increasing participation levels in such activities among older people.

REFERENCES

Achenbaum, W. A. (1995). *Crossing frontiers.* New York: Cambridge University Press.

Aldous, J. (1987). New views on the family life of the elderly and the near-elderly. *Journal of Marriage and the Family, 49* (2), 227–234.

Bass, S. A., & Barth, M. C. (1992). *The next educational opportunity: Career training for older adults.* New York: The Commonwealth Fund.

Bass, S. A., & Caro, F. G. (1996). Theoretical perspectives in productive aging. In W. H. Crown (Ed.), *Handbook on employment and the elderly* (pp. 265–275). Westport, CT: Greenwood.

Bass, S. A., Morris, R., & Oka, M. (1996). *Public policy and the old age revolution in Japan.* New York: Haworth.

Bass, S. A., Quinn, J. F., & Burkhauser, R. V. (1995). Toward pro-work policies and programs for older Americans. In S. Bass (Ed.), *Older and active: How Americans over 55 are contributing to society* (pp. 263–294). New Haven: Yale University Press.

Bengston, V. L. Rosenthal, C., & Burton, L. (1990). Families and aging: Diversity and heterogeneity. In R. H. Binstock & L. George (Eds.), *Handbook of aging and the social sciences* (3rd ed.). San Diego, CA: Academic.

Brudney, J. (1990). *Fostering volunteer programs in the public sector.* San Francisco: Jossey-Bass.

Brudney, J., & Duncombe, W. (1992). An economic evaluation of paid, volunteer, and mixed staffing options for public services. *Public Administration Review, 52,* 474–481.

Butler, R. N., & Gleason, H. P. (1985). *Productive aging.* New York: Springer.

Butler, R. N., & Schechter, M. (1995). Productive aging. In G. Maddox (Ed.), *The encyclopedia of aging* (2nd ed., pp. 763–764). New York: Springer.

Campbell, J. C. (1992). *How policies change.* Princeton: Princeton University Press.

Caro, F. G., & Bass, S. A. (1995). Dimensions of productive aging. In S. Bass (Ed.), *Older and active: How Americans over 55 are contributing to society* (pp. 204–216). New Haven: Yale University Press.

Caro, F. G., & Bass, S. A. (1997). Receptivity to volunteering in the immediate post-retirement period. *Journal of Applied Gerontology, 16* (4), 427–441.

Caro, F. G., Bass, S. A., & Chen, Y.-P. (1993). Introduction: Achieving a productive aging society. In S. A. Bass, F. G. Caro, & Y.-P. Chen (Eds.), *Achieving a productive aging society* (pp. 1–25). Westport, CT: Auburn House.

Chambre, S. M. (1987). *Good deeds in old age: Volunteering by the new leisure class.* Lexington, MA: Lexington Books.

The Chronicle of Higher Education. (1998, August 28). *Almanac Issue, 64* (4), 18.

The Commonwealth Fund. (1993). *The untapped resource: The final report of the Americans over 55 at work program.* New York: The Commonwealth Fund.

Cross, K. P. (1981). *Adults as learners.* San Francisco: Jossey-Bass.

Crown, W. H. (1996). The political context of older worker employment policy. In W. H. Crown (Ed.), *Handbook on employment and the elderly* (pp. 391–404). Westport, CT: Greenwood.

Doty, P. (1995). Older caregivers and the future of informal caregiving. In S. Bass (Ed.), *Older and active: How Americans over 55 are contributing to society* (pp. 97–121). New Haven: Yale University Press.

Eggebeen, D. J., & Hogan, D. P. (1990). Giving between generations in American families. *Human Nature, 1,* 211–232.

Eggebeen, D. J., & Wilhelm, M. (1995). Patterns of support given by older Americans to their children. In S. Bass (Ed.), *Older and active: How Americans over 55 are contributing to society* (pp. 122–168). New Haven: Yale University Press.

Ellis, S., & Noyes, K. (1990). *By the people: A history of Americans as volunteers.* San Francisco: Jossey-Bass.

Eurich, N. P. (1990). *The learning industry.* Princeton: Princeton University Press.

Fischer, L. R., & Schaffer, K. B. (1993). *Older volunteers: A guide to research and practice.* Newbury Park, CA: Sage.

Gelfand, D. E. (1993). *The aging network.* New York: Springer.

Harden, A. W., Clark, R. L., & Maguire, K. (1997). *Informal and formal kinship care.* Washington, DC: U.S. Department of Health and Human Services.

Hareven, T. K. (1994). Family change and historical change: An uneasy relationship. In M. White Riley, R. L. Kahn, & A. Foner (Eds.), *Age and structural: Society's failure to provide meaningful opportunities in work, family, and leisure* (pp. 130–150). New York: Wiley.

Herzog, A., Kahn, R., Morgan, R., Jackson, J., & Antonucci, T. (1989). Age differences in productive activities. *Journal of Gerontology: Social Sciences, 44B,* 129–138.

Holstein, M. (1993). Women's lives, women's work: Productivity, gender, and aging. In S. Bass, F. Caro, & Y.-P. Chen (Eds.), *Achieving a productive aging society* (pp. 235–248). Westport, CT: Auburn House.

Jackson, J. S., Antonucci, T. C., & Gibson, R. C. (1993). Cultural and ethnic contexts of aging productively over the life course: An economic network framework. In S. Bass, F. Caro, & Y.-P. Chen (Eds.), *Achieving a productive aging society* (pp. 249–268). Westport, CT: Auburn House.

Kaffenberger, K. R. (1998). *Nursing home ownership and public policy: An historical analysis.* Dissertation. Boston: University of Massachusetts Boston.

Lambdin, L. (1997). *Elderlearning.* Phoenix, AR: Oryx.

Lowy, L., & O'Connor, D. (1986). *Why education in the later years?* Lexington, MA: Lexington Books.

Lugaila, T. (1998). *Marital status and living arrangements.* Washington, DC: Bureau of the Census, Current Population Reports (Series P-20, No. 560).

Moody, H. R. (1988). *Abundance of life: Human development policies for an aging society.* New York: Columbia University Press.

Morris, R., & Bass, S. A. (1986). The elderly as surplus people: Is there a role for higher education? *The Gerontologist, 26* (1), 12–18.

Morris, R., & Bass, S. A. (1988). *Retirement reconsidered: Economic and social roles for older people.* New York: Springer.

Morris, R., & Caro, F. G. (1996). Productive retirement: Stimulating greater volunteer efforts to meet national needs. *Journal of Volunteer Administration, 14* (2), 5–13.

Morris, R., Caro, F. G., & Hansan, J. A. (1998). *Personal assistance: The future of home care.* Baltimore: Johns Hopkins University Press.

Mutschler, P. H. (1996). Early retirement incentive programs (ERIPs): Mechanisms for encouraging early retirement. In W. J. Crown (Ed.), *Handbook on employment and the elderly* (pp. 182–193). Westport, CT: Greenwood.

Ogburn, W. (1964). *On culture and social change: Selected papers.* Chicago: University of Chicago Press.

O'Reilly, P., & Caro, F. (1994). Productive aging: An overview of the literature. *Journal of Aging and Social Policy, 6* (3), 39–71.

Peterson, D., & Wendt, P. (1995). Training and education of older Americans as workers and volunteers. In S. Bass (Ed.), *Older and active: How Americans over 55 are contributing to society* (pp. 217–236). New Haven: Yale University Press.

Pruchno, R. A., & Johnson, K. W. (1996). Research on grandparenting: [Review of *Current Studies and Future Needs*]. *Generations, 20,* 1, 65–70.

Quinn, J. (1998). Employment and the elderly [Review of *Handbook on Employment and the Elderly*]. *The Gerontologist, 38,* 254–259.

Quinn, J., & Burkhauser, R. (1994). Retirement and the labor force behavior of the elderly. In L. G. Martin & S. H. Martin (Eds.), *The demography of aging* (pp. 50–101). Washington, DC: National Academy Press.

Riley, M. W. (1998). [Letters to the Editor]. *The Gerontologist, 38,* 151.

Riley, M. W., Kahn, R. L., & Foner, A. (1994). *Age and structural lag.* New York: John Wiley & Sons.

Riley, M. W., & Riley, J. W., Jr. (1994). Structural lag: Past and future. In M. Riley, R. Kahn, & A. Foner (Eds.), *Age and structural lag* (pp. 15–36). New York: John Wiley & Sons.

Robertson, J. F. (1995). Grandparenting in an era of rapid change. In R. Blieszner

& V. H. Bedford (Eds.), *Handbook on aging and employment*. Westport, CT: Greenwood.

Rosow, I. (1985). Status and role change through the life cycle. In R. H. Binstock & E. Shanas (Eds.), *Aging and the social sciences*. New York: Van Nostrand Reinhold.

Rossi, A., & Rossi, P. (1990). *Of human bonding: Parent-child relations across the life course*. New York: Aldine de Gruyter.

Rowe, J. W., & Kahn, R. L. (1998a). *Successful aging*. New York: Pantheon.

Rowe, J. W., & Kahn, R. L. (1998b). [Letters to the Editor]. *The Gerontologist, 38,* 151.

Schooler C., Caplan, L., & Oates, G. (1998). Aging and work: An overview. In K. Schaie & C. Schooler (Eds.), *Impact of work on older adults* (pp. 1–19). New York: Springer.

Schulz, J. (1992). *The economics of aging* (5th ed.). Dover, MA: Auburn House.

Schwartz, J., & Waldrop, J. (1992). The growing importance of grandparents. *American Demographics, 14,* 10–11.

Sterns, H., & Sterns, A. (1995). Health and employment capability of older Americans. In S. Bass (Ed.), *Older and active: How Americans over 55 are contributing to society* (pp. 10–34). New Haven: Yale University Press.

Taylor, H., Bass R., & Barnett, S. (1992) *Productive aging*. New York: Louis Harris and Associates.

Taylor, H., & Leitman, R. (1989). *Older Americans: The untapped labor source.* Program sponsored survey. New York: The Commonwealth Fund.

Thornstam, L. (1992). The quo vadis of gerontology: On the scientific paradigm of gerontology. *The Gerontologist, 32,* 318–326.

Turner, J. A., & Doescher, T. (1996). Pensions and retirement. In W. J. Crown (Ed.). *Handbook on employment of the elderly* (pp. 165–181). Westport, CT: Greenwood.

Weisbrod, B. A. (1988). *The nonprofit economy*. Cambridge, MA: Harvard University Press.

II

DISCIPLINARY PERSPECTIVES

ON PRODUCTIVE AGING

4

BIOMEDICAL PERSPECTIVES ON PRODUCTIVE AGING

Alvar Svanborg, M.D., Ph.D.

In a biomedical perspective, the state of knowledge about aging per se in humans has advanced noticeably during recent decades. It is, however, still limited for a scientifically based estimation of the productive capacity of present and coming generations of old people.

One of the aims of this chapter is to illustrate methods and research results distinguishing between manifestations of aging in itself and dysfunction caused by disease. The main objective, however, is to provide evidence that certain functional impairments related to aging in itself are not only genetically determined but in fact markedly influenced by exogenous factors such as personal lifestyle, living circumstances in general, and availability of adequate medical care. Consequently, a change in such exogenous factors would influence functional aging and allow a postponement of dysfunction, which threatens the ability to stay productive. Central to this discussion is the notion of possibilities for "reactivation"—the existence of reserve capacity at old age that would allow recovery of functioning following periods of debilitating medical or social events. And there is potential for helping frail older persons to maintain and regain functional capacity. Furthermore, a better understanding of ongoing trends in productive capacity of current age cohorts of older adults might allow for prediction of possibilities for future, even longer living, cohorts to stay productive.

A definition of productive aging might differ from a geriatric biomedi-

cal perspective or a more general sociological viewpoint. A biological definition of aging implies morphological change, lowered physical strength,
progressive stiffness in most organs, lowered stability of the skeleton, sensory loss, change in speed, and the like. Age-related risks for morbidity
and dysfunction caused by disease often add to aging-related functional
decline. This makes predictions for health and vitality of coming generations of older persons even more complex.

Furthermore, in a geriatric/gerontological view, an extension of the part
of life when the older person would be allowed or encouraged to contribute professionally might lead not only to a country's socioeconomic gain
through professional contributions, but also to a prolongation of the
individual's own vitality and a postponement of expensive needs for sociomedical support. Is it really true that rest and retirement from work would
prolong life, and its quality, for most people?

One research question that geriatric medicine and gerontology must
deal with is to predict the extent to which countries like the United States
can at least partially compensate for the projected imbalance between the
relative constancy in the proportion of younger people at productive ages,
compared to the rapidly increasing proportion of older people now considered to be unable to be productive because of their age or unwillingness to work professionally anymore. This foreseeable imbalance calls for
research producing at least "potentials for theory development." How
much do we really know about the ability and willingness of the present
generation of older persons to be and stay productive? Are we underusing
them? Are we under- or overestimating their vitality and capacity? And
how much do we know retrospectively about ongoing trends, positive or
negative, between recent age cohorts that might allow predictions for coming generations?

The remarkable medical achievements of recent decades have been
important for the older patient—often even more so for the old person
with a combination of aging-related dysfunction and disease. At the same
time, however, the cost of medical care, especially in hospitals, has increased dramatically. This has led to a shortening of length of stay and an
earlier discharge of old and frail patients, even when their own reserves of
strength do not allow them to regain preadmission level of functional
performance without help. These individuals need help not only to cure
or ameliorate their disease but to regain function. They need *reactivation,*
an attempt to help them to regain at least their habitual, premorbid level
of performance.

With respect to older persons' ability to stay productive, it is important to consider not only present performance but also to make an accurate assessment of the reserve capacity. One important aspect is to understand how functionally aged they are, and to what extent their waning reserve capacity means that they still have the potential to regain function by themselves after episodes threatening their vitality. Many require help to be brought back to a level of productive ability.

Longevity-Productivity in Historical Perspective

William Shakespeare is considered to have understood and portrayed human nature and function with an exceptional futuristic foresight—to be a man of vision. In *As You Like It* he described aging: "The last scene of all, that ends this strange eventful history, is second childishness and mere oblivion, sans teeth, sans eyes, sans taste, sans everything." He did not foresee potentials of coming generations to live longer and to enjoy a meaningful participation in an increasingly productive environment. Old persons in Shakespeare's day might have been looked upon as being in their upper middle age today. Many trends indicate that longevity will increase further in coming generations.

It is difficult to find reliable statistics on population longevity in Shakespeare's generation. The oldest reliable statistics I know of come from Sweden, and from the middle of the eighteenth century and onward. It is well known that total life span has been increasing in many populations, to a great extent due to lowering of infant and child mortality. It might for our discussion be more relevant to examine further life expectancy when a person already is considered to be old. Figure 4.1 shows further life expectancy at age 65 in Sweden from 1750 and onward. In certain populations the demonstrated lengthening of further life expectancy at age 65 contributes today more to the increase in total life span than a decline in infant mortality or change in mortality in the middle part of life.

This positive trend in lengthening of further life expectancy at a time when we are considered to have become old already is a reality in many populations and subpopulations, and even in many developing countries. If one expects to hypothesize and generalize about the future productivity of older people, it is important to be aware that longevity over recent years has not only increased in many countries but also declined in certain populations, such as many in Eastern Europe. Table 4.1 shows previous and recent differences in longevity between two contrasting European populations, Hungary and Sweden. This comparison shows not only that Hungarian males live more than 10 years less than Swedish males, but it also reveals a shortening of longevity in Hungarian males during recent decades, at the same time as a prolongation has occurred in Sweden and in many other countries. Such observations limit our ability to generalize about health, vitality, and productivity to international populations.

Many indirect observations, mainly obtained through comparisons of longevity in different populations as well as between subgroups within populations, indicate that differences in longevity among populations are related to differences in not only morbidity and availability of medical care but also functional consequences of aging in itself. A comparison of the Nordic populations of Denmark, Finland, Iceland, Norway, and Sweden shows significant differences in longevity. In 1995 the longevity at birth varied no less than 3.5 years in both males and females, given similar socioeconomic standards, incidence and prevalence of disease, and availability of medical care. Although it is always risky to rely on diagnosis entered on death certificates, these Nordic countries have similar traditions for diagnostic criteria and ways of confirming causes of death. As expected, certain variations in the reported causes of death exist among these five countries, but a superficial comparison reveals no explanation for the observed differences in longevity. Although a real scientifically based, detailed examination of possible differences in morbidity pattern

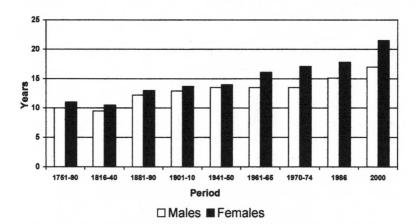

Figure 4.1   Life expectancy at 65 years in Sweden, 1751–2000
SOURCE: Mellström, D. (1988). Retrospective identification of further life expectancy and estimations for the ninth decade of this century. Prepared by Dr. Dan Mellström in collaboration with demographers at the National Statistic Office in Sweden.

explaining variations in longevity would be necessary for a definite conclusion, the existing data might arouse a suspicion that population difference in longevity might not only depend on diseases and their treatments but also on differences in manifestations of aging in itself. Indeed, some populations and population subgroups might grow old faster than others due to nongenetic factors such as lifestyle and living circumstances influencing the rate of functional aging.

Longevity-Productivity in Prospect

Some fear that an even further prolongation of our life span might imply a socioeconomic stagnation, as discussed for example in 1998 at a UNESCO council (Jasmin & Butler, 1999). A graying of nations implies that more people will become incapacitated and require medical service, social care, and support produced by those still of "productive" ages. Optimists counter, on the other hand, with a prediction of "compression of morbidity" (i.e., with extended life span we would also stay vital and healthier longer in life and consequently shorten the period we live with dysfunction and medical need). Some postponements of dysfunction have been reported in certain populations, but the life span of these groups is also increasing. A proven shortening of the period with dysfunction does not seem to have been demonstrated in representative population samples.

In a biomedical perspective, how much is known about the possible influence of exogenous factors such as lifestyle and living circumstances

TABLE 4.1   Life Expectancy at Birth in Hungary and Sweden

	Years	Males	Females
Hungary	1980–1985	65.3	73.0
	1990–1995	64.8	73.9
Sweden	1980–1985	73.4	79.3
	1990–1995	75.5	80.8
Maximum difference	1980–1985	8.1	6.3
	1990–1995	10.7	6.9

SOURCE: Data from United Nations. (1998). *World population prospect, 1998 revision.* Vol. 1, *Comprehensive tables.* New York: Author.

on aging in itself, or at least about factors with an impact on the functional manifestations of aging? And consequently, would it, through changing one's lifestyle or living situation, be possible to stay productive and independent in life, or even retain professional work, longer than what is usually considered to be relevant for both individuals and society today?

Biomedical Aspects on Functional Capacity

One difficulty in studies of human aging is the length of the average life span. The current trend toward further increase in life span in so many populations obviously will not reduce that methodological challenge. Longitudinally tracking vitality and health indicators for individuals over their entire lifetimes with unchanged methodology seems extremely difficult, almost unrealistic. Another challenge is that disease conditions commonly cause functional changes similar to those related to aging, especially at a point when manifestations of aging per se really take their toll. A crucial prerequisite for biomedical studies was, therefore, the improvement of diagnostic criteria of diseases, which allowed a better differentiation between aging and morbidity.

The major successful research focused directly on human aging has been based on longitudinal (and expensive) population studies in which representative samples are followed over long periods of time. Remarkable improvements for meaningful outcomes of longitudinal studies were obtained through the many-fold recent developments of noninvasive examination techniques, allowing detailed morphological, functional, and sometimes even biochemical analyses of single organs, organ systems, and distinct functions within an organ. Many of these noninvasive studies can be performed without inconvenience or risks for the participant.

Through such population studies, accumulated evidence has shown that at least certain aging-related manifestations are influenced by exogenous factors and not totally dominated by our genes. Conversely, we now understand that certain forms of aging-related functional decline are mainly genetically influenced and not significantly influenced by such exogenous factors as lifestyle. What, then, are the theoretical possibilities for keeping aging individuals productive even longer in coming generations?

The biomedical literature on studies of aging in animals with a shorter life span than humans is also accumulating, adding important illustrations of the impact of exogenous factors on functional aging. A survey of such findings relevant to the topic of productivity during aging goes beyond the reach of this chapter.

The following section will give *examples* of influences of exogenous factors, such as lifestyle and living circumstances, and their impact on the functional consequences of aging on key organ systems, and, furthermore, on functional changes that seem to be primarily regulated by genetics. Most of the research results presented here are based on findings of longitudinal studies, or interventions, performed in human populations. Several such studies have mainly focused on disease pattern over shorter or longer periods within the life span; fewer have undertaken the challenge to identify and examine manifestations of aging in itself separately from disease. There are, however, now available several important contributions illustrating aging per se through longitudinal population studies, like the Duke Longitudinal Study, the Baltimore longitudinal study, the functional assessment of men in Jyvaskyla, Finland, and the Göteborg longitudinal study of 70-year-olds. (For reviews of these studies, see Maddox, 1995, and Birren, 1996.)

The main basis for a differentiation between aging and morbidity are findings in such longitudinal studies, as well as from age cohort comparisons and medicosocial interventions in, for example, the studies of 70-year-old people in Göteborg, Sweden. A crucial question in the evaluation of population studies is the representativeness of the sample(s) studied. To what extent do the observations allow generalization to a population as a whole, or at least to a definable part of a population? In the Göteborg study of 70-year-old people, the original samples were shown to be generally representative for the population of 70-year-olds in that city. The first age cohort sample has been followed since 1971, and includes a detailed study of health, need for medical service and care, and functional performance. The study includes also a comparison of hitherto three 70-year-old age cohorts born at five-year intervals (i.e., 1901–1902, 1906–1907, or 1911–1912) (Rinder et al., 1975; Svanborg, 1977, 1993). Because the longitudinal follow-ups and the comparisons between the two first age cohorts indicated that exogenous factors played a significant role not only for health but also even for functional aging, a broad sociomedical intervention study was added to the third age cohort. This intervention study aimed to identify the extent to which certain statistical relationships observed in the longitudinal follow-ups really were causatively related. Other aims of the intervention were to see to what extent it might be too late to postpone aging-related decline when the participants were already as old as 70 years, and to explore to what extent the participants were at all interested in changing the lifestyle they had practiced for 70 years (see Eriksson et al., 1987; Svanborg, 1993, 1996).

Many disciplines participated in the longitudinal studies and in the intervention project, including most medical clinical specialties, dentistry, nutritional science, occupational therapy, physical therapy, medical social work, psychology, statistics, and in the intervention study even architecture, economics, history, and sociology.

To evaluate an old individual's ability to remain productive, decide if further extension of productive activity (e.g., professional work) would be good for that individual, and then recommend measures to postpone aging-related functional decline is challenging. In the same organ or organ system, certain functions might be influenced by exogenous factors, others not. Stimulating one function but not another might then put the organ as a whole, and the individual, in an undesired situation.

The Aging Heart

When the heart grows old, it undergoes certain morphological changes that increase its volume. This change is partly due to a widening of mainly the left atrium and chamber, and partly due to a thickening of the wall of the left chamber and of the septum between the chambers. The strength and speed of contraction of the heart muscle fibers decrease. At the same time the heart becomes stiffer, and subsequently it fills less efficiently. However, both direct and indirect evidence show that heart muscle strength even under these conditions can be "trained," through physical activation, to expel an increased amount of blood per stroke (for review, see Saltin, 1986). Current knowledge indicates that the strength of the heart muscle can be trained to compensate to a certain extent for the dysfunction caused by the stiffening of the heart.

During aging, changes occur also in the important neurohormonal and neuroconduction systems within the heart. These systems regulate heart rate, as well as how the atria and chambers work together. As far as is known, and contrary to the trainability of the heart muscle strength, the aging heart's neuroconductive system does not seem to be influenced by physical activity regimes or other lifestyle factors. Yet, engaging in a moderate level of physical activity seems to be good for the majority of older people, although the risk for unwanted changes in their heart rhythm might be higher. Good myocardial function should, however, generally be positive in the majority of situations, even if rhythm disturbances, caused or facilitated by aging in itself, develop. This example, among many, points to the urgent need for geriatricians and gerontologists with real knowledge about aging to advise and coach older people who wish to postpone unnecessary functional decline.

Blood Pressure and Aging

An individual's blood pressure commonly rises from childhood up to age 70 to 75, and then usually declines. It is influenced by several factors, like body weight, intake of certain nutrients, and physical activity habits. Changes in lifestyle might, thus, be of therapeutic and preventive significance. The dynamics of the common increase in blood pressure during aging is further illustrated by the fact that blood pressure at the age when it reaches its top level varies among age cohorts (Table 4.2). The findings from the Göteborg study revealed a declining trend among the generations in the study.

TABLE 4.2   Arterial Blood Pressure in Three Age Cohorts of 70-year-olds (without drugs 2D, 2E, or 2F)

	Women			
	1	2	3	Significance
SBP	168	166	160	$p < 0.000$
DBP	93	90	85	$p < 0.000$
	Men			
	1	2	3	Significance
SBP	159	160	157	$p < 0.361$
DBP	96	92	84	$p < 0.000$

SOURCE: Svanborg, A. (1989). Blood pressure change with aging: The search for normality. In C. Cuervo, B. Robinson, & H. Sheppard (Eds.), *Geriatric hypertension* (pp. 5–17). Tampa, FL: International Exchange Center on Gerontology, University of South Florida.

NOTE: SBP = systolic blood pressure; DBP = diastolic blood pressure; 2D, 2E, and 2F represent blood pressure–lowering drugs and diuretics available at that time.

For the individual, unwanted changes in blood pressure is known to be a risk factor for cardiovascular complications and strokes. Certain changes in lifestyle can, thus, be expected at least to delay some incapacitating events that would have a negative effect on the old person's ability to stay productive. Recommended interventions, especially in the many older persons with borderline hypertensive values and no clear evidence of a syndrome of a real hypertensive disease, might include at least systematic and well-planned physical activity and a lowering of body weight in over-weight people. More knowledge is needed in order to clarify how much physical activity an old individual requires to significantly lower blood pressure.

Striated Muscle Performance and Aging

Striated muscle seems to retain a greater functional reserve much later in life than earlier believed. The initial observations showed that, at least up to age 75, training could improve muscle strength (Aniansson & Gustafsson, 1981). Through studies of isolated muscle fibers, indirect evidence indicated that to a certain extent the speed of muscle contraction also could be stimulated. Both strength and speed of contraction can be essential not only for mobility in general but to guard against falls and fractures, which are common, serious, and potentially debilitating events for old people. Several groups in the United States have undertaken extended studies of muscle function as it relates to the possibility of training old people. It has been reported that reserves can be mobilized to strengthen extremity muscles through systematic physical training even in those over age 80 (Fiatarone et al., 1990). It should be emphasized, moreover, that the relative improvement achieved through strength training has been reported to be approximately the same in healthy younger and older adults (Grimby & Saltin, 1983). In absolute terms, the young person starts at a higher level of muscle strength and will reach a higher level through training than an old person will be able to do. Nevertheless, these findings demonstrate that it is possible to stimulate improvements in the muscle strength through strength training of older persons. One would, however, expect that reserves to mobilize muscle strength become almost depleted in the terminal phase of life.

Unfortunately, not even strength training has been shown to slow down the rate of decline in the number of muscle fibers. Furthermore, and in the same way as in the heart, the nerve supply to striated muscles degenerates. Therefore, the muscle fibers have to share nerve fibers to a greater extent in the old individual, a phenomenon called sprouting. The extent to which the degree of sprouting of nerves to multiple muscle fibers, happening as a consequence of aging per se, has a negative effect on fine motor coordination (i.e., the precision in function) has not been clarified.

Aging of the Connective Tissue

Another tissue influenced markedly by aging is connective tissue, which not only stabilizes organ structure but also influences compliance and elasticity, and aids in the function of many organs. Aging-related alterations of this tissue are of main importance for the decline in compliance and elasticity, and the progressive stiffening of the lungs, the heart, blood vessels, tendons and joint capsules, the skin, and the like. Important components of the connective tissue (e.g., the fibrous proteins collagen and elastin) undergo aging-related quantitative and qualitative changes. These changes contribute to tissue stiffening, which, in some tissues like the skeleton, causes a decline in stability.

Findings indicate that physical activity might postpone the rate of stiffening, at least in certain tissues like striated muscles and tendons (Suominen & Heikkinen, 1975). In general, however, stiffening of many of the abovementioned tissues seems to be one of the manifestations of aging that might be difficult to markedly postpone through a change in exogenous lifestyle factors. The consequences of tissue stiffening for human are directly evident in its effects on physical performance and indirectly in changes in the function of the central nervous system (impact of oxygenation in the lungs and the efficacy of the circulatory system).

Skeletal Stability and Function in Aging Joints

Productivity based on physical strength and mobility obviously does not depend solely on muscle power and circulatory and respiratory conditions but also on skeletal stability and joint function. Although, in general, joint disorders are common in older people, aging in itself does not usually influence the range of motion of joints to a point at which the functionality of arms and legs is significantly limited. In the back, however, the range of motion is often restricted in older people, and progressive stiffness will cause functional limitations.

Osteoporosis (low bone density), although often exaggerated by exogenous factors, must be considered an inevitable consequence of aging whether or not it reaches a level at which the skeleton becomes fragile. Osteoporosis is often a contributing factor to compression fractures of vertebrae in the spine, hip fractures, and arm and leg fractures. Many lifestyle-related habits, like tobacco smoking and too little physical activity, have been shown to be risk factors for hip fractures. On the other hand, a reasonable mechanical loading, for example, in the form of regular daily walking, seems capable of slowing fragility of the skeleton. Too heavy loading of an old skeleton would, of course, increase risks for injuries. The most important message is that aging-related osteoporosis can be influenced and postponed, even if not prevented. Nutritional intake of calcium, certain vitamins, and the like reduces the rate of development of osteoporosis. In recent decades, a slowing of skeletal fragility through substitution therapy with certain hormones (e.g., estrogen for females) that decline during aging has also been intensely studied.

Cognition and Aging

A key question at the evaluation of an old person's ability to be productive regards cognitive function (e.g. psychomotor speed, intelligence, memory, creativity, etc.) and that person's performance changes over time. Research in this area obviously is another example of the necessity of a thorough differentiation between abnormal brain conditions and physiological manifestations of aging, as brain morbidity leading to dementia is common. Several research groups have found a decline in psychomotor speed starting early in adult life (Berg, 1980; Baltes, 1993; Schaie, 1994). At the same time, in detailed longitudinal studies of older adults, participants without any definable morbidity have been reported to maintain cognitive abilities other than psychomotor speed well into old age (Berg, 1980). Some psychologists have explored the possibility of improving older people's cognitive function and found that being intellectually active might postpone functional decline (Schaie & Willis, 1986). Restoring cognitive ability after inactivating events might also be a possibility in advanced age.

Sensory Loss

The well-known aging-related declines in vision and hearing are examples of areas where technical advances have contributed to compensation for aging-related dysfunction. Sensory deprivations during our lifetime have, to a certain extent, other causes than aging per se, like exposure to certain factors now believed to contribute to muddiness in the eyes and noise damaging hearing. Such exogenous forms of damage will hopefully be less common in future generations. Declines in vision and hearing are, however, also a consequence of aging in itself, and can clearly become an obstacle for continued productivity in certain professions. Unfortunately, there seems to be no evidence in the literature indicating that the visual and hearing decline caused by aging itself can be prevented or postponed.

Efficient illumination allows many older persons to compensate for the forms of vision problems caused by aging per se. One example on aging-related vision impairments that seems to be inevitable and difficult to compensate for is the lengthening of the time it takes to adapt to changes in amount of ambient light. To come into a dark room or to drive into a dark tunnel means, for the old person, a much longer period of "darkness" before an adaptation takes place than in a young individual. Obviously, such impairment would be a hindrance for productivity in certain professions. Certain improvements are expected to come; for example, car manufacturers have ambitions to include technical aids that can help older persons to drive more safely.

Aging-related hearing impairments are common and cause not only a clear impairment of productivity in certain professions but also increased risks for social isolation, inactivity, and accidents. The understanding of the manifestations of presbycusis (aging-related hearing loss) has increased markedly in recent years. Reports describe that some forms of impairment are dominated by high-frequency hearing loss, others by reduced ability to discriminate sounds (e.g. speech). Some impairments do not considerably impair speech discrimination, but cause a generalized hearing loss over the audiometric spectrum. It might not be possible to influence some of these impairments, such as the marked, predominantly high frequency loss of hearing capacity and resultant decline in the ability to hear high tones. The present availability of hearing aids has contributed to a lengthening of the productive period in many older persons' lives. Statistics, however, indicate that only a relatively limited part of the population with presbycusis pass hearing examinations, and an astonishingly low percent of older persons wear their hearing aids. Research to make even better functioning hearing aids available is intense.

One practical consequence of presbycusis that often is neglected is the old person's inability to localize sounds. The ability of the two ears to register short differences in the time when a sound reaches first one and then the other ear is excellent in the young person. Unfortunately, it degrades during aging. This can have severe practical consequences, such as increasing the risk of accidents and impairing productivity in many professions when working in teams is essential.

Functional Reserves and Aging

Whether or not dysfunction has become obvious in everyday life, aging produces diminution in important functional reserves. Too many old and frail people do not receive adequate help with regaining functional performance after episodes threatening their vitality. There are several indications that such a lack of assisted intervention has become an increasing threat. One is the shortening of length of stay in hospitals due to economic concerns. Acute curable diseases and conditions are addressed, and the patient is hopefully healed, only to be sent home functionally disabled. Many of these old patients may not be able to regain their previous level of functioning through a mobilization of their own strength reserves. Figures illustrating population aging in functional terms usually show smooth curvilinear declines that describe the average downhill trends. But in an individualized perspective many older persons go downhill step-by-step with sudden declines after episodes of diseases that were curable. Help with reactivation usually implies a recovery of functional ability. Such a functional recovery is in itself important, not only for the individual's future level of performance but also for that person's future rate of functional decline.

From a societal perspective, a cost-benefit analysis of better reactivation programs for frail older adults must be scientifically approached (Figure 4.2). A potential gain of such research would be the identification of situations in which older people would be stimulated more often to postpone retirement and stay professionally productive. Due to legal changes, a formal barrier to an extension of professional activities above traditional retirement age no longer exists in the United States. Ability to stay productive, as it relates to a sense of control over one's own life, is more difficult to measure in economical terms.

Gender Differences in Longevity

Research on productive aging must account for the apparently basic biomedical phenomenon that females live longer than males. This longevity difference has, in many populations, increased during several recent decades, but has shown no evidence of progression in certain populations over the past 10 years. A prediction of future productive contributions by old people in different graying nations must take into account such gender differences not only in total life expectancy, but also with respect to further life expectancy from the age presently considered to be retirement age. Although this gender difference favors females, average retirement age is reported to be lower in certain countries for the longer-living females than for the shorter-living men.

Concluding Remarks

This chapter focuses on examples of aging-related change and dysfunction, emphasizing that even in the biomedical sciences, there is a clear need for a better understanding of aging itself and its impact on longevity and productivity. It does not aim to cover trends in morbidity patterns, which obviously markedly influence vitality and functional performance. It is difficult to speculate on the extent to which developments in therapeutic methods within clinical medicine have increased the ability of older people to be productive, but this extent is remarkable. It should be emphasized that, even with this perspective, there is still need for better understanding of the aging process itself if we are to obtain the best possible outcomes from new treatment resources for the growing number of graying people.

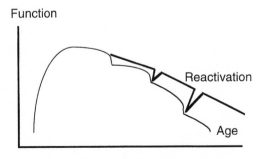

Figure 4.2   Reactivation curve

This chapter has given examples of aging-related decline in functional ability in humans. In a biomedical perspective, would it be possible to postpone negative consequences of aging to such an extent that a theory could be developed about how many old individuals would be able, and willing, to stay productive significantly longer in life than is common today? The examples given indicate that the answer concerning possibilities for an influence is yes for certain important biomedical functions, for other manifestations of aging, no. In general, however, possibilities for postponement of many manifestations of aging through a change in lifestyle factors, found to influence aging per se, seem to be better than previously considered. Expected future progress in the development and utilization of technology, as well as medical advances, will hopefully minimize the practical consequences of aging-related dysfunction. Would combinations of such predicted advancements allow an extension of the productive period beyond traditional age limits and be recognized politically in our societies? And would the older voter accept such changes in a world where resting has been considered to be good, and activity more or less dangerous? Perhaps only a few individuals might consider it better to burn down than to rust down.

On the other hand, are there any other alternatives than a mobilization of older people's capacity to avoid, or at least minimize, socioeconomic stagnation in populations, such as the United States, where a rather stable proportion of middle-aged people and a rapidly increasing proportion of old people in the nearest decades will cause an imbalance between those established to be productive and those traditionally considered to be in need of resting? The production of reliable theories about future productivity of people over traditional retirement ages will require a challenging combination of biomedical, psychological, and socioeconomic research. From what we know now, not to take action in this field of research would be the only unacceptable action.

In a clinical perspective, more knowledge of aging means improved diagnostic and therapeutic criteria. It was not too long ago when upper limits for advanced interventions in intensive care units were restricted to younger and generally healthier individuals. A deeper and more extensive knowledge about aging itself, not only in geriatrics but also in the majority of other medical disciplines, has and will allow a more detailed utilization of advances in medicine to improve care to older patients. One essential issue is how to mobilize reserve capacities necessary for a reactivation of functions essential for a meaningful life, including productive ability of old persons. It is also important to restore "indirect" productivity (i.e., to help frail older persons postpone a threatening inability to cope with life independently and care for themselves). Because of the special nature of these measures—to help with not only one function, but with the whole picture of lowered functional performance that is a part of aging itself—the term *reactivation* seems to be warranted.

This chapter also illustrates the complexity and variability of how aging can influence functional "fitness" in different organs. In order to significantly improve muscle strength, a combination of endurance and resistance training seems to be required; if the goal is to also increase muscle volume, real strength training seems to be needed. In the heart, myocardial strengthening can be achieved, but physical activation does not seem to have been proven to influence the neuroregulatory mechanisms within the heart. Multidisciplinary knowledge about aging itself and enhanced geriatric and gerontological cooperation in the development of effective coaching and training programs are prerequisites for the provision and improvement of safe and meaningful training and reactivation for especially frail old people.

REFERENCES

Aniansson, A., & Gustafsson, E. (1981). Physical training in older men with special reference to quadriceps muscle strength and morphology. *Clinical Physiology, 1,* 87–98.

Baltes, P. B. (1993). The aging mind: Potential and limits. *The Gerontologist, 33,* 580–594.

Berg, S. (1980). Psychological functioning in 70- and 75-year-old people. A study in an industrialized city. *Acta Psychiatrica Scandinavica, 288* (Suppl.), 1–47.

Birren, J. (Ed.). (1996). *Encyclopedia of gerontology: Age, aging, and the aged.* San Diego: Academic.

Eriksson, B. G., Mellström, D., & Svanborg, A. (1987, December). Medical-social intervention in a 70-year-old Swedish population. A general presentation of methodological experience. *Comprehensive Gerontology, 1,* 49–56.

Fiatarone, M. A., Marks, E. C., Ryan, N. D., Meredith, C. N., Lipsitz, L. A., & Evans, W. J. (1990). High-intensity strength training in nonagenarians. Effects on skeletal muscle. *Journal of the American Medical Association, 263* (22), 3029–3034.

Grimby, G., & Saltin, B. (1983). The ageing muscle. *Clinical Physiology, 3* (3), 209–218.

Jasmin, C., & Butler, R. (Eds.). (1999*). Worldwide revolution in longevity and quality of life: Opportunities, challenges, and responses.* Reports from the 3rd International Council for Global Health Progress. Paris: UNESCO. (Available in French; English version in press.)

Maddox, G. L. (Ed.). (1995). *The encyclopedia of aging* (2nd ed.). New York: Springer.

Rinder, L., Roupe, S., Steen, B., & Svanborg, A. (1975). Seventy-year-old people in Göteborg. A population study in an industrialized Swedish city. *Acta Medica Scandinavica, 198* (5), 397–407.

Saltin, B. (1986). The aging endurance athlete. In J. R. Sutton & R. M. Brock (Eds.), *Sports medicine for the mature athlete* (pp. 59–80). Indianapolis, IN: Benchmark.

Schaie, K. W. (1994). The course of adult intellectual development. *American Psychologist, 49* (4), 304–313.

Schaie, K. W., & Willis, S. L. (1986, March). Can decline in adult intellectual functioning be reversed? *Developmental Psychology, 22,* 223–232.

Suominen, H., & Heikkinen, E. (1975). Enzyme activities in muscle and connective tissue of M. Vastus lateralis in habitually training and sedentary 33- to 70-year-old men. *European Journal of Applied Physiology, 34,* 249–254.

Svanborg, A. (1977). Seventy-year-old people in Göteborg: A population study in an industrialized Swedish city. II. General presentation of social and medical conditions. *Acta Medica Scandinavica, 611* (Suppl.), 5–37.

Svanborg, A. (1993). A medical-social intervention in a 70-year-old Swedish population: Is it possible to postpone functional decline in aging? *Journals of Gerontology, 48* (Suppl.), 84–88.

Svanborg, A. (1996). Conduct of long-term cohort sequential studies. In E. Shah & A. Kalache (Eds.), *Epidemiology in old age* (pp. 57–65). London: British Medical Journal Publishing Group in Collaboration with the World Health Organization.

United Nations. (1998). *World population prospect, 1998 revision.* Vol. 1, *Comprehensive tables.* New York: Author.

Recommended Readings

GENERAL

Butler, R. N., & Brody, J. A. (1995). *Delaying the onset of late-life dysfunction.* New York: Springer.

Rowe, J., & Kahn, R. (1998). *Successful aging.* New York: Pantheon.

POPULATION STATISTICS

The International Database maintained and updated by the International Programs Center, U.S. Bureau of the Census.

Manton, K. G., & Vaupel, J. W. (1995). Survival after the age of 80 in the United States, Sweden, France, England, and Japan. *New England Journal of Medicine, 333* (18), 1232–1235.

Manton, K. G., & Vaupel, J. W. (1996). Comments. *New England Journal of Medicine, 334* (8), 537–538. (Discussion, p. 538)

Vaupel, J. W., & Jeune, B. (1994). *The emergence and proliferation of centenarians* (Population Studies of Aging, No. 12). Odense, Denmark: Aging Research Unit, Center for Health and Social Policy, Odense University Medical School.

LONGITUDINAL STUDIES OF AGING IN HUMANS:
DESIGN, PROCEDURE, AND EXAMPLES OF RESULTS
Population Intervention Studies

Heikkinen, E., Arajärvi, R. L., Era, P., Jylha, M., Kinnunen, V., Leskinen, A. L., Leskinen, E., Masseli, E., Pohjolainen, P., Rahkila, P., et al. (1984). Functional capacity of men born in 1906–10, 1926–30, and 1946–50. A basic report. *Scandinavian Journal of Social Medicine, 33* (Suppl.), 1–97.

The Aging Heart: Blood Pressure and Aging

Folkow, B., & Svanborg, A. (1993). Physiology of cardiovascular aging. *Physiology Review, 73* (4), 725–764.

Lakatta, E. G. (1993). Cardiovascular regulatory mechanisms in advanced age. *Physiology Review, 73* (2), 413–467.

Landahl, S., Bengtsson, C., Sigurdsson, J. A., Svanborg, A., & Svardsudd, K. (1986). Age-related changes in blood pressure. *Hypertension, 8* (11), 1044–1049.

Staessen, J., Amery, A., & Fagard, R. (1990). Isolated systolic hypertension in the elderly. *Journal of Hypertension, 8* (5), 393–405.

Whelton, P. K., Appel, L. J., Espeland, M. A., Applegate, W. B., Ettinger, W. H., Jr., Kostis, J. B., Kumanyika, S., Lacy, C. R., Johnson, K. C., Folmar, S., & Cutler, J. A. (1998). Sodium reduction and weight loss in the treatment of hypertension in older persons. A randomized controlled trial of nonpharmacologic interventions in the elderly (TONE). *Journal of the American Medical Association, 279* (11), 839–846.

Striated Muscle

Harridge, S., Magnusson, G., & Saltin, B. (1997). Life-long endurance-trained elderly men have high aerobic power, but have similar muscle strength to nonactive elderly men. *Aging (Milano), 99* (1–2), 80–87.

Klitgaard, H., Mantoni, M., Schiaffino, S., Ausoni, S., Gorza, L., Laurent-Winter, C., Schnohr, P., & Saltin, B. (1990). Function, morphology, and protein expression of ageing skeletal muscle: A cross-sectional study of elderly men with different training backgrounds. *Acta Physiologica Scandinavica, 140* (1), 41–54.

Sensory Dysfunctions

Rees, T. S., Duckert, L. G., & Milczuk, H. A. (1994). Auditory and vestibulary dysfunction. In W. R. Hazzard, E. L. Bierman, & J. P. Blass, et al. (Eds.), *Principles of geriatric medicine and gerontology* (3rd ed.). New York: McGraw-Hill.

Rosenhall, U., Pedersen, K., & Svanborg, A. (1990). Presbycusis and noise induced hearing loss. *Ear & Hearing, 11,* 257–263.

Connective Tissue Aging

Labat-Robert, J., & Robert, L. (1988). Aging of the extracellular matrix and its pathology. *Experimental Gerontology, 23* (1), 5–18.

Verzard, F. (1956). Das alterns des collagens. *Helvetica Physiologica et Pharmacologica Acta, 14,* 207–220.

Viidik, A. (1982). Age-related changes in connective tissues. In A. Viidik (Ed.), *Lectures on gerontology,* Vol. 1, *On biology of ageing* (pp. 173–211). London: Academic.

Skeletal Stability and Function in Aging Joints

Cummings, S. R., Nevitt, M. C., Browner, W. S., Stone, K., Fox, K. M., Ensrud, K. E., Cauley, J., Black, D., & Vogt, T. M. (1995). Risk factors for hip fracture in white women. Study of Osteoporotic Fractures Research Group. *New England Journal of Medicine, 332* (12), 767–773.

Mellström, D., Rundgren, Å., Jagenburg, R., Steen, B., & Svanborg, A. (1982). Tobacco smoking, ageing and health among the elderly: A longitudinal population study of 70-year-olds and an age cohort comparison. *Age and Ageing, 11* (1), 45–58.

Rundgren, Å., Aniansson, A., Ljungberg, P., et al. (1984). Effects of training programme for elderly people on mineral content of the heel bone. *Archives of Gerontology and Geriatrics, 3,* 243–248.

Seeman, M., Hopper, J. L., Bach, L. A., Cooper, M. E., Parkinson, E., McKay, J., & Jerums, G. (1989). Reduced bone mass in daughters of women with osteoporosis. *New England Journal of Medicine, 320* (9), 554–558.

Suominen, H., Heikkinen, E., Vainio, P., & Lahtinen, T. (1984). Mineral density of calcaneus in men at different ages: A population study with special reference to life-style factors. *Age and ageing, 13* (5), 273–281.

Functional Reserves

American Medical Association. (1990). American Medical Association white paper on elderly health. Report of the Council on Scientific Affairs. *Archives of Internal Medicine, 150* (12), 2459–2472. [published erratum appears in *Archives of Internal Medicine,* 1991;151(2): 265].

5

PSYCHOLOGICAL IMPLICATIONS
OF PRODUCTIVE AGING

James E. Birren, Ph.D.

It is a challenge to comment on a complex topic that has developed a sizable literature and sophistication both conceptually and empirically. The topic is broad and important and I admire the motives of the researchers and scholars who have attempted to estimate the productivity of older persons who are out of the labor force.

Origins of the Term *Productive Aging*

The concept of productive aging is not an ancient one. Use of the phrase appears to have emerged in the mid-1980s (Butler & Gleason, 1985) and since then considerable effort has been given to defining productive aging and discussion of the topic has reached a high level of sophistication (Bass & Caro, 1996). The purpose of this chapter is to point out some of the implications of the concept and its measurement from a psychological point of view.

In the background of the discussions of age and productivity, there seems to be a view that older persons are undervalued for their past, present, and potential future productivity. The other side of this coin is the viewpoint that older people in American society consume more than they produce and are more cared for than caring. Older persons have had negative images and been stereotyped (Featherstone & Hepworth, 1996). For these reasons, the motive behind many of the efforts to characterize the retired population appears to be to demonstrate their hidden or potential productivity (Butler, Oberlink, & Schechter, 1990; Caro & Bass, 1993). Recognizing their contributions to society would raise the status of older persons in a society that heavily evaluates efforts and products in monetized terms. In part, the use of the term *productive aging* is to encourage the development of a brighter picture of old age and to counteract the negative images of the greedy geezers. In a similar way, with perhaps the same underlying motive, recent publications have used the concept of successful aging. Both productive aging and successful aging seem to have at their roots a desire to raise the status of older persons as significant contributors to society and not solely as consumers of resources.

One use for terms such as *productive aging, successful aging,* and *vital aging* appears to be to raise the aspirations of older persons. Moody said that "to speak of productive aging at all is to set forth an ideal image for the last stage of life" (Moody, 1988, p. 38). He also said that "productive aging, inevitably, has connotation of a mode of existence that is active, successful, vitally engaged, and contributive to the wider community. Like *successful aging,* the term *productive aging* means to assign a positive value and connotation to age, quite in contrast to stereotypical ideas that associate old age with decrepitude, passivity, or decline" (Moody, 1988, p. 38).

Definitions and Directions

A major agenda in research on productive aging has been to provide evidence of the relative contributions of older persons. However, there is reason to examine the motives of the use of the terms and metaphors surrounding productive aging. The intent, as Moody has pointed out, is to put a positive image on being old and the processes of aging. Perhaps placing a positive image on older persons will honor them and cause more of them to aspire to the model. This perhaps has roots in religious motivation like honoring good schoolchildren.

This raises issues of definition. If we want to honor good children, we have to define what good children are and how to measure their qualities. If we were successful we could determine how many good children there are at any age, whether there are more good girls than boys, and something about the underlying processes. In this case we would be immediately sensitive to the implicit and explicit values in the concept of the "good child." Is a good child one who doesn't cheat in school, goes to church or synagogue regularly, and is respectful to elders? Similarly, is the productive older person one who continues to create a product or service, has useful ideas, participates in the community, and helps raise grandchildren? The processes of developing into a good child would seem to be exposure to good schooling, good parenting, and good peers. We might also ask the question whether older men and women are equally productive and also what processes lead to productive aging.

Key research questions are the validity of the measurements of the good child or the productive older person, and by extension, the identification of the underlying processes whereby one becomes a good child or a productive older person. Whether an image change is justified is a matter of interaction of science and the values of society. Societies and their institutions can create honors for any subgroup it wishes (e.g., war veterans, scientists, space explorers, movie actors, writers, martyrs for causes, and sports figures). The establishment of honors and desired images is a broad social process and reflects a competition of values. This appears different from the process of science in the exploration of productive aging, although values are clearly involved in the process of evaluating what is productive. The primary task of science is to determine in a reliable manner *what is,* not *what should be,* which is the domain of religion, philosophy, and ethics (Minkler & Estes, 1991).

If there is productive aging, presumably there is unproductive aging; and if there is successful aging, there is unsuccessful aging. Productive aging seems to reflect a desire to call attention to the underrecognized value of older persons and perhaps to create a positive image of them as actual and potentially greater contributors to society. In the context of published papers on productive aging, an implicit question is being asked: To what extent are older persons active or potential *sources* or *sinks* of economic value to society (Sterns, Sterns, & Hollis, 1996; Glass et al., 1995)?

As in comparing countries according to their gross national product (GNP), individuals of different ages might be compared for their productivity. To this might be added the value placed on individuals for their past productivity, present productivity, and perhaps their unexpressed or potential productivity. This is parallel to the question about when a child becomes productive, no longer a sink into whom resources flow. A child may help with housework that represents a productive contribution and become partially productive to offset the inflow to him or her of information, time, energy, and family income. Can we determine when the total contribution exceeds the total inputs?

Dimensions and Levels of Productivity

This discussion attempts to point out some of the concepts of productivity—economic, social, and psychological. Each of these views of productivity involves different definitions, values, and measurements. A purely economic definition of productivity would define it as the activities that produce commodities or services that have exchangeable value as measured by their monetary attractiveness. Thus if someone is productive, he or she has a product that is exchangeable for money or bartered products or services. The individual's productivity would simply be measured by the amount of money or bartered goods and services. A society's productivity is commonly measured by the size of its GNP. This makes it possible to express not only the total productivity but also to express it in terms of the values of goods and services produced per capita.

A social concept of productivity would expand to include recognition of social values beyond monetary value. Thus a society that produces monetary exchanges for prostitution, selling of young girls for such services, or producing drugs that have debilitating effects would not be regarded as highly socially productive. Social productivity might be defined in terms of the level of education, life expectancy, disability level and morbidity, and level of personal autonomy.

A psychological definition of productivity would depart further from an economic one whose focus was on activities that produce wealth or commodities of exchangeable value. A psychological definition might include the extent of an individual's engagement in activities that improve his or her physical and mental health, increase the effectiveness of personal relationships, increase the effectiveness of decision making, and increase the probability of insight and creativity that can reduce the level of dependency in the self or others and contribute to raising the quality of their lives. For example, the encouragement of creativity can not only result in reducing the cost of commodity production but also the production of artistic products (e.g., music, art, and literature) that add to individual growth whether or not they can be monetized.

Each of the above concepts of productivity is potentially expressible in measurements of societies, institutions, and individuals for comparative purposes. Comparisons might be made, for example, of the relative productivity of men and women in different societies. The measurements of course involve the recognition of the values of a society beyond those expressed in terms of monetary value of salable goods and services.

As mentioned, the comparison of the productivity of countries, institutions, and individuals involves measurements that invoke values that should be articulated. In each of these domains there are implicit or explicit values that make evaluations of productivity complex. Is a retired person who repairs and decorates a house more or less productive than an apartment dweller who does volunteer work at a local library? Is a retired person who writes poetry more or less productive than a sedentary person who watches much television in leisure hours?

The comparative evaluation of creative pursuits in later adult life is particularly difficult because they are so difficult to specify in monetary value. Yet if we consider the value to the individual, the activity may be of very high personal value and it may maximize the individual's self-esteem and health and perhaps minimize physical disability.

Thus the use of the concept of productive aging leads us down a pathway that has several branches. Its definition will vary depending on the intended reference level: (1) society, (2) institution, (3) business or employer, (4) family or social network, and (5) the individual (Bass, Caro, & Chen, 1993; Birren, 1985).

Corresponding to the definition of productivity and its reference level, there are matters of measurement to consider if comparisons of groups or individuals are wanted, such as monetary costs of replacement, amount of cooperation, physical health and disabilities, mental health, life satisfaction, and contentment.

Can We Integrate Different Views of Productive Aging?

To some extent psychologists and sociologists seem to want to get their noses under the tent of economics, and to some extent the economists are inviting them (Cutler, Gregg, & Lawton, 1992; Earl, 1988; Swedberg, 1993). Also there seems to be a growing recognition that economics is only a partially rational subject matter (Thaler, 1994). Perhaps the multi-billion-dollar losses in 1998 of the Long Term Capital Management Fund, guided to crisis by the investment models of two Nobel Prize winners in economics, make one more skeptical about the universal nature of narrow economic laws and principles. Behavioral and social sciences may have something to offer the interpretation of the productivity of society and individuals, particularly when attempting to estimate the productivity of older persons outside the labor force. Here the issue is whether we should be heavily guided by concepts and measurements generated by a narrow range of scholarship and research or encourage a broader approach.

An expanded criterion of productive aging would seem to lie in a profile or portfolio of individuals' investment in the activities of life. Some portfolios have larger payoffs than others. In the book, *Where to Go from Here,* Linda Feldman and I described the option of redefining one's life portfolio of how time, energy, and concerns are invested (Birren & Feldman, 1997). Presumably one's life portfolio is somewhat modifiable to maximize productivity, successful aging, or the elements of some other concepts of the output of individuals.

A useful next step in studying the dynamics of the distribution of time and effort may consist of conducting focus groups with persons of diverse backgrounds to identify how they value different activities in their lives, including being useful to others. Such groups might include workers and retirees, men and women, and persons of different socioeconomic backgrounds.

Thinking more broadly still, instead of comparing individuals, we may want to compare nations and ask how countries rank in their productivity in relation to age of the members of their populations. In this regard, the United States has a relatively high per capita GNP but it is exceeded on other key measures of productivity by small Iceland, which has a 100 percent literacy level, a lower infant mortality rate, and longer life expectancy.

Protests might be made that the criterion should only be per capita GNP, analogous to monetized individual productivity. However, more variables might be used to rank nations, institutions, and individuals according to some agreed-on criteria apart from their monetary value. As a psychologist, I would rank a country high if it had long-lived people, low morbidity and disability, low crime, high education, and high levels of health care and pensions (Preston & Taubman, 1994). Education in particular enters as a general value since, as discussed below, it contributes to other outcomes, such as health and consumer effectiveness.

Level of education and life expectancy are elements of present and future productivity that might be used for both societies and individuals. Long-lived healthy and educated persons are more likely to be productive than the short-lived and less educated. If one compares the United States to other developed countries solely on the basis of GNP, it has the highest per capita of any country, suggesting a high rating for productivity. However, it is less favorable in terms of literacy, life expectancy, and other possible criteria of quality of life and productivity. In 1966 life expectancy at birth in the United States was 73 for men and 79 for women. Comparable data for Japan were 77 and 83, and for Canada 76 and 83. Literacy in those countries was judged to be 100 percent whereas in the United States it was 96 percent. Infant mortality in America was 7 out of 1,000 live births, compared with 6 in Canada and 4 in Japan. Iceland exceeds all developed countries in life expectancy, 78 for men and 83 for women; although it has a lower GNP per capita than many of the countries, it exceeds them in health and education (World Almanac Books, 1997). Thus life expectancy, while correlated with productivity, neglects much that would be desirable in comparing countries. Similarly, major omissions accompany comparisons of the productivity of people by age and gender, using only a monetized index of their uses of time.

Serious attempts have been made to evaluate the activities of older persons in terms of their contributions to society. Typically this is done by estimating the replacement value of the time given to the activity. However, there is a limit to this approach since the productive value of the activity is restricted to efforts that others gain from it. Its value depends on the estimates of its replacement costs by others (e.g., for baby sitting, driving someone to a shopping center, or volunteering for a community service).

Herzog and Morgan (1992) did a comprehensive study of the relative productivity of persons of different ages and genders. They pointed out that women might engage in as many activities as men but typically engage in fewer paid activities. This contributes to the image of women as being of lower productivity. Herzog and Morgan contributed significantly to the methods of estimating the monetary value of unpaid work. Their sophisticated methodology allowed differential market values to be placed on such efforts as home maintenance, volunteering, child care, and informal help. Using their analysis as a basis, further measures might be devised to expand the notion of valued productivity.

The task of estimating the productivity of people from an economic point of view is to secure a cost estimate of the things they do if they were purchased. A criterion is the amount of work a person does that is sought or valued by others, such that it can be given a monetary value. While it is relatively easy to measure hours of employed work and their costs, it is not as easy to measure volunteer time and family caregiving, although several studies have done this. One avenue is to evaluate volunteer time by its replacement cost by employed persons. Such attempts have produced rather impressive economic value of the volunteer activities of older persons. These analyses represent a gain in knowledge about the contribution of older adults to society but they do not resolve all of the issues of definition and evaluation problems.

An older adult may choose to cease from some volunteer effort in order to follow an exercise routine. Presumably an exercise program contributes to the health of the individual and may reduce future health care costs covered by insurance or Medicare. In a similar vein of reasoning, we might question whether an older worker in a cigarette factory is more or less productive in comparison with the nonemployed older person engaged in daily exercise. The productivity of the older worker in a cigarette factory or distillery is measured easily in terms of the salary paid but it avoids the matter of the costs to society of resulting health and social problems of the worker's output. An example of the manufacture of cheap handguns could be added.

Thus, in addition to the problems of comparing monetized and non-monetized activities, there is the issue of the value of the activity in the present or future for society, an institution, an employer, a family, or the individual himself or herself. The value issue is not an easy one to skirt, and the courts have been attempting to evaluate the negative contribution of cigarette manufacturing and truck motor emissions by leveling fines. In the latter case, the fines were over $1 billion but it leaves unmeasured the negative value of the workers who produced the emissions evading truck motors. Their efforts are included in the GNP. Do they have a higher productivity value than a sedentary retired worker?

The dependent variables are implicit in the above categories. Perhaps less clear are the independent variables. In the case of economic productivity, there is the matter of producing the most valuable product with the lowest energy and manpower. Presumably this expresses the law of least effort, in which the greatest product is encouraged from the least physical effort or energy expenditure. We may observe this law in effect when we see paths cutting diagonally across fields and lawns where individuals take short cuts to save time and energy. In other contexts, the same individuals may disregard the law of least effort and extend the time they spend in physical effort to raise their physical fitness and reduce the probabilities of untoward events and illnesses (Svanborg, 1985).

Market-oriented business decisions concentrate on the law of least effort (i.e., the application of minimum effort to generate products that have economic value). But the well-being of the individual depends on the amount and balance of physical effort per day more than does the economic value of the product. If an agricultural worker sits on a large tractor eight or more hours a day, he or she may be producing a bountiful harvest but perhaps contributing to a decline of personal health. Future physical disabilities may also arise in a white-collar worker from sitting, viewing, and using a key board for long hours.

The concept of productivity implies a gradient of effectiveness and efficiency. If I am highly productive, then it is reasonable that I use my time efficiently as well as for recognized useful purposes. One of the neglected elements is consideration of the distribution of productivity over time. Many years ago, several social psychologists followed individual children throughout a day and analyzed their activities. This gives rise to the idea that we might compare the life profiles of time distribution of persons in relation to age, gender, and other variables such as education and ethnicity.

If this reasoning is extended further, it might be said that the productivity of the individual depends less on the economic value of the output than it does on the balance of physical effort, the cognitive load, and the social network in which the individual functions. The evaluation of individual productivity may also be placed in the context of its contribution to the physical and mental health of society as well as to its gross national product. Such issues arise in conjunction with legalized gambling whose activities contribute billions to the GNP but lead to the unproductive ruin of many retired persons' lives.

The reasoning is that the simplification of productive aging to solely a monetary criterion may result in measures that are of marginal relevance in a changing society. The replacement costs of an activity do not seem to offer enough sophistication in our postindustrial society (Martin & Preston, 1994). Perhaps we should consider several criteria of productivity and compare them for their usefulness. One might compare countries by their gross national product without regard to what they produced; however, it is likely that we would want to include in our judgments of productivity whether workers are producing nuclear weapons, germ warfare products, or addicting drugs. One might say that any worker engaged in a product that is legal in a society is productive. However, this leaves us with some uncertainty in evaluating the productivity of gambling in Las Vegas or

Atlantic City that is legal there but not elsewhere. Are employed older Black Jack dealers in Las Vegas productive?

In addition to the short-term productivity of employees and whether the products of their activities add to or subtract from the well-being of society, a question might be raised about the long-term effects of the productive activities on the employed individual. Some activities may lead to late-life dependency, such as black lung disease from mine work. Also, there are legacies of the productive life on cognitive structure and motivation to engage in further work or retirement volunteering. A lifetime of routine work may lead to boredom and disinterest in undertaking new tasks. Also, the long-term effects of nonstimulating work and a restricted stream of information in which the individual is embedded may lead over the course of work life to simplified decision making. By analogy, the long-term effects of products and services have consequences for the productive potentials of a society (e.g., environmental pollution and the waste of resources such as future land use). Thus the approaches to defining and measuring productivity have the time dimension to consider. Not only the productivity as measured today but the longitudinal effects on a society and individuals must be considered in the evaluation of economic, social, and psychological productivity.

Sources and Sinks

An individual may contribute money, time, effort, and information to others or to society, or absorb one or more of these and become a productive sink into which such resources flow. This equips us, up to a point, to decide if an individual is a *source* or *sink* in society. An important issue arises and should be discussed; this is the question of whether the concept of productivity should be extended to self-directed efforts (e.g., for personal health maintenance). Workers who are in sedentary occupations, consume a large amount of alcohol, and smoke are potential candidates for expensive medical therapies and liver transplants and thereby a major economic sink while still employed or later in life when retired (Evans, Barer, & Marmor, 1994).

A worker who is contributing to the deterioration of his or her health will become a future sink into which resources will flow in terms of costs of medical care, but there are also the less explicit costs of co-workers' drop in efficiency and attention and family care. Babies are sinks of resources that we accept as dependents until they are mature. Child care requires money, effort (energy), information, attention, and affection if the child is to grow up and be a producer in family life and society. An alcoholic family member is a sink into which money, effort, information, attention, and affection flow. If rehabilitative efforts are successful, then such a person may become a source providing resources to others, or in the broader concept, a productive person. In a sense the individual is like a capital investment of many types of resources. As an individual grows older, he or she may shift in the balance of resources flowing in and out and may give care, attention, and affection to grandchildren that are difficult for working parents to provide, but are valuable investments in the future of the children. Incorporating such elements as the flow of attention, affection, and information into an economic view of individual productivity is difficult. However, they would appear to be important elements of productivity. From such reasoning arises a picture that remains to be painted in the future of the time course of a life in which at different periods a person is more or less productive, a sink or source for others and society.

Information and Ideas

Unfortunately, time and effort are more easily monetized than information, which is the germ cell of the adapting society or individual. The transformation of our society from an agricultural one to an industrial one and now to an information one has been marked by the generation of ideas. In 1800 an agricultural field worker could cut a half-acre of grain a day with a hand sickle and later, with the invention of the scythe, could increase his productivity to an acre. Later in the nineteenth century, the field worker using a tractor could cut a hundred acres. This released millions of workers in America from agriculture as the primary employer to other occupations. The transfer was primarily a source of an idea that was not patented but passed on to workers. Here the potency of ideas and their effect on productivity is raised but also the difficulty in estimating their potential economic value. If a man developed the hand sickle, which contributed so much to the productivity of a past agricultural economy, is the productive contribution to be regarded as a lifetime contribution of the individual or only if it is translated into money or exchangeable goods?

The human species is remarkably adaptable. It has the advantage over other species in that its adaptations, discoveries, and ideas can be passed on through the use of language and other symbols that it creates. Each day individuals make discoveries that reduce the effort required to yield a product, improve a product, or reduce risk to body and health. Many of the ideas occur in relatively simple environments, in the kitchen, garden, or shopping mall. Ideas are passed among family members and raise their productivity. A thoughtful member of a family may through ideas save money, reduce work effort, and enhance the safety of other members. Ideas also occur in more complex environments and give rise to the uses of steam power, electricity, other sources of energy, and communication systems that raise the productivity of a society almost by incalculable amounts. One of the most difficult aspects of productivity to assess is the productive and potential power of ideas, but it should be kept in mind as an element of the productivity of an individual, a group, a society, or a young or elderly person. Estimating the productive value of an idea is perplexing but relevant to productivity of individuals or societies.

Presumably a society underwrites the cost of much of higher education with the view that the productive potentials of individuals are expanded. University graduates have a higher probability of contributing new ideas to science, medicine, or patents that are useful in everyday life. Important ideas may be passed along to family members by an older person (e.g., I think you should see a doctor, or a lawyer). A grandparent may sense that a grandchild would profit from having a break from the family by attending a summer camp and provide the camp fee. The camp experience may turn out to be a large contribution to the child's maturation. This line of reasoning touches on the concept of wisdom, a combination of experience, emotional maturity, and creativity whose benefits are transferred to other generations by the elderly.

Intergenerational Contributions

It has often been noted that grandparents may have a special relationship with grandchildren. This relationship may include the exchange of thoughts about the grandchild's meeting school obligations or parental demands. It may also include affective elements of attachment and trust that support the child's present and future "productivity."

To a psychologist, assessing the productive value of the cognitive and affective exchanges between generations is a task of the future. However, research can be conceived that would assess the intergenerational transfers of not only money and time but the complex of factors that enters into raising the young. This should include the contribution of elders to influencing the well-being of children who become parents and helping them in periods of marital discord or employment opportunities.

Informal mentoring of students by professors has a recognized but unevaluated status. Older professors may be more productive in such relationships because of diminished need for career contributions as well as their experience in recognizing what may be good for the student.

Few would doubt that having loving grandparents increases the likelihood of productive generations. In this context, the contributions of older adults might well be broadened to consider the affective quality of relationships. The supportive character of relationships is certainly a factor in the productivity of the individuals involved, whether it is in the work environment, family and home life, or community and neighbor interactions. There are certainly many individuals who, by their behavior, diminish the productivity of others. In considering the relationship of productivity to age, it would be useful to explore the age differences in the proportion of supportive versus critical persons, who by the character of their interactions, enhance or diminish the productivity of others.

Unfortunately, like younger adults, not all older persons are wise or constructive in their relationships. Some become emotional and time-consuming drains on the resources of others. One writer has characterized such older persons as "toxic older adults" and offers guidelines to coping with difficult elders (Davenport, 1999). Thus, at any age, there are individual differences in the productive contributions that individuals make to their families, the institutions with which they are affiliated, and the societies in which they live.

Productivity Effects of Education and Decision Style

Education has strong correlates with health and economic variables. Persons of high education tend to have higher incomes, have fewer hospital days, and have longer life expectancy (Preston & Taubman, 1994). An exploration of answers to the question, "Why are some people healthier than others?" led to consideration and identification of many elements that contribute to health (Evans, Barer, & Marmor, 1994). Clearly genetic background is a factor, but it is surprising how much social status indicators are related to health outcomes over the life span (Evans, Barer, & Marmor, 1994). In particular education is a ubiquitous variable that relates to health across the life span. In part, education's pervasive relationship to health may have correlates in economic level and access to health care. However, other features of education may help shape decision-making styles that conserve resources and expand a constructive, successful, or productive lifestyle. That is, a productive older person will tend on average to have an education that will maximize the generation of new information and the effective uses of time and energy that will add to health and a valued quality of life for himself or herself and other persons as well.

My colleagues and I conducted two research studies that add to this picture (Birren, 1994). Under the title of "Consumer Decision-Making and Age: Maintaining Resources and Independence," a research survey was carried out on a national sample of 1,723 persons from age 20 to above 70 years. Education was more highly correlated with consumer knowledge than was chronological age in three areas surveyed: health knowledge, financial knowledge, and knowledge about everyday consumer affairs.

Educated persons apparently live in a richer daily stream of information, which furnishes a higher likelihood of having up-to-date information on which to base a decision to spend money or take other actions. They tend to read consumer reports and other sources that provide comparative information about products and services. They are more likely to belong to AARP, read material related to health promotion, and adopt new technical products. New products may offer features that make them more efficient and add to the quality of life.

Perhaps more significant than education's relationship with consumer knowledge is its relationship to decision style. How people go about making decisions in their daily lives is greatly influenced by their education level. We interviewed university alumni ($N = 30$), participants in a senior center program ($N = 54$), and residents in a public housing project ($N = 49$). Each individual interview took about an hour and a half. We asked about how the individual had gone about a recent health, consumer, or financial decision in his or her life. After transcribing the interviews, they were rated on three qualities: (1) information seeking, (2) integration of information, and (3) awareness of the consequences of the decision.

In each of the three categories of decision making, the university alumni scored highest, the senior center participants in the middle, and the public housing residents lowest. The interpretation of these findings rests on the proposition that the most effective decision makers seek more information, consider more consequences, and attempt to integrate the information, including subjective as well as objective sources. The interviews also suggest that educated people tend to discuss information more readily with experts and with family and persons in their social networks.

It is possible that, because of the association of lower economic status with low education, low education groups tend to have less experience with complex decisions and related information sifting. Although education gives emphasis to information seeking, it may also result in making individuals more at ease with highly educated experts. That is, least educated persons may be more timid about asking technical questions and base their decisions primarily on trust in an expert with whom they have contact.

In the consumer knowledge survey, 10 questions were asked about consumer attitudes of potential importance in shaping effective consumer behavior. These questions involved a passive versus an active outlook on consumer behavior, cynicism, and utilization of resources. The fact that being a highly knowledgeable consumer is related to a bit of cynicism may be of significance in helping consumers avoid being victims in purchases or even frauds. There may be a clue in this research that the public has less knowledge about financial affairs than other areas. This makes such issues as the privatization of Social Security a somewhat perilous public policy course of action. The least educated persons would be the most vulnerable to inefficient decision making in this area.

Contemporary research on consumer economics is showing a trend toward incorporating concepts and methods from psychological and social research. The results may be an emerging economics of behavior that offers promise of greater understanding of the factors influencing consumer effectiveness. If we are to maximize the productivity of our population, it seems necessary to increase the general educational level of the population so people can not only be productive employees but also be able to retain and maximize their resources in retirement to their own advantage and to the advantage of others dependent on them.

Educated people in general appear to acquire a decision style that leads to the conservation of their resources of relationships, health, and finances. In part this may be a product of intelligence level, but it also seems likely that education brings with it a style of information seeking, evaluation, and discussion with others that leads to more efficient decisions. Not the least of the related products of higher education is increased likelihood of the generation of new information that is a large part of the productive contributions of persons across the life span. As we move farther into the information age, the inclusion of ideas and the generation of information would seem to be a large factor in individual productivity.

Summary and Conclusions

The published literature on productive aging has introduced many topics that should be explored in more detail as we face the age revolution of the twenty-first century. We are living longer, and are more active, and there will be millions more older persons. How can the extra days and years be used to best advantage? In this sense science can be a feedback loop that offers some new options in the process of social change, not only presenting evidence of what retired persons do, but what they can do, and the values underlying the alternatives.

The concept of productive aging appears to be a fertile one. It has led to research illuminating the fact that older persons are more useful in society than commonly appreciated. In turn this leads to a greater appreciation of older adults and raises their image in a society that emphasizes economic values. In addition to monetized productivity, however, additional measures of productivity should be developed that relate to values such as contribution to one's health and quality of life or that of other persons.

Conceptually, an individual, family, institution, community, or nation is a sink or source of information, time, energy, attention or concern, and affection. Difficult to assess, but important, is the flow of information. Information and ideas can be the most effective tools of productivity since they can lead to higher output of desired goods, solve technical or social problems, or calm an emotionally needy person. The transfer of productive ideas, information, and results of experience across generations needs further exploration. For example, the philanthropy of older persons is a large feature of contemporary American society and the assessment of its productivity needs to be explored. Behind the financial contributions are the ideas to be pursued by the money. The question might be raised, for example, whether the productive value of philanthropy is solely based on the money transfer or on the results of the target of the philanthropy.

One source of productivity in developed societies is education that leads to increased idea generation, better health, and consumer effectiveness that generally reduces present and future costs of society and caregivers. Multiple criteria should be encouraged that reflect more fully the distribution of time, energy, and information and how their uses are evaluated by society, families, and individuals. Advances in our understanding of the productive contributions of retired persons, or persons of any age, would seem to depend on collaborative interdisciplinary research by economists, sociologists, psychologists, and others. An economic view of the productive contribution of persons of different ages is a useful beginning. However, the contributions of older persons to family, society, and institutions does not seem fully assessed by monetary indices alone since their contributions may also be important in terms of the passage of ideas, care, affection, and the elusive quality of wisdom involved in intergenerational transfers.

References

Bass, S. A., & Caro, F. G. (1996). Theoretical perspectives on productive aging. In W. H. Crown (Ed.), *Handbook on employment and the elderly* (pp. 262–275). Westport, CT: Greenwood.

Bass, S. A., Caro, F. G., & Chen, Y.-P. (Eds.). (1993). *Achieving a productive society.* Westport, CT: Auburn House.

Birren, J. E. (1985). Age, competence, creativity, and wisdom. In R. N. Butler & H. P. Gleason (Eds.), *Productive aging: Enhancing vitality in later life* (pp. 29–36). New York: Springer.

Birren, J. E. (1994). *Consumer decision-making and age: Maintaining resources and independence.* Boettner Lecture, Boettner Center of Financial Gerontology, University of Pennsylvania, Philadelphia, PA.

Birren, J. E., & Feldman, L. (1997). *Where to go from here.* New York: Simon & Schuster.

Butler, R. N., & Gleason, H. P. (Eds.). (1985). *Productive aging: Enhancing vitality in later life.* New York: Springer.

Butler, R. N., Oberlink, M. R., & Schechter, M. (Eds.). (1990). *The promise of productive aging: From biology to social policy.* New York: Springer.

Caro, F. G., & Bass, S. A. (1993). *Patterns of productive activity among older Americans.* Boston: University of Massachusetts Boston.

Cutler, N. E., Gregg, D. W., & Lawton, M. P. (Eds.). (1992). *Age, money, and life satisfaction: Aspects of financial gerontology.* New York: Springer.

Davenport, G. M. (1999). *Working with toxic older adults: A guide to coping with difficult elders.* New York: Springer.

Earl, P. E. (Ed.). (1988). *Psychological economics: Development, tensions, prospects.* Boston: Kluwer Academic.

Evans, R. G., Barer, M. L., & Marmor, T. R. (Eds.). (1994). *Why are some people healthy and others not?* New York: Aldine de Gruyter.

Featherstone, M., & Hepworth, M. (1996). Images of aging. In G. L. Maddox (Ed.), *Encyclopedia of gerontology* (pp. 743–751). San Diego: Academic.

Glass, T. A., Seeman, D., Herzog, A. R., Kahn, R., & Berkman, L. F. (1995). Change in productive activity in late adulthood: MacArthur Studies of Successful Aging. *Journal of Gerontology: Social Sciences, 50B* (2), S65–S76.

Herzog, A. R., & Morgan, J. N. (1992). Age and gender differences in the value of productive activities. *Research on Aging, 14* (2), 169–198.

Martin, L. G., & Preston, S. H. (Eds.). (1994). *Demography of aging.* Washington, DC: National Academy Press.

Minkler, M., & Estes, C. L. (1991). *Critical perspectives on aging: The political and moral economy of growing old.* Amityville, NY: Baywood.

Moody, H. R. (1988). *Abundance of life: Human development policies for an aging society: The political and moral economy of growing old.* New York: Columbia University Press.

Preston, S. H., & Taubman, P. (1994). Socioeconomic differences in adult mortality and health status. In L. G. Martin & S. H. Preston (Eds.), *Demography of aging* (pp. 279–318). Washington, DC: National Academy Press.

Sterns, A. A., Sterns, H. L., & Hollis, L. A. (1996). The productivity and functional capacities of older adult workers. In W. H. Crown (Ed.), *Handbook on employment and the elderly* (pp. 276–303). Westport, CT: Greenwood.

Svanborg, A. (1985). Biomedical and environmental influences on aging. In R. N. Butler & H. P. Gleason (Eds.), *Productive aging: Enhancing vitality in later life* (pp. 15–27). New York: Springer.

Swedberg, R. (Ed.). (1993). *Explorations in economic sociology.* New York: Russell Sage Foundation.

Thaler, R. H. (1994). *Quasi-rational economics.* New York: Russell Sage Foundation.

World Almanac Books. (1997). *World Almanac, 1997.* Mahwah, NJ: Author.

6

SOCIOLOGICAL PERSPECTIVES
ON PRODUCTIVE AGING

Brent A. Taylor, Ph.D., and Vern L. Bengtson, Ph.D.

Within the past few years, gerontologists have developed the concepts of productive aging and successful aging as desired outcomes to the aging process for two reasons: first, they view aging in a positive light, and second, they suggest the potential of an aging population (Baltes & Baltes, 1990; Butler & Gleason, 1985; Caro, Bass, & Chen, 1993; Rowe & Kahn, 1998). These are welcome alternatives to the stereotype of frail elders and the view of the elderly as dependent members of our population. But while this emphasis on productive or successful aging has generated much interest, it has not led to a cumulative body of empirical research; nor has it resulted in useful applications in gerontological practice or policy. The reason for this, as we suggest in this chapter, is that insufficient attention has been given to the conceptual and theoretical development underlying these desired outcomes—the "what" and the "why" behind productive or successful aging.

Our primary purpose in this chapter is to urge researchers in productive aging to pay more attention to theory-based attempts to explain and understand their empirical results. A second goal is to provide a summary of recent theoretical developments in social gerontology, including both micro (individual) and macro (society) levels of social theory. We argue that, to develop a cumulative knowledge base of productive aging, gerontologists must present empirical findings within a theoretical framework;

furthermore, practitioner interventions should be based on theory as well as research.

We want first to define some terms and indicate why their conceptual and theoretical development has been inadequate thus far.

Successful Aging is the title of a recent bestseller by Rowe and Kahn (1997) as well as the theme of the 1998 Gerontological Society of America's Annual Meeting. For Rowe and Kahn (1997), the definition of successful aging is "the many factors which permit individuals to continue to function effectively, both physically and mentally, in old age" (p. xii). They emphasize the "positive aspects of aging—which had been terribly overlooked" (p. xii) in contrast to the "problems of the aged" approach. Their approach focuses on the power of individuals to shape their lives and the powers of aging—what sociologists call "human agency." Their message is that older people have significant abilities to prevent illnesses, to minimize losses in physical and mental function, and to enhance their engagement in life. They provide a relatively simple prescription for individuals who want to experience successful aging: exercise body and mind; eat nutritiously; maintain close relationships; and stay involved.

This conceptualization of successful aging has generated several critiques (Riley, 1998; Schmeeckle & Bengtson, 1999). First, Rowe and Kahn ignore the intellectual and theoretical tradition of other scholars who have developed more comprehensive perspectives on successful aging. The term *successful aging* was first introduced to the gerontological research community by Havighurst (1958) as a conceptual framework for the landmark Kansas City Study of Adulthood and Aging. Research based on the Kansas City study led Cumming and Henry (1961) to propose a disengagement theory of aging in contrast to what they described as activity theory (Havighurst's implied perspective). We find it interesting that most of Rowe and Kahn's prescriptions for successful aging follow the activity theory format proposed almost four decades ago: stay active, keep involved, keep striving. Unfortunately, no subsequent research over the past four decades has provided empirical support for the activity theory of aging. Thus Rowe and Kahn's central hypothesis—that maintaining the level of performance and activities of middle age will provide for a successful aging—is unsupported by research evidence to date.

Second, successful aging ignores the effects of social structure, the macrosocial context in which individuals grow up and grow old, in a society that is obviously stratified in terms of income, race, and gender. Following this reasoning, successful aging appears irrelevant for the majority of America's aged today and tomorrow—those who are poor, members of racial and ethnic minorities, immigrants, and particularly older women.

Productive aging has been defined by Caro, Bass, and Chen (1993) as "any activity by an older individual that produces goods and services, or develops the capacity to produce them, whether they are to be paid for or not" (p. 6). This definition provides a more economic and sociological perspective to desired outcomes in aging. The image is of the capacity of an individual or an entire population to serve in the paid workforce, to serve in volunteer positions, to assist in family matters, and to maintain himself or herself as independently as possible (Butler & Gleason, 1985).

The term was developed as a response to ageism, the negative stereotyping of the elderly, emphasizing that it is the responsibility of both society and the individual to help older persons reach their potential. This perspective suggests that society needs to reduce and eliminate the barriers that older people face in being productive. Individuals need to be responsible and take part in society's functioning on multiple levels, including work for pay, community service, and family.

Past research on productive aging has focused on four institutional sectors and the barriers that older adults face in productive aging: employment and retirement, volunteering for organizations, informal caregiving, and education and training (O'Reilly & Caro, 1994). Unfortunately, the term *productive* has connotations that imply Weber's Protestant ethic of striving for material capital as a measure of one's worth. Robinson (1994) notes that the term is often "more confusing than clarifying, more amorphous than specific, and leaves itself open to constant reinterpretations in such a way that its meaning can easily be perceived as anything anyone wants it to be" (p. 6).

Unfortunately, there is relatively little empirical evidence to support any linkage between productive aging and quality of life for elderly individuals. This promising concept, a way of emphasizing the positive potentials of aging in contrast to images of progressive and inevitable decline, has not yet led to the development of a sound base for research or applications in gerontological practice or policy. Why?

The Need for Theory

At present, both "successful aging" and "productive aging" appear to be buzzwords in gerontology, not yet adequately defined by researchers yet increasingly popular among advocates, practitioners, and older persons themselves. The terms reflect "popular level theories of aging," which contain value-laden assumptions about what is successful, what is productive, and how these lead to an enhanced quality of life in our later years. The conceptual and theoretical foundations for these assertions are as yet underdeveloped.

We argue the importance of theoretical contributions to the future development of a productive aging perspective. Scholars, social policy makers, practitioners, and advocates need to pay more attention to theory and utilize existing social gerontological theories to inform research on a productive aging society. While theory is sometimes dismissed as abstract and esoteric, we argue that theory provides relevant insights on the problems being addressed by professionals and that theory is crucial for an examination of productive aging.

We have briefly discussed the background and limitations of productive aging. Next we illustrate how a sociological perspective can shed light on understanding a productive aging society. We respond to C. W. Mills' call for the "sociological imagination." We also explicate the importance of evaluating underlying assumptions, and the crucial role of theory in developing a knowledge-base of productive aging. Then we will show how three sociological frameworks, symbolic interactionism, conflict, and functionalism, can inform discussion on the benefits and limitations of productive aging. Following the explanation of the frameworks, we articulate how several social gerontological theories have significantly contributed to the aging literature and how these theories can be applied to a productive aging society. We address theories that attempt to explain social behavior on the micro, meso, and macro levels of society. Next, we illustrate the promises and pitfalls of conceptualizing age and aging in terms of productive aging. While there are many positive attributes to a productive aging society, we contend that there are also potential problems that may develop with the increasing usage of this term. Finally, we conclude with suggestions about how incorporating a more sociological examination of productive aging will lead to interventions grounded in theory which will result in the desired effect—a more productive and successful aging population.

The Sociological Examination of Productive Aging

The Sociological Imagination

One shortcoming with many approaches to productive or successful aging is that they do not adequately address the effects of social contexts on individual behaviors. Productive aging is a more comprehensive term than successful aging because it is less individualistic and considers institutional barriers and the effects these have on individuals (Bass & Caro, 1996). C. Wright Mills, a classic sociologist, coined the term *sociological imagination* to explain the importance of examining individual behavior and life events in the context of the social forces and institutional arrangements that shape them. This can be a useful concept that sheds light on the possibilities of being productive in later life. Both the macro- and microsocial dimensions are critical to consider when attempting to ameliorate "problems of aging," a consideration that is often lost by practitioners and advocates in gerontology. We suggest in this essay how theories at both the macro and micro levels can inform our knowledge about problems with productivity and the possible solutions.

The sociological imagination allows us to go beyond the surface level of an issue by illuminating the importance of values and theories underlying all social issues. Social contexts, such as populations, social structures, social class, and social roles, greatly affect people's choices and their chances to be productive. The context in which people become "old" is constantly changing, thus making it difficult to produce long-lasting, effective policies. A person's propensity to be productive also depends on many individual characteristics, as Butler and Gleason (1985) noted, such as health, cognitive capability, and disease prevention. What is not articulated by Butler and proponents of productive aging is that certain groups or classes of people, such as the poor and minorities, do not have access to the same information regarding disease prevention or compensations for disabilities that are available. Characteristics such as socioeconomic status, race, citizenship status, gender, and sexual orientation are some indicators of social inequality that affect people's opportunities to be productive.

The Importance of Values

It is also imperative that as social scientists and theoreticians we examine the underlying values and assumptions of what we study and propose.

The term *productive aging* in itself connotes an Occidental orientation of equating success with productivity. Values can be defined as standards of the desirable, and in Western society the salience of certain values, such as the Puritan work ethic, are crucial to an understanding of such terms as *success* or *productivity*. One weakness of productive aging is the value contexts of the definition. The underlying values implicit in any definition of productive or successful must be brought forward and articulated. Definitions of successful or productive are diverse among members of American society, depending on people's location among social strata and groups reflecting majority and minority subgroups. It may not be desirable for some cultures to want to be productive, and we may inadvertently discriminate against alternative lifestyles to productivity. What does it mean if people choose not to be productive? And by whose definition of productivity?

The Importance of Theory

This leads to the importance of basing our work in a strong theoretical perspective. By theory we mean the construction of explicit explanations in accounting for empirical findings (Bengtson, Burgess, & Parrott, 1997). Within the relatively short history of the social sciences and aging, our field has accumulated many findings, and we have by now begun to establish several important traditions of theory. Much recent research in gerontology, including articles published regarding productive aging, appear to have disinherited theory (Bengtson, Burgess, & Parrott, 1997). Researchers need to integrate their empirical findings within a larger explanatory framework, connecting their results to established explanations of social phenomena. Theory plays a crucial role in research on aging by building a cumulative knowledge base that can be readily understood and applied. We now have multiple theories representing various aspects of the aging process that provide different lenses through which to view and explain phenomena of aging.

Theories are an attempt to explain what we see in the empirical world around us. Theories are like lenses of different colors or magnification that reveal something different about the object being viewed; each lens views the same object yet sees it in a different light. Theories help us to integrate knowledge by summarizing empirical findings and providing linkages between concepts and empirical results. Theory also explains how and why observed phenomena are related and also allows us to make predictions about what is not yet known or observed. A good theory summarizes the many discrete findings from many empirical studies and incorporates them into a brief statement that summarizes linkages between concepts and empirical results. Pursuing theory related to productive aging will be a fruitful endeavor.

Researchers in aging should create theoretical models to help inform public discourse and policy making on aging issues. Overcoming the pitfalls in thinking that early social gerontologists demonstrated (e.g., too-grand theories, or homogeneous, linear models of aging focused on averages) requires turning a critical lens on basic assumptions about aging, and actively promoting theories that reflect the diversity of experiences, behaviors, and assumptions about human aging. Productive aging has hints of a grand theory. The ubiquitous quality of this approach can be dangerous since it has the potential to marginalize alternative aging styles.

An Examination of Productive Aging through Three Sociological Frameworks

There are three main sociological frameworks that sociologists utilize to interpret social phenomena: structural-functionalism, symbolic interactionism, and conflict theory. Each framework provides different interpretations of society and social problems. Each of these offers a useful perspective on productive aging.

The Structural-Functionalism Framework

From the framework of structural-functionalism, society is viewed as a self-correcting, orderly system. Its various parts work together to bring the whole into equilibrium. Each part performs a function (hence, the term *functional analysis*) and makes a contribution to the system. In short, functional analysis examines the relationship between the parts and the whole of a social system (Merton, 1968). This notion dates back to the 1850s, when Emile Durkheim (1893) developed his classical conceptualization of society, suggesting that a system is constructed of various parts that work interdependently to create the whole social system. Society is based on the division of labor, where interrelated parts of society work together to create solidarity. When one part of the system breaks down, the whole system breaks down. Parsons formalized the functional perspective in the 1950s by providing empirical evidence and a formal theory on the importance of structures, social roles, and social norms (Parsons, 1951). Manifest functions are the intended and expected goals of a social pattern or system. Latent functions are the unexpected and unintended consequences that result from social pattern. While productive aging may have some useful manifest functions, such as contributing to the productivity of society, we must also examine the latent functions that this concept may incur. From a structural-functionalist perspective, productive aging replaces the view that aging is a dysfunction and supplants it with a view that aging can be seen as a time of prosperous productivity.

The Symbolic Interactionism Framework

Symbolic interactionists view symbols as the essence of human interaction and social life. Our interpretations of life come from the symbols that we use. If we use different symbols, we understand our experiences differently (Mead, 1934). As our symbols of aging and the aged change, so do our interpretation of the elderly. The ideas of symbolic interactionism are nearly as old as those proposed by structural-functionalists. This approach is more reflective than structural-functionalism and examines the meanings and symbols that are the essence of social life. Our symbols of aging have changed remarkably over the past 100 years. There has been a phenomenal restructuring of the life course over the last century as the life expectancy has doubled since 1900. This leads to the question, who is aged? Do we use late-twentieth-century notions of aging or those from the beginning of history? Children born in the twenty-first century will spend one-third of their life outside the traditional workplace. Productive aging provides the opportunity to establish a new set of symbols regarding the elderly. Instead of viewing the elderly as frail and weak, the elderly may symbolize a potential working force that will significantly contribute to society. Whatever the new set of symbols will be, they will provide guidelines for how we think about and act toward old people. Productive aging is an important framework to change perceptions of the elderly. Productive aging has the potential to both shape people's attitudes and reflect the changing reality of older people's lives.

The Conflict Theory Framework

Conflict theorists, based in a Marxian tradition, emphasize that power, privilege, and whatever other resources a society offers are limited. These resources are unequally distributed among the various groups that make up a society. As these groups interact with each other and compete over these limited resources, they inevitably come in conflict with one another (Marx & Engels, 1846/1976; Simmel, 1904/1966). Max Weber (1945) discussed the three P's—Power, Privilege, and Prestige—which cause an unequal distribution of resources. Weber alerts us to ask whose interest is being served. From this perspective, whenever we examine a social issue such as aging, we should look at the distribution of power and privilege, for social issues always center on the conflicting interests of a society's groups. The resources available to each group are limited, and the gains of one will be resented by the other.

Conflict theory is likely to be critical of the concept of productive aging. Does society offer opportunities for every member to be productive? There may be underlying biases in productivity that would allow men to be more productive than women. The lower-class population may already be productive in older age, due to the necessity of working to provide means for themselves and family members. Throughout late life many people are unable to retire due to no pension, others are extensively involved in caregiving since they cannot afford professional services. Productive aging theories must realize that people in power will have more opportunities to be productive than the oppressed who have limited options throughout their life course.

SYMBOLIC INTERACTIONISM, FUNCTIONALISM, AND CONFLICT will serve as the organizing principles around which each of the social theories that follow will be discussed. These three frameworks have led to much of the theorizing that has taken place in the past 50 years in sociology. The first theories in social gerontology (such as disengagement theory and activity theory) were what we consider "grand theories" because they attempted to explain everything about aging at both the micro and macro levels of analysis. Disengagement and activity theories have been heavily criticized; nonetheless they have played important roles in the history of theoretical development.

Disengagement theory, one of the first formal theories on aging, started with the assumption that disengagement is an inevitable process in which many of the relationships between an aging person and other members of society are severed, and those remaining are negatively altered in quality. Activity theory, another classic gerontological theory, proposed the opposite: if people remain active in later life, this will result in a higher sense of well-being and successful aging. Unfortunately, these theories did not hold up under the scrutiny of the scientific method and there is not sufficient empirical data to support their hypotheses.

Productive aging appears to represent a resurgence of activity theory in that the underlying assumption is that people should be productive in later life. While we agree people should have the option to be productive, there is a danger that it can become a new standard in which to exclude alternative ways of competent aging.

Micro-Level Analysis of Productive Aging

We consider first two micro-social level theoretical perspectives that have great potential in developing an understanding of productive aging: social constructionism and social exchange theories. These theories stem from very different theoretical traditions. Social constructionism tends to employ interpretive frameworks in order to understand the problems of aging, often using qualitative research techniques. This lends itself to being most closely identified with the symbolic interactionist perspective. In contrast, social exchange theory, which is rooted in the functionalist paradigm, relies more heavily on the positivist tradition found in the scientific method by using quantitative analyses of interactions that occur as individuals age.

Social Constructionist Perspectives

What has recently become known as the social constructivist perspective of aging reflects a long tradition of micro-level analysis in the social sciences, focusing on individual agency and social behavior within larger structures of society: symbolic interactionism (Mead, 1934), phenomenology (Berger & Luckmann, 1966), and ethnomethodology (Garfinkel, 1967). Following an even earlier tradition pioneered by Max Weber (1905/1955), social constructionism uses hermeneutic approaches, the science and methods of interpretation.

It may be argued that few of the emerging social constructionist theories have built explicitly on earlier micro-level gerontological theories, and only recently have social constructionist theories gained recognition in gerontology (Neugarten, 1985). Kuypers and Bengtson's (1973) social breakdown theory called attention to the process of "labeling" older individuals as incompetent at both the micro and macro levels of social mechanisms. This theory has received attention primarily as an intervention strategy for practitioners.

Researchers who employ social constructionist theories emphasize their interest in *understanding,* if not *explaining* (a distinction that is important to many scholars in this tradition), individual processes of aging as influenced by social definitions and social structures. By examining the social construction of age and aging, these researchers link individuals to social-structural contexts. For example, labeling the elderly as dependent, asexual, or deviant is defined socially, as can be seen by examining attitudes toward aging and stereotypes of the aged.

Productive aging provides a new prism in which to view the elderly. This term connotes activity and independence. "Productivity" was developed as a way of aging in direct response to the stereotype of "dependency." The first mention we see in the literature regarding productive aging was at the Salzburg Seminar in 1982. Butler proposed that health and productivity "go hand in hand and deteriorate together" (Butler & Gleason, 1985, p. xii). Productivity has the potential to enhance health and well-being among older adults and prevent the devalued status of the elderly. By introducing this term, the *meanings* that we attribute to being old can change since, according to social constructionists, knowledge comes out of language. Social constructionism explores the "situational, emergent and constitutive features of aging" (Passuth & Bengtson, 1988, p. 345) by examining how social meanings of age and self-conceptions of age arise through negotiation and discourse.

Productive aging advocates are attempting to change the attributions of old age by introducing new ideas into the discourse of equating age with decline. Social constructionist theories of aging also emphasize that social reality shifts over time, reflecting the differing life situations and social roles that come with maturation (Dannefer & Perlmutter, 1990; Kuypers & Bengtson, 1973). The productive aging literature has not adequately addressed how productivity may be dependent on societal circumstances which may change at any time and the different life situations of each individual. The social constructionist perspective provides useful insight into the construction of the term *productive aging*, why it came about, and where researchers need to go from here. Productive aging theories need to more closely examine the context and situation-based circumstances in which people age.

Social Exchange Theories

Applied to aging, this perspective attempts to account for exchange behavior between individuals of different ages as a result of the shift in roles, skills, and resources that accompany advancing age (Hendricks, 1995). A second function of social exchange theories of aging is to offer explanations of the balance (or lack thereof) in what is received and given between generations. In the case of unbalanced social exchanges, the analysis turns to the perceived costs and benefits of the exchange and whether the calculations are rational and self-interested or altruistic. A third concern of social exchange theories of aging is to understand how exchange behaviors reflect the changing circumstances of the elderly and those with whom they interact, such as family members or others who are in their social support network.

A central tenet in the social exchange framework is that each person brings resources (which are not necessarily material) to the interaction, and that these resources usually are unequal. A second tenet is that people will only continue to engage in exchanges for as long as the benefits are greater than the costs and no better alternatives readily exist (Hendricks, 1995). Third, it is assumed that exchanges are governed by norms of reciprocity (Gouldner, 1960): when we give something, we trust that something of equal value will be reciprocated. This is the premise behind the "Golden Rule": do unto others as you would want them to do toward you.

One aspect of productive aging is caregiving to family members. Social exchange theory provides a useful lens in which to examine caregiving issues. Bass and Caro (1996) state that the family is one of the central institutions in which we can use ideas of productive aging to measure the contribution that the elderly make to families. This is most apparent in the dramatic increase in recent years of grandparents taking primary responsibility for raising grandchildren (U.S. Bureau of the Census, 1999).

In exchange theory terminology, old people lose status as they become increasingly older, leaving them with little bargaining power. Their major claim to society's resources is based on the expectation of reciprocity for the contributions they previously made to society. The hopeful message of productive aging is that, as society shifts views on the elderly by seeing this population as potentially productive, the elderly will likely have greater access to many aspects of society.

Theories at Both the Micro- and Macro-Social Levels of Analysis

Bridging both the micro- and macro-social levels of analysis, the life course perspective and feminist theories incorporate the dynamics and social processes of aging that occur at *both* levels of analysis. Each perspective simultaneously highlights aspects of social interaction and social structure in order to understand and explain research findings in aging. Feminist theory is strongly opposed to the functionalist perspective on society. Much of the ideas surrounding feminism are built from a Marxian tradition, out of which grew conflict theory. Recent developments in feminist theory have relied more heavily on postmodernism and fit into the symbolic interactionist framework.

Feminist Theories and Perspectives

The origins of feminist theories in social gerontology reflect the diverse tradition of feminist theorizing in sociology and the social sciences (Connell, 1987; Hess & Ferree, 1987; Smith, 1987). Since the 1970s, feminist theorists have highlighted the importance of gender by recognizing the absence of women in social scientific research, rethinking the differences between women and men, and examining gender biases within the social sciences (Ferree & Hess, 1987). Feminist theorists argue that gender is a crucial consideration in attempts to understand aging and the aged. Gender is an organizing principle for social life across the life span (Rossi, 1985) that significantly alters the experience of aging (Ginn & Arber, 1995; Hess, 1985). Feminist theorists argue that current theories and models of aging are insufficient because they fail to include gender relations or the experience of women in the context of aging (Blieszner, 1993; Reinharz, 1986).

Applying a feminist perspective to a "productive aging society" leads to some important questions. Productivity is often equated with traditional male activities and has the tendency to devalue relational activities that are more commonly a part of the female role. To their credit, Bass and Caro do claim the importance of family—yet some feminists would view their quantifying of relationships as reductionistic. Holstein (1992) notes that even the strongest proponents of productive aging "easily slip into equating productive aging with employment" (p. 21). A productive aging society cannot be divorced from the historical and political context and the gender-based distributions of power and prestige that exist in this context. Many women have faced inequality in the workforce throughout their life and this exploitation would likely continue in older age. Is this a goal that we want as a society? Why would women want to continue in this type of environment? Holstein (1992) also mentions that productive aging could be used politically against the elderly to dismantle government programs that are in place to help them. By framing the elderly as productive, some could argue that "handouts" are not needed.

Aging and the Life Course Perspective

The intellectual origins of the life course perspective are rooted in the nineteenth-century theory developed by social economist B. S. Rowntree (1901) that provided explanations of poverty in terms of stages in family structure; early anthropologists' analyses of age-grading (Mead, 1934; Van Gennep, 1908/1960); the seminal analysis by Cain (1964) concerning the life course and social structure; and the work of Riley and her associates culminating in the age stratification perspective (Riley, Johnson, & Foner, 1972).

It is debatable whether the life course perspective should be considered a theory, a model, or a paradigm (Bengtson & Allen, 1993; Dannefer, 1984a, 1984b; Marshall, 1995). This perspective represents a convergence of thinking in sociology and psychology about processes at both macro- and micro-social levels of analysis and for both populations and individuals over time. Researchers who incorporate the life course perspective in their work are attempting to explain the following: (1) the dynamic, contextual, and processual nature of aging; (2) age-related transitions and life trajectories; (3) how aging is related to and shaped by social contexts, cultural meanings, and social structural location; and (4) how time, period, and cohort shape the aging process for individuals, as well as for social groups (Baltes, 1987; Bengtson & Allen, 1993; Elder, 1992a, 1992b; George, 1993).

A life course analysis can be applied to examine how earlier productivity may affect the propensity to be productive in later life. Is there a cumulative effect that occurs regarding people's opportunities throughout life? Consider, for example, the "multiple jeopardy" hypothesis. This suggests that if someone has faced institutional barriers, such as racism, throughout life it is less likely that she or he will take the opportunity to be productive late in life. Ethnic and racial minorities often suffer social, psychological, and economic disadvantages that have negative effects in older age (Dowd & Bengtson, 1978; Jackson, Antonucci, & Gibson, 1993). An opposing theory suggests that age serves as a leveler and that the vicissitudes of old age make up for the advantages that nonminority individuals had in earlier life. Jackson has urged a life course perspective stressing the importance of an individual's early experiences with the labor force as influencing later opportunities for productivity.

Theories at the Macro-Social Level of Analysis

At the macro-social level of analysis, three perspectives—age stratification, political economy of aging, and critical theory—provide understanding of how social structures influence experiences and behaviors. Age stratification is rooted in the theoretical tradition of structural-functionalism and largely approaches the study of divisions among groups and cohorts from a positivist framework. Political economy of aging is theoretically rooted in Marxian traditions, but takes mainly a structural and economic approach to questions of aging, relying on both interpretive and positivist techniques in pursuit of understanding or prediction and control. Critical theory also has its roots in Marxian theoretical traditions but follows the path of hermeneutic and cultural analysis, which relies almost exclusively on interpretive approaches to theorizing. Hence, both political economy of aging and critical theory fit within the conflict framework.

The Age Stratification Perspective

Over the past 25 years Riley and her colleagues have put forth a uniquely sociology-of-aging perspective, one that focuses on the role of social structures in the process of individual aging and the stratification by age in the society. Recently Riley (1994) has suggested that these efforts are better described under the label of the "aging and society paradigm." Certainly the age stratification perspective represents one of the oldest traditions of macro-level theorizing in social gerontology. Riley, Foner, and Waring (1988) note three main components to this "paradigm": (1) studying the movement of age cohorts across time in order to identify similarities and differences between them, (2) examining the asynchrony between structural and individual change over time, and (3) exploring the interdependence of age cohorts and social structures.

Recently Riley and her associates have applied the age and society perspective to the concept of structural lag (Riley, Kahn, & Foner, 1994; Riley & Riley, 1994). Structural lag occurs when social structures cannot keep pace with the changes in population dynamics and individual lives (Riley & Loscocco, 1994), of which the most obvious example is the increase in average life expectancy beyond age 65 and the lack of available societal structures to accommodate or utilize postretirement elders. Productive aging is a useful concept to address the asynchrony between aging and the capability of older adults to aid society. Riley and Loscocco (1994) discuss how policy changes such as extended time off for education or family can bring social structures in balance with individuals' lives, by restructuring the social institutions of work, education, and the family. Structural lag has caused many older citizens to be less productive.

A second application of the age stratification perspective concerns the influences of social change on the family. Riley and Riley (1993) argue that contemporary social change has created a new dimension to extended family relationships, which they call a latent matrix of kin connections. Because each new generation has a greater life expectancy, individuals will have more family ties over the life course that may provide possible support. These scholars suggest the age stratification perspective explains how kinship patterns among younger cohorts suggest a shift toward a latent kin matrix of support.

This theoretical perspective can be useful in showing how older persons can contribute to extended family relationships. Riley's age-integrated model also suggests how society can develop policies to overcome many of the institutional barriers (due to structural lag) that the elderly face in being productive.

The Political Economy of Aging Perspective

Political economy perspectives applied to aging maintain that socio-economic and political constraints shape the experience of aging; they result in the loss of power, autonomy, and influence for older persons. Life experiences are seen as being patterned not only by age, but also by class, gender, and race and ethnicity. These structural factors, often institutionalized or reinforced by economic and public policy, constrain opportunities, choices, and experiences of later life.

The political economy perspective emphasizes influences that social structure, economics, and public policy have on elderly individuals, and the limits these place on the options available to the elderly. When combined with a critical theory analysis, the political economy perspective suggests that the experience of aging is variable, based on such structural constraints as social class or minority group status. Political economy of aging can also be linked with social constructionist perspectives to point to the ways in which structural forces manage and control the social construction of aging and how old age is experienced.

A relatively new twist in the political economy perspective has been to combine it with a "moral economy of aging" approach, a development that deals with the criticism that political economy is too focused on economics and social control. By examining the "shared moral assumptions about reciprocity and fairness" (Minkler & Cole, 1991, p. 45), a more thoughtful analysis of oppressive and emancipated situations is yielded. The political economy of aging lens leads to a careful analysis of the larger sociocultural issues that affect people's opportunities to be productive. The moral economy of aging perspective also can help view the underlying moral assumptions that productive aging promotes. This is a theoretical orientation that is related to critical theory, reviewed next.

The Critical Theory Perspective

Discussing the humanistic discourse, Moody (1988) identified four goals of critical gerontology: (1) to theorize subjective and interpretive dimensions of aging; (2) to focus not on technical advancement but on praxis, defined as action or involvement in practical change (such as public policy); (3) to link academics and practitioners through praxis; (4) to produce "emancipatory knowledge." Another perspective from Dannefer (1994) suggests that critical gerontology should not merely critique existing theory but create positive models of aging, emphasizing strengths and diversity of age, which is what scholars discussing productive aging have attempted to do. Here the focus is on the critique of knowledge, culture, and the economy. Critical gerontology questions traditional positivistic assumptions and prefers to examine concepts or ideas from a multidimensional perspective.

Tornstam (1992) applied the perspectives of critical gerontology to the field itself and argued that conventional gerontology is based on limited positivist notions of knowledge and science, producing a model of aging based only on social problems. By contrast, a more humane gerontological approach would allow the aged themselves to define the research questions—for example, Tornstam's (1992, 1996) own theory of "gerotran-scendence."

Critical theory causes us to question the economic valuation of activities, such as volunteering, that is often utilized by researchers in productive aging. Theorists from this paradigm are critical of quantifying the contributions of the elderly. Critical theory also causes us to ask who benefits from using the term *productive aging*. Moody aptly acknowledges that there can be more than one meaning to later life. Other alternatives to productivity need to be considered which are addressed elsewhere in this volume. The importance of the arts and humanities also seems to be denied in a "productive aging society."

Promises and Pitfalls of Productive Aging

There are several areas of promise where scholars in productive aging can significantly contribute to the gerontological literature: (1) the term *productive* reflects a healthy and hopeful approach to aging; (2) productive aging has the capability to quantify the contributions of the elderly; (3) there may be greater interface between theories and intervention attempts in gerontological practice and policy with the use of productive aging as a framework; and (4) this perspective is less individually based than successful aging. At the same time, we see several kinds of pitfalls in recent research on productive aging: (1) productive aging is a fluid concept, with varying definitions depending on the researcher; (2) productive aging has a slippery meaning and the underlying assumptions surrounding the term must be examined; (3) there appears to be a lack of looking at larger social forces that affect structure: many opportunities for productivity are based on a particular economic condition, and macro forces and historical context need to be more readily examined; and (4) this perspective has hints of a grand theory, which tries to accomplish too much by seeking to develop similar explanations at the micro-social as well as the macro-social level.

What productive aging attempts to do may actually have a paradoxical effect. While attempting to illustrate the contributions that the elderly can provide to society, it may be ignoring or pathologizing many elderly who choose not to be productive or may not even have the choice to be productive. There are many macro forces influencing aging, such as dramatic changes in demography and the labor market supply that dictates retirement policies. The opposite of the term *productivity* implies "unproductivity" or "laziness," which in our capitalist society means "failure."

An Agenda for Research on Productive Aging

Before any research begins, it should have a theoretical basis. The emerging research on productive aging has not yet molded itself within a specific theoretical framework. We find much of the literature regarding productive aging confuses the micro- and macro-social levels of analysis. Productive aging as a model allows for a wide range of analyses and purposes. It can be adopted at both the micro and macro levels of analyses. However, researchers must articulate which type of analysis they are attempting to conduct and not mix the two different levels.

Theory development is a dialectical process that is only accomplished through careful analysis and much mental exertion. We recommend that before embarking on a research project, researchers first consider existing theories and decide which applies best to their focus of study. By looking at each theory, it is possible to eliminate concepts that do not apply and to adopt ideas that lend understanding to the issues under examination.

We have presented several different theoretical positions, some of which are diametrically opposed to each other. We think it might be helpful to the novice researcher for us to conclude with our own suggestions about the most useful theories to be applied to productive aging. The researcher must distinguish between the micro and macro levels of analysis. At the micro level, we suggest looking first at social exchange theory since it is the theory that most readily applies to productive aging. Second is the social constructionist perspective that can readily lead to an understanding of people's definition of or reaction to productive aging. Finally, the life course model may be considered; however, this is very abstract and difficult to operationalize. At the macro level of productive aging we suggest beginning with the political economy perspective on aging since it reveals the underlying societal inequalities that determine whether people are productive or not. Follow this with a examination of the age stratification model, which has the implied intent of helping people having access to all opportunities throughout the life cycle; then consider the feminist perspective, and finally critical gerontology.

Summary

In this chapter we have argued that researchers should be giving more attention to the process of cumulative theory development in research on productive aging in the social sciences. Contrary to what many recent contributors to social gerontology journals seem to assume, theory is not a marginal, meaningless, esoteric exercise. First, the systematic progression of knowledge (explanations) over time is the standard by which any field of scholarly or scientific research is judged (Brown, 1986). Second, the way in which a research field deals systematically and explicitly with problems of epistemology and explanation determines its future progress in knowledge-building (Hagstrom, 1965). Third, understanding or discovery of phenomena is seldom achieved by the solo investigator, but rather is a social process within a community of investigators involving discussion and criticism between new and previous theories and explanations (Kuhn, 1962). Fourth, only in the context of such theory-driven debates about empirical findings do "anomalies" surface—findings that cannot be explained or understood within the current body of knowledge. These anomalies (and their emergent explanations) are the basis for "paradigm shifts" and "scientific revolutions" which can leapfrog the progress of knowledge forward (Kuhn, 1962). For this reason, we applaud the opportunity to share insights as scholars in this volume to produce an agenda for productive aging research in the twenty-first century.

In gerontology today, however, we find ourselves "data-rich but theory-poor" (Birren & Bengtson, 1988, p. ix). What Bromley (1974) observed about our field is still relevant two decades later: "much of what we have learned consists of detailed, low-level, empirical observations, lacking system and explanation. It is not sufficient merely to observe that certain age changes take place; we need to know why they take place" (p. 372).

Too seldom in recent years have research articles in the productive aging literature addressed the challenge of theory development. But when researchers have made the effort to utilize theoretical perspectives in predicting relationships and explaining findings, the knowledge base of the field has grown. And a rich diversity of explanatory frameworks at the micro and macro levels of analysis has emerged. Thus, whether we consider productive aging as a part of "science" (within the positivistic paradigm) or a "field of inquiry" (in the constructivist or humanistic tradition), we should be giving more attention to theory—the cumulative development of explanation and understanding about observations and findings—

as we publish the results of our empirical investigations. We must also pay attention to the underlying assumptions that are implied by productive aging.

Our purpose in this chapter has been to urge researchers to pay more attention to theory-based attempts to explain and understand empirical results in productive aging. A second goal has been to provide a summary of recent theoretical developments in social gerontology, including both micro- and macro-level theoretical problems. Third, we have argued that the most credible way for such findings to add to the cumulative development of knowledge is through theory building. Despite the relatively short history of productive aging, it has already been influential.

A major theme of this chapter is that the societal context is crucial to understanding productive aging. We have argued that there must be a balance of human agency and social forces in understanding productive aging. By analyzing the productive aging society through multiple frameworks, we will underscore the variability of the elderly and consider that there are different realities for each subgroup of the elderly. And the reality is that some subgroups may not want to be productive at all.

We want to close on a note of caution. We are concerned about the applications so far of this potentially useful concept of productive aging. This concept needs to be applied with careful attention to theory. Empirical application without a basis in theory is dangerous ground to tread on. For example, it is sometimes not clear if productive aging research is really studying phenomena as they actually exist or if they are attempting to change the current reality by introducing this concept. Greater attention to the sociological significance of productive aging will allow for more useful applications to the increasingly diverse elderly population in the twenty-first century.

References

Baltes, P. B. (1987). Theoretical propositions of life-span developmental psychology: On the dynamics between growth and decline. *Developmental Psychology, 23*, 611–626.

Baltes, P. B., & Baltes, M. M. (1990). Psychological perspectives on successful aging: The model of selective optimization with compensation. In P. B. Baltes & M. M. Baltes (Eds.), *Successful aging: Perspectives for the behavioral sciences* (pp. 1–34). New York: Cambridge University Press.

Bass, S. A., & Caro, F. G. (1996). Theoretical perspectives on productive aging. In

W. H. Crown (Ed.), *Handbook on employment and the elderly* (pp. 262–275). Westport, CT: Greenwood.

Bengtson, V. L., & Allen, K. R. (1993). The life course perspective applied to families over time. In P. G. Boss, W. J. Doherty, R. LaRossa, W. R. Schumm, & S. K. Steinmetz (Eds.), *Sourcebook of family theories and methods: A contextual approach.* New York: Plenum.

Bengtson, V. L., Burgess, E. O., & Parrott, T. M. (1997). Theory, explanation, and a third generation of theoretical development in social gerontology. *Journal of Gerontology: Social Sciences, 52B* (2), S72–S88.

Berger, P. L., & Luckmann, T. (1966). *The social construction of reality.* New York: Doubleday.

Birren, J. E., & Bengtson, V. L. (Eds.). (1988). *Emergent theories of aging.* New York: Springer.

Blieszner, R. (1993). A socialist-feminist perspective on widowhood. *Journal of Aging Studies 7,* 171–182.

Bromley, D. B. (1974). *The psychology of human ageing.* Middlesex, England: Penguin.

Brown, H. (1986). *The wisdom of science.* New York: Random House.

Butler, R. N., & Gleason, H. P. (1985). *Productive aging: Enhancing vitality in later life.* New York: Springer.

Cain, L. D., Jr. (1964). Life course and social structure. In R. E. L. Faris (Ed.), *Handbook of modern sociology.* Chicago: Rand McNally.

Caro, F. G., Bass, S. A., & Chen, Y.-P. (1993). Introduction: Achieving a productive aging society. In S. A. Bass, F. G. Caro, & Y.-P. Chen (Eds.), *Achieving a productive aging society* (pp. 1–25). Westport, CT: Auburn House.

Connell, R. W. (1987). *Gender and power: Society, the person and sexual politics.* Stanford, CA: Stanford University Press.

Cumming, E., & Henry, W. E. (1961). *Growing old: The process of disengagement.* New York: Basic Books.

Dannefer, W. D. (1984a). Adult development and social theory: A paradigmatic reappraisal. *American Sociological Review, 49,* 100–116.

Dannefer, W. D. (1984b). The role of the social in life-span development, past and future: Rejoinder to Baltes and Nesselroade. *American Sociological Review, 49,* 847–850.

Dannefer, W. D. (1994, July). Reciprocal cooptation: Some reflections on the relationship of critical theory and social gerontology (Rev.). Symposium conducted at the meeting of the International Sociological Association, Bielefeld, FRG.

Dannefer, W. D., & Perlmutter, P. (1990). Development as a multidimensional process: Individual and social constituents. *Human Development, 33,* 108–137.

Dowd, J. J., & Bengtson, V. L. (1978). Aging in minority populations: An examination of the double jeopardy hypothesis. *Journal of Gerontology, 33* (3), 427–436.

Durkheim, E. (1964). *The division of labor in society.* New York: The Free Press. (Originally published 1893)

Elder, G. H., Jr. (1992a). Life course. In E. F. Borgatta & M. L. Borgatta (Eds.), *The encyclopedia of sociology.* New York: Macmillan.

Elder, G. H., Jr. (1992b). Models of the life course. *Contemporary Sociology: A Journal of Reviews, 21* (5), 632–635.

Ferree, M. M., & Hess, B. B. (1987). Introduction. In B. B. Hess & M. M. Ferree (Eds.), *Analyzing genders: A handbook of social science research.* Newbury Park, CA: Sage.

Garfinkel, H. (1967). *Studies in ethnomethodology.* Englewood, NJ: Prentice-Hall.

George, L. K. (1993). Sociological perspectives on life transitions. *Annual Review of Sociology, 19,* 353–373.

Ginn, J., & Arber, S. (1995). Only connect: Gender relations and aging. In S. Arber & J. Ginn (Eds.), *Connecting gender and aging: A sociological approach.* Philadelphia: Open University.

Gouldner, A. W. (1960). The norm of reciprocity: A preliminary statement. *American Sociological Review, 25,* 161–178.

Hagstrom, W. O. (1965). *The scientific community.* New York: Basic Books.

Havighurst, R. J. (1943). *Human development and education.* New York: Longman.

Havighurst, R. J. (1958). *Disengagement and patterns of aging. Middle age and aging; a reader in social psychology.* Chicago: University of Chicago Press.

Hendricks, J. (1995). Exchange theory in aging. In G. Maddox (Ed.), *The encyclopedia of aging* (2nd ed., pp. 348–350). New York: Springer.

Hess, B. B. (1985). Aging policies and old women: The hidden agenda. In A. S. Rossi (Ed.), *Gender and the life course.* New York: Aldine de Gruyter.

Hess, B. B., & Ferree, M. M. (Eds.). (1987). *Analyzing gender: A handbook of social science research.* Newbury Park, CA: Sage.

Holstein, M. (1992). Productive aging: A feminist critique. *Journal of Aging and Social Policy, 4* (3–4), 17–33.

Jackson, J. S., Antonucci, T. C., & Gibson, R. C. (1993). Cultural and ethnic contexts of aging productively over the life course: An economic network framework. In S. A. Bass, F. G. Caro, & Y.-P. Chen (Eds.), *Achieving a productive aging society* (pp. 249–268). Westport, CT: Auburn House.

Kuhn, T. (1962). *The structure of scientific revolutions.* New York: Norton.

Kuypers, J. A., & Bengtson, V. L. (1973). Social breakdown and competence: A model of normal aging. *Human Development, 16,* 181–201.

Marshall, V. W. (1995). Social models of aging. *Canadian Journal on Aging, 14* (1), 12–34.

Marx, K., & Engels, F. (1976). *The German ideology.* New York: International Publishers. (Originally published 1846)

Mead, G. H. (1934). *Mind, self, and society.* Chicago: University of Chicago Press.

Merton, R. K. (1968). Manifest and latent functions. In *Social theory and social structure* (rev. ed.). New York: The Free Press.

Minkler, M., & Cole, T. R. (1991). Political and moral economy: Not such strange bedfellows. In M. Minkler & C. L. Estes (Eds.), *Critical perspectives on aging: The political and moral economy of growing old* (pp. 37–49). Amityville, NY: Baywood.

Moody, H. R. (1988). Toward a critical gerontology: The contributions of the humanities to theories of aging. In J. E. Birren & V. L. Bengtson (Eds.), *Emergent theories of aging.* New York: Springer.

Neugarten, B. L. (1985). Interpretive social science and research on aging. In A. S. Rossi (Ed.), *Gender and the life course.* New York: Aldine de Gruyter.

O'Reilly, P., & Caro, F. (1994). Productive aging: An overview of the literature. *Journal of Aging and Social Policy, 6,* 39–71.

Parsons, T. (1951). *The social system.* New York: The Free Press.

Passuth, P. M., & Bengtson, V. L. (1988). Sociological theories of aging: Current perspectives and future directions. In J. E. Birren & V. L. Bengtson (Eds.), *Emergent theories of aging.* New York: Springer.

Reinharz, S. (1986). Friends or foes: Gerontological and feminist theory. *Women's Studies International Forum, 9* (5), 503–514.

Riley, M. W. (1994). Aging and society: Past, present, and future. *The Gerontologist, 34,* 436–446.

Riley, M. W. (1998). Response to successful aging. *The Gerontologist, 38* (2), 151.

Riley, M. W., Foner, A., & Waring, J. (1988). Sociology of age. In N. J. Smelser (Ed.), *Handbook of sociology* (pp. 243–289). Beverly Hills: Sage.

Riley, M. W., Johnson, M., & Foner, A. (1972). *Aging and society* Vol. 3, *A sociology of age stratification.* New York: Russell Sage Foundation.

Riley, M. W., Kahn, R. L., & Foner, A. (Eds.). (1994). *Age and structural lag: Societies' failure to provide meaningful opportunities in work, family and leisure.* New York: John Wiley & Sons.

Riley, M. W., & Loscocco, K. A. (1994). The changing structure of work opportunities: Toward an age-integrated society. In R. P. Abeles, H. C. Gift, & M. G. Ory (Eds.), *Aging and quality of life* (pp. 235–252). New York: Springer.

Riley, M. W., & Riley, J. W. (1993). Connections: Kin and cohort. In V. L. Bengtson & W. A. Achenbaum (Eds.), *The changing contract across generations* (pp. 169–190). New York: Springer.

Riley, M. W., & Riley, J. W. (1994). Age integration and the lives of older people. *The Gerontologist, 34,* 110–115.

Robinson, B. (1994). In search of productive aging: A little something for everyone. *Aging International, 21,* 33–36.

Rossi, A. S. (Ed.). (1985). *Gender and the life course.* New York: Aldine de Gruyter.

Rowe, J. W., & Kahn, R. L. (1998). *Successful aging.* New York: Pantheon.

Rowntree, B. S. (1901). *Poverty: A study of town life.* London: Longmans, Green.

Schmeeckle, M., & Bengtson, V. L. (1999). Conclusions from a longitudinal study: Cross-national perspectives. [Review of Rowe, J., & Kahn, R. (1998). *Successful Aging*]. *Contemporary Gerontology, 5* (3), 87.

Schutz, A. (1967). *Collected papers* (M. Natanson, Ed.). The Hague: Martinus Nijhoff.

Simmel, G. (1966). *Conflict* (K. H. Wolff, Trans.). Glencoe, IL: The Free Press. (Original work published 1904)

Smith, D. (1987). *The everyday world as problematic: A feminist sociology.* Boston: Northeastern Press.

Tornstam, L. (1992). The *quo vadis* of gerontology: On the scientific paradigm of gerontology. *The Gerontologist, 32,* 318–326.

Tornstam, L. (1996). Gerotranscendence—A theory about maturing in old age. *Journal of Aging and Identity, 1,* 37–50.

U.S. Bureau of the Census (1999). *Coresident grandparents and grandchildren* (Current Population Reports, Series P23-198). Washington, DC: U.S. Government Printing Office.

Van Gennep, A. (1960). *The rites of passage* (M. B. Vizedom & G. L. Caffee, Trans.). Chicago: University of Chicago Press. (Original work published 1908)

Weber, M. (1930). *The Protestant ethic and the spirit of capitalism* (T. Parsons, Trans.). New York: Charles Scribner's Sons. (Original work published 1904)

Weber, M. (1945). *Max Weber: Essays in sociology* (H. H. Gerth & C. W. Mills, Eds.). New York: Oxford University Press.

Weber, M. (1955). *Economy and society.* New York: Bedminister. (Original work published 1905)

7

PRODUCTIVE AGING

An Economist's View

James H. Schulz, Ph.D.

Productive aging is basically about the roles of people in later life.* Preceding its introduction into the social science literature there had already developed a rich body of theory and research related to the roles of individuals at various stages of the life cycle. In this regard, the discipline of economics has been mainly concerned about why people stop working in the paid labor force and the alternatives to work that are available to provide individuals with economic support. Economists have had little interest in the nonwork roles of people over their life and, therefore, little interest in what people do when they retire. But, yes, economists have always been interested in "work incentive" questions and the *productivity* of workers.

At first glance, then, there may seem to be a basic synergy between the productivity interests of economists and the productive aging interests of gerontologists. However, this is not true. As indicated above, the economist is concerned primarily about work activities *before* retirement, and the productive aging researchers are concerned primarily with work (and other "things") *after* retirement.

---

*The definition of productive aging assumed in this chapter is the definition used by Caro and Bass in their later publications: "The term productive aging is used to refer to any activity by a older individual who produces goods or services, whether paid or not, or develops the capacity to produce them."

Another important caveat relates to the audience being addressed when discussing productive aging. No one is likely to deny older people the opportunity to be economically productive if it is their choice, and almost everyone would be agreeable to there being a wide range of choices (with regard to activities and roles) available to people wanting to work. But many people, especially researchers in various fields of gerontology, find the productive aging framework too narrow and restricting in discussing the roles and activities of people in the later years.

In this regard, it is important to keep in mind the origins of the writings on productive aging. While too narrow for some researchers, the restricted focus of the productive aging concept is probably quite adequate to respond to the political concerns that stimulated its initial development. The concept of productive aging developed in part as a reaction to the limited view of work as defined by economists and the resulting structure of the national income and product accounts that measure the aggregate economic output of the nation. Given present practices, many of the activities and contributions made after (and also before) retirement are not counted in the official statistical reckonings of *economic* activity.

Now why would anyone care how government statistics classify various activities of life—economic or noneconomic? Of course, the answer is obvious: statistics have an impact and generate power in the political arena. Thus, the concept of productive aging, as originally developed in the United States, was motivated in large part by a perceived need to provide a political response to political attacks on the elderly. As Bass and Caro put it, "productive aging is a concept that refocuses the political debate and discussion about social welfare and programs for the elderly. It provides a different perspective from which to view the elderly and their needs. It changes the way we think of aging and our images of older people" (1992, p. 78). It is no accident that the origins of the concept coincided with a change from a public image of the elderly as a group of "deserving poor" *unable* to work to a much more negative image of them as a well-off group of "greedy geezers" who are *unwilling* to work (see Butler, 1994).

The Changing Political Face of Aging

What caused this change in image? There are five major developments that have supported the shift: (1) rising economic status and decreased work incentives; (2) older workers being "not needed"; (3) the costs of the baby boom; (4) the threat of global competitiveness; and (5) low productivity.

Rising Economic Status and Decreased Work Incentives

Historically there has always been a consensus in the United States that its norms, policies, laws, and acts of retribution should be designed to encourage individuals to work hard. The concern has been to maximize work effort in order to maximize economic growth.

Special, new concerns with regard to work incentives were first generated in the eighteenth and nineteenth centuries when a radically new form of economic organization came into being, coordinated and driven by market forces and entrepreneurial organizers ("capitalists"). However, in the early days of the industrial revolution this concern about lazy workers and work incentives had little relevance for aging policy. Demographically the country was young, with relatively few people who were old in the labor force. To the extent that older people worked, they were largely self-employed on farms.

But as economic production mushroomed with the new manufacturing methods and technology, the nature of the old age experience also changed in a fundamental way. Almost 50 years ago, Eugene Friedmann and Robert Havighurst, pioneers in the field of social gerontology, expressed it this way: "Thus, retirement is not a rich man's luxury or an ill man's misfortune. It is increasingly the common lot of all kinds of people. Some find it a blessing; others, a curse. But it comes anyway, whether blessing or curse, and it comes often in an arbitrary manner, at a set age, without direct reference to the productivity or the interest of the individual in his work" (1954, p. 2).

What Friedmann and Havighurst were referring to was the fact that retirement is a product of the industrial revolution. Older people before then were not retired people, and there was no retirement role (Donahue, Orbach, & Pollack, 1960). Industrialization created a new problem. In contrast to the farm, where people could almost always work (even if it was at reduced levels), industry was characterized by a large amount of job insecurity. Recurrent recessions and depressions and shifts in employment opportunities increased competition for the available jobs. Job obsolescence was a certain reality, as technology continued to change rapidly. And pensions were created to facilitate, encourage, or force older workers to leave the workforce (Schulz, 1974). Older workers in this environment were not viewed as critical to the production process. In fact, they were often viewed as excess baggage.

In recent years, however, the economic environment has changed. The negative views of private industry toward older workers have not changed significantly. But the attitudes of government with regard to pension and retirement policies have. As the economic status of the elderly has increased dramatically (in large part due to liberalization of Social Security), their labor force participation has declined, creating new concerns. With the increase in elderly incomes and the higher costs arising out of the maturation of the Social Security system, more people became aware of the large size of economic transfers projected for the future. Moreover, there was concern about the possible negative impact on economic growth of the now mammoth public pension program (i.e., Old Age, Survivors, and Disability Insurance [OASDI]). Increasingly, it was argued that the transfers between workers and the "nonproductive" elderly should be reduced and that the aged should work more.

Older Workers Are "Not Needed"

Paradoxically, as far as the economies of industrialized countries are concerned, there is no need for the elderly to be productive, that is, to remain in the formal labor force. The United States has gone through a dramatic transformation of its productive capacity. Under the familiar title of "the industrial revolution," we can group the breathtaking array of transformations in technology, human capital, and the organization of the production process that have occurred. The result has been a gigantic rise in production potential, creating many new opportunities in the twenty-first century for society.

One of the opportunities or problems (we have had trouble over the years deciding which it was) is the potential for spending less time in the paid labor force over one's lifetime. The expansion of productive potential has brought with it the opportunity either to increase the amount of goods and services available or to produce a specified amount of output but with less hours of labor. Historically, of course, industrializing countries have opted for both. Some of the rising productive potential has been used to raise output, incomes, and standards of living (as measured by consumption levels). Simultaneously, the rising economic potential has permitted a dramatic reduction in the number of hours a particular worker spends in the paid labor force. In the United States, for example, the workweek has declined from approximately 60 hours in 1879 to about 38 hours in 1995.

When viewed from this perspective, the question of whether societies need older workers to work longer is very complex. Assuming full employment, one way a society can deal with the higher costs of Social Security and medical care for the aged, for example, is by raising the nation's output potential. A way of doing that would be to increase the size of the *employed* labor force by encouraging or requiring older workers to retire at later ages. But the assumption of full employment necessary to make this option viable is not consistent with historical reality. The chronic unemployment that has plagued nations has actually produced the opposite policy response; workers have been encouraged to leave at increasingly early ages (Myles & Quadagno, 1991). As economist Juanita Kreps pointed out as early as 1977, "retirement, a relatively new life stage, has quickly become a device for balancing the numbers of job seekers with the demand for workers at going rates of pay. . . . [Given the continuing problems of unemployment], there is no incentive to prolong work life in general" (p. 1427).

Some argue, given demographic trends and the resulting smaller numbers of younger people entering the workforce, that countries will need the services of older workers to keep their economies growing. But this conclusion ignores the fact that it is possible for industries to respond to labor shortages in a number of ways; hiring older workers is only one of many ways. Companies can: (1) invest in more physical capital that reduces labor needs; (2) encourage liberalization of immigration policies favoring applicants with needed skills; (3) encourage more women with children to stay in the labor force; or (4) shift production processes to developing countries where there are labor surpluses and cheaper wages.

The design of retirement age policy is not as easy as some make it out to be. At the heart of the matter is the extent to which a nation (and its people) wish to use their increasing growth potential to produce a higher standard of living (more goods and services per capita) or, alternatively, whether they wish to allow workers to spend more time out of the formal workforce to pursue other activities (travel, grandparenting, community service, etc.). Given a choice for more leisure, the issue then becomes one of deciding how to take it—more retirement, more vacations, a shorter workweek, and so on—and what to do with the free time.

The Costs of the Baby Boom

Given changing demographic patterns arising from the baby boom and the consequent increase, early in the twenty-first century, in the proportion of the population who are elderly, concern about economic burden and lagging growth increased even more. Would the economy of the future be able to sustain the costs of the high pension benefits going to such a large numbers of nonproductive older people? And would the demographic aging of the population be a drag on the economy?

Again, the argument was made that it is necessary for the elderly to work until later retirement ages to help offset the costs of adversely changing demographic situation. To see the new heights to which criticism of the elderly reached, we need only look to the recent actions of former Colorado governor, Richard D. Lamm. In an unprecedented and almost unbelievable act, Lamm mounted a bid for the presidency in 1996 with a campaign based almost solely on attacking the elderly for their unreasonable economic drain on the nation, now and especially in the years to come.

The calamities predicted by such prophets of doom have fallen on receptive ears because they argue that the survival of some of our most important social and economic ideals are at stake. They predict that population aging will seriously undermine our efforts to compete in the new global marketplace, threatening future economic growth and, hence, the "American Dream" that each generation will have a standard of living better than its predecessor. And, as if that were not enough, they predict that one of America's most popular institutions, Social Security, is unsustainable and will become a bad deal for future generations—if it is able to survive at all.

No wonder these prophets of doom have gotten our attention. Who can ignore, for example, the recent statement of the well-known economist Lester Thurow: "A new class of people is being created. . . . It [the elderly class] is a revolutionary class, one that is bringing down the social welfare state, destroying government finances, altering the distribution of purchasing power and threatening the investments that all societies need to make to have a successful future" (1996, p. 46).

Almost every prediction of demographic doom starts with one basic statistic of growing dependency: for example, in the year 2030, given current Social Security law, there will be only 2.0 workers per Social Security recipient—in contrast to the current level of 3.3 workers per recipient.*

---

*The ratios vary, depending on the projection assumptions chosen and the start/end years used. The numbers in the text are from the Social Security trustees' *Annual Report* and published in Joseph F. Quinn. (1996). *Entitlements and the federal budget: Securing our future.* Washington, DC: National Academy on Aging.

It is now commonplace to read about such "dependency ratio" statistics. The numbers represent an attempt to measure the number of persons in the society not engaged in producing economic output relative to those in the labor force who are. The aged dependency ratio measures the relationship between, for example, Social Security old-age recipients and those workers paying Social Security taxes based on their labor force participation. The truth is that aged dependency ratios are one-sided and very misleading. In almost all industrial countries of the world, the total dependency ratio (i.e., measuring both young and old) is actually quite low, much lower than in the past and much lower than the ratios in developing nations today (for a good explanation, see Cowgill, 1986).

There have been all sorts of demographic statistics presented in the population aging discussions to date. Most of them are worthless in assessing the economic impact of an aging population. Demographic analysis without economic analysis is a kind of voodoo demographics with regard to the issues in question (a good example is Wattenberg, 1987).

Compare, for example, the economic situations of different generations. The parents of the baby boomers shared a per capita GDP of $12,195 in 1964. Assuming less than 2 percent annual growth, the retired boomers and their children will share in the year 2030 a per capita income (inflation adjusted) that is almost three times greater ($35,659).*

Analyzing the impact of population changes on the economy is a far more difficult challenge than presenting simplistic demographic dependency ratios. So what if the demographic decline in children offsets the increase in older people? What does that mean economically? Is the amount of the economic resources consumed in a year by various individuals the same for both babies and old people? For preschoolers, for teenagers, for college students, or for mothers at home with their children? Obviously not.

Very little research has been done on this question of economic equivalency with regard to population aging. In one of the few economic studies to date, Schulz, Borowski, and Crown (1991) weighed the demographic data to reflect the "private support costs" associated with different age groups of nonworking persons. They also looked also at the potential effect of future economic growth.

---

*These per capita estimates, of course, ignore income distribution issues (which are serious). The estimates were made by economist Robert Eisner and reported in Richard C. Leone. (1997, January–February). Why boomers don't spell bust. *The American Prospect, 68–71.*

In another study, analyzing economic data over the past 100 years for the United States and 10 European countries, Richard A. Easterlin finds little support for predictions that population aging will have a negative impact on economic growth and the economic welfare of future generations (1995). He finds a generally consistent inverse relationship between trends in economic growth and population growth—economic growth rising while population growth is falling. As he points out, this "is just the opposite of what one would have expected if declining population growth were exerting a serious drag on the economy" (Easterlin, 1995, p. 78). Moreover, based on the historical data, "one would be hard put to argue that dependency had much to do with the dramatic post-1973 drop in economic growth rates, and, not surprisingly, it is never mentioned in scholarly attempts to explain this decline" (Easterlin, 1995, p. 80). Yet it is that threat that colors much of the discussion that creates the new economic image of the elderly today.

The Threat of Global Competitiveness

The world has witnessed in recent years new patterns of global competition. One major change has been that fewer producers in the United States are insulated from foreign competitors by geographic distances and trade protection provided by government. Hence there is more concern with regard to the large employee benefits paid to workers in industrialized countries relative to the costs of production in developing countries. It is argued that "excessive" costs to employers of these employee benefits, especially for health and retirement benefits, make it more difficult for firms to compete with low-wage countries in global markets.

Low Productivity

Despite much evidence to the contrary, the standard assumption of most employers is that the productivity of workers declines in the later years. Even if productivity does not fall, the higher wages paid to older workers (ignoring other factors) put them at a competitive disadvantage with regard to younger employees receiving lower salaries. The result is that many employers, especially those in highly competitive markets, view older workers negatively. The result is a bias in favor of hiring younger workers and encouraging employed older workers to retire. (This issue is discussed below in greater detail.)

Public Policy Ambiguity

One main theme of this chapter is policy ambiguity. The economic images of the elderly presented above show the ambiguity in our attitudes and policies with regard to the appropriate roles in society of older people:

- On the one hand, we have generally accepted the notion that in old age many people would not be able to work, so that the promotion of a strong "work ethic" to support economic growth has not been as big an issue regarding employment of older persons. On the other hand, as elderly incomes and assets have increased, more and more people have begun to wonder whether the elderly should be viewed differently with regard to work incentives and whether they should be given more encouragement to work.

- On the one hand, it is seen as appropriate to take some of the gains of economic growth potential in the form of leisure (i.e., less work in the formal labor force), especially at older ages. On the other hand, the demographic crunch of the baby boom has resulted in increasing efforts to help solve government budgetary problems by keeping older workers in the labor force longer—at the expense of decreased leisure time relative to what might have been.

- On the one hand, longer life expectancy and healthier older workers suggest that more people can work longer, raising the nation's economic growth potential and, at the same time, keeping down pension costs for employers and government. On the other hand, chronic unemployment in industrialized countries results in both employers and government designing mandatory retirement rules and attractive pension schemes to move older workers out of the labor force at earlier ages.*

- On the one hand, employers would like to reduce their employee benefit costs (discouraging retirement) to meet the challenges of global competition. On the other hand, they liberalize retirement options (e.g., early retirement schemes) "to get rid of high cost labor."

- On the one hand, many employers perceive older workers to be less flexible in their work habits, not as well educated, often limited by health conditions, technologically obsolete, and not easy to retrain

---

*In the United States, legislation to abolish mandatory retirement rules was enacted in 1977, and its scope was expanded to cover most workers in 1986.

(AARP, 1989; Barth, McNaught, & Rizza, 1993). On the other hand, other employers find that the older workers who are employed by them are as creative, more dependable, and far more experienced than younger workers, with research showing that "there is an exceedingly weak relationship between age and performance" (Sterns & McDaniel, 1994, p. 31).

Four Frames to View the Issues

To deal with this confusion in attitudes and private/public policy actions, we need to clarify the options confronting nations in the twenty-first century. There are four major frames that can assist in this clarification (Schön & Rein, 1994). They allow us to separate the various conflicting problems, goals, and objectives that people bring to the discussion of future economic policies for the elderly. I call them:

1. the aged as buffer
2. economic growth *über Alles*
3. lifelong productive aging
4. a reflective old age

Too often the political debate and many economic discussions have focused on whether the aged should work more or not. What research has shown is that this is far too simplistic a question. The more we study when, how, and why people work, the more complex the picture becomes. The frames listed above provide us with a way to help explicate the complexity.

The Aged as Buffer*

With the market incentives of industrialized countries—incentives that promote efficiency, innovation, and economic growth—also come unemployment, bankruptcy, social disruption, and inequality. Thus, competi-

---

*The discussion in this section is based on James H. Schulz. (1991). Epilogue: The "buffer years": Market incentives and evolving retirement policies. In John Myles & Jill Quadagno (Eds.), *States, labor markets, and the future of old-age policy* (pp. 295–308). Philadelphia: Temple University Press.

tive markets, reacting to technological change, shifts in consumer preferences, new sources of productive inputs, and so forth, create tremendous economic instability. Both workers' jobs and firms' profits are threatened.

The issue of the trade-offs between economic efficiency and social stability has been discussed many times over the years (Okun, 1975; Putterman, Roemer, & Silvestre, 1998). What has not been given sufficient attention is the extent to which manpower policies for older workers have been shaped by this more general issue of economic policy.

Historically, the problems arising from markets have had a powerful impact on evolving pension and retirement policies. Empirically we see that countries that have not been able to follow an effective full-employment policy have tried to balance labor supply and demand by moving older workers out of the labor force. As Dan Jacobson has expressed it, "more and more governments and unions have . . . come to recognize that adopting employment *buffering* strategies or developing worker-oriented adjustments and job-replacement strategies are a vital and, indeed, expedient element in human resource policies" (Jacobson, 1988, p. 287 [emphasis added]).

Thus retirement policies in market-oriented, industrialized countries have reflected in a significant way the changing views in these countries with regard to labor force needs and the changing macroeconomic situations in each country. And the early retirement phenomenon that dominated almost all industrialized countries in the 1970s and 1980s should be viewed as primarily a result of government and employer policies reacting to macroeconomic considerations (Kohli et al., 1991). The early retirement phenomenon witnessed in all Western countries is part of an uncoordinated market solution to economic periods of (1) chaotic disruptions in banking and other financial institutions, (2) depressions during the first half of the twentieth century, and (3) the recessions, stagflation, and generally low-growth environment that has dominated most countries' economies in the years following the OPEC oil crisis.

The need for some sort of buffer mechanisms will not go away. In fact, given the new global competitive environment, the need may increase. If older workers and retirement policy are not to be one of the primary buffers, other mechanisms will need to be found.

One such approach (that also involves older workers) would be to give new meaning to the idea of lifelong learning (Schulz, 2000). There could be much more effective education and retraining of workers later in life. By helping workers meet the skill requirements of the expanding sectors of the economy, such learning would help reduce one source of unemployment—unemployment arising from job obsolescence.

But lifelong learning does not deal with unemployment arising from a lack of sufficient labor demand arising out of macroeconomic events: cyclical downturns or a general inability of a country to effectively compete with foreign competition at home or in world markets outside the country. As long as countries experience serious unemployment problems, there is likely to be strong pressures on and by unions, employers, and governments to use older workers as a buffering tool. This means that for the foreseeable future, we can expect a large proportion of the older population to be out of the formal labor force. And if currently proposed increases in pension retirement ages actually occur, we can expect a relatively small impact from them. Most countries are likely to allow sufficient flexibility in the provisions so that workers can still leave at early ages—probably with lower pension incomes.

From the aged as buffer perspective, the questions and issues many people raise with regard to productive aging take on added political significance. Moreover, the question of what roles for people in old age (given the continuing decline in "the work role") is likely to increase in importance.

Economic Growth *über Alles*

An alternative frame that drives much of contemporary discussion about pension policies is one dominated by its focus on growth economics (Schulz, 1999). In an article entitled "The Paradox of Productive Aging," Martin Sicker observes: "The whole industrialized world, with the United States in the lead, seems to be ensnared in the throes of an obsession with economic efficiency" (1994, p. 12). Associated with this frame is the view that if the market is allowed to operate with minimum interference and growth is promoted, most social problems (poverty, unemployment, discrimination, etc.) of the nation will eventually be solved.

Using this frame, the main criterion applied to work and pension policies is the impact such policies will have on work incentives and the amount of a nation's saving and investment. Out of this perspective comes the view that policies should encourage work over retirement and that major emphasis should be given to promoting personal saving to facilitate greater investment.

For most of modern history, as we observed above, older people were not seen as a relevant consideration in advancing the cause of growth. There were not many of them, and they were not seen as an important factor in the growth process. But today that has all changed. The growing numbers of elderly in various nations are now very much a part of the economic growth discussion and that discussion is almost entirely negative. As Paul Pierson puts it in his review of Reagan–Thatcher policies during the 1980s, "For the first time since before World War II, political executives in Britain and the United States were now openly critical of central features of social policy. For Reagan and Thatcher, the welfare state was not simply a victim of poor economic performance but one of it principal causes" (1994, p. 4).

The biggest set of programs, and hence the biggest cause of poor economic performance, are thought to be Social Security programs for older people. The potential impact of Social Security on economic growth has been a major issue for many decades. Contemporary calls for privatization of Social Security are motivated in part by a desire to ensure that retirement pension programs do nothing to diminish saving and growth. In fact, the current emphasis is on encouraging pension programs that may increase saving.

There are two ways Social Security may affect saving: (1) Social Security programs may encourage people to save less on their own, resulting in a net decrease in total saving; or (2) if individuals when old generally save less and consume more of their income than other age groups, an aging population could reduce aggregate saving.

Economists consider saving vitally important for growth. As summarized by James M. Buchanan: "The act of saving allows for a release of resources into the production of capital rather than consumer goods. The increase in capital expands the size of the economy and this, in turn, allows for an increased exploitation of the division and specialization of resources. This then may result in the economic value of output per unit of input expanding. This result (if it occurs) then ensures that many persons—whether they are workers, savers, or consumers—will be economically better off" (1993, p. 276).

However, despite the assertion of everyone being better off, this outcome is in fact by no means as certain as Buchanan implies. The saving, investment, and growth literatures in economics are large, complex, sophisticated, highly controversial, and generally inconclusive. The complexity and inconclusiveness of economic theory and empiricism in this area are generally ignored, however, in contemporary policy pronouncements. Many economists today advocate for an increase in the personal saving of individuals in order to deal with the need to promote economic growth. In their minds, low saving translates into slow growth and lower living standards, and it follows, therefore, that Social Security in its present form represents a threat to growth.

In another essay I have shown that a strong case can be made against this viewpoint, however (Schulz, 1999). Current macroeconomic theory assumes and related research indicates that there is not just one factor (saving) or two factors (saving and investment) that are the key determinants of growth. While saving and investment are necessary, they are not alone sufficient for a nation to be sure that the rate of growth will be adequate to achieve any set of economic goals. There are many other factors that are as important—perhaps more important. These factors are:

- successful macroeconomic policies promoting full employment and low inflation
- the quantity and quality of labor
- technological change
- the prevalence of entrepreneurial initiative and risk-taking
- managerial skills and work structures
- government provision of infrastructure
- investment in human and business capital

Research indicates that the number of people and their ages (i.e., the typical dependency ratio) pales in importance to most of these other factors on the above list. To see why this is true, we can look at the role played by one of these factors, the labor force.

Of course, to produce and expand the economic output of a nation, there must be workers. But as far as production is concerned, there is no required number of workers (or work hours) needed to produce some specified amount of economic output.* And a declining number of workers does not necessarily mean declining output. For example, everyone knows that agricultural output has risen dramatically in many countries while, at the same time, the number of workers in agriculture has dramatically declined. What is true for agriculture is true for the economy as a whole.

---

*Factors of production are substitutable—such as more machines for fewer people.

Similarly, the productivity of workers is not solely (or primarily) related to their numbers. Nor is it primarily related to worker education
and skills or to their motivation and work ethic. These things are certainly relevant and important. However, economists appropriately define
productivity as the joint product of the quantity and quality of all the
factors that work together to produce output, including factories, machines, land, other natural resources, and the like.

Thus, to assess the impact of population aging on economic growth,
one has to take into account the impact of all the factors, not just the
quantity of labor. Below we focus on three of them that are key: the quality of labor, technological change and workforce aging, and the role of
saving.

The Quality of Labor. "All over the world it is taken for granted that
educational achievement and economic success are closely linked—that
the struggle to raise a nation's living standards is fought first and foremost
in the classroom" (*The Economist*, 1997, p. 15). That is, it is not just that
a nation needs workers; a nation needs "the right" workers. Most types
of output require workers with specific skills—as basic as knowing how
to read or as sophisticated as knowing how to write software that will
enable computers "to read." Thus, for most purposes the quality of labor
is much more important than its quantity. And workers command different wages in part because they bring to the job different talents and skills.
Moreover, differentials in wages between countries are often the result of
not just the relative quantities and skills of workers but also the nature of
the other factors of production (such as capital equipment) they have to
work with.

How do age differences of workers and variation in age cohorts impact
the economy? We only discuss a few important issues that arise; there are
many others. From the standpoint of the quality of the labor force, one of
the most important matters is the question of worker skill obsolescence
with age and what should be done about it.

Technological changes are constantly making jobs obsolete. Shifting
preferences of consumers as a result of new products, and shifting relative
prices for all products also make some jobs obsolete. Moreover, the changing of what economists call "comparative advantage," that is, changes in
the competitive advantage of different regions or countries, also makes
jobs obsolete in other regions and countries. Together these three sources
of change (technology, consumer preference, and comparative advantage)
mean no skill or job is really secure in market-oriented countries. No

worker can predict what will happen in his or her lifetime. Nor can workers easily shield themselves and their families from the insecurities generated.

Unions, government, and business think it is cheaper to terminate workers at early ages than to retrain them for the new jobs being constantly created. It is often asserted—with little, if any, proof—that as a result of this phenomenon and other factors, older workers generally have lower productivity than younger workers.* Much research exists to call this generalization into question (Schulz, 1995, pp. 84–86). This is not to say, however, that job obsolescence does not occur; clearly it does (and frequently among older workers). As we said above, that is one major reason why the issue of lifelong learning is often raised in policy discussions.

What does the research to date in this area have to say about the productivity of the aging workforce that is associated with an aging population? A recent comprehensive review of the literature by British economist Richard Disney concludes that

> a younger workforce may be more adaptable, and quicker to learn, but it will embody less training, and will not yet be sorted into jobs and into grade positions within jobs appropriate to the relative productivity differences among individuals. An older workforce will have had some depreciation of its skills, and may well be harder to retrain when the economy goes through rapid structural change, but the greater "experience" of a mature tenured workforce does embody high productivity. The net effect of these factors is not clear; however, there is no support for the view of "aging pessimists" that an older workforce must necessarily be less productive, or that it will earn high wages inconsistent with its level of productivity. (1996, p. 187)

Technological Change and Workforce Aging. Another assertion that is frequently made is that creativity and invention reside primarily in the younger mind. A corollary to this is that organizations, including economic institutions, require "young blood" to keep development and growth going at a rapid pace. Again, this view of older workers is too simplistic and conveys too negative a view of the productive contributions people are able to make when they get older.

Early research indicated that "marked declines in old age occur only in

---

*This is a very complicated issue; our discussion here only touches on the relevant substantive matters.

certain types of creative activity and may affect quality more than quantity of output" (Riley & Foner, 1968, p. 435). One classic study of this question by Wayne Dennis for the United States found that a large part of the lifetime contribution to scholarship, science, and art was made by men in their later years (Dennis, 1966). In fact, the period of life after age 50 accounted for the major portion of output in most scholarly and scientific fields, with ages 70 to 79 alone accounting for 20 percent of the output in the fields of scholarship (such as history and philosophy) and 15 percent in the sciences.

More recent research, however, has been less positive, indicating that creativity may decline in the later years (Sterns, Sterns, & Hollis, 1996; Kausler, 1992). For example, Alpaugh and Birren (1967) studied factors affecting creativity across the life span. They found age differences favoring younger adults with regard to originality, adaptive flexibility, functioning "strategies," fluency of ideas, and preferences for more complex situations.

How does age affect performance (as opposed to creativity)? Again, gross generalities are unwarranted (Sonnenfeld, 1988). There are many studies on performance by occupation, with the research showing very little relationship between age and performance (other factors held constant). And the literature contains many examples of companies that never introduced mandatory retirement policies because they found that most workers in their 70s and 80s did exemplary work.

Certainly it is true that there are *some* declines in mental and physical functioning of *some* people as they grow older. Research shows, however, that many people remain productive in spite of these functional limitations or chronic diseases, finding ways to compensate for the problems.

Another issue that arises is age differences in reaction to the introduction of new technology and other economic changes in the production process. This is a very complex issue intimately related to the ongoing controversies surrounding management style, worker participation, and work conditions in general. It can be argued that whether workers at any age are resistant to technological change is not so much a function of age but of these other factors. Moreover, as a recent survey (Sterns, Sterns, & Hollis, 1996) of research in the area of older worker productivity points out:

> Older adults bring experience and extensive skills to any job. They have had a lifetime of communicating, overcoming hardships, solving problems,

and acquiring lessons learned. Older employees have had years to integrate their knowledge with practical experience to develop efficient methods of accomplishing their work. When new techniques arise, open-minded older workers are often the best source to determine how successful new ideas will be and how best to implement them. (Sterns, Sterns, & Hollis, 1996, pp. 290–291)

What Role for Saving? The point is not that saving has an unimportant role to play in growth or that policies to encourage saving are inappropriate. Rather, we need to put the issue of large numbers of older people and their impact on aggregate saving in proper perspective. Currently we are continually confronted with pronouncements that make it seem that the impact of population aging and Social Security saving is the most, or one of the most, important factors in evaluating policy options relating to growth. But the significance of population aging and Social Security in the determination of savings rates is certainly small in relation to many of the other factors.

Even if Social Security reduces saving (and many economists have pointed out that conclusion has not been proven), people worried about future economic growth and the "economic pie" available to share should look elsewhere for factors determining the outcome. All one has to do is look around at businesses that succeed and those that fail to see that saving is only one of many factors important for growth.

Over the years, economist Richard R. Nelson, for example, has pointed out the complexities of growth and the key role played by factors other than saving. Unfortunately, many economists' models treat businesses like machines, ignoring empirical research clearly documenting the fact that businesses are social systems that are often resistant or unresponsive to management commands. Thus, management style, for example, can make a big difference in the success or failure of a firm.

And what about knowledge—the education of the workforce and the development of a scientific base for facilitating and stimulating the use of new technologies? As pointed out by one of the "fathers of economics," Alfred Marshall, it is vitally important to spend sufficient society resources on improving the quality of the workforce (human capital).

Again, it is not that economists have ignored the role of knowledge, technology, risk-taking, and entrepreneurship. Rather it is that the importance of these factors is almost always missing from, or downplayed, in most policy discussions about issues related to economic growth and, in our case, the specific issues related to population aging and Social Security. Instead, the focus is on older persons as a drag on economic growth through their retirement and saving behavior.

Lifelong Productive Aging

This frame emphasizes that almost all individuals are engaged in productive activities throughout their entire life and focuses on ways to promote and facilitate the enrichment and improvement of these activities. As Butler (1989, p. 63) has commented: "Life is really of one piece, a whole series of marvelous transformations throughout the cycle, a great gift, and a remarkable opportunity for joy and warmth and creativity." This statement does a great job of setting the tone for the lifelong productive aging frame.

As we discussed above, political issues were a major reason for the original development of the conception of productive aging. Over the years, however, many researchers have found the concept useful as an appropriate framework for discussing one of the first big debates in the young field of social gerontology: the changing nature of the roles of older people in an industrial society and the personal problems that might arise from role loss.

The lifelong productive aging frame accepts the economic paradigm that focuses on activities that have "value." But it seeks to expand the definition of economically valuable activities beyond those whose value is determined by economic markets. Herzog and Morgan (1992), for example, argue that "social reporting efforts aimed at monitoring productivity and how it might change as a function of the age of the person are biased by the way productivity is operationalized in most available social statistics" (1992, p. 173). In the spirit of expansion of productiveness, O'Reilly and Caro's review of the productive aging literature indicates the wide range of topics that the concept has grown to encompass: employment/retirement, volunteer activities, informal caregiving, and education/training (O'Reilly & Caro, 1994).

Matilda White Riley's writings provide a systematic discussion and challenging agenda of policy recommendations related to viewing life as an integrated, whole process. For Riley, as for all economists exploring the issues surrounding the "work-leisure choice" decisions, the focus is not so much on whether people are productive or not; rather, one of the benefits of a society realizing high economic growth is the ability to reallocate over all ages some of the leisure now accruing in retirement. Riley sees older people assuming some of the work responsibilities of the middle-aged, thereby releasing these younger people from stresses of that period arising from their labor force and family roles. She argues: "Tremendous numbers of capable and potentially productive older people cannot long co-exist with empty role structures, while younger adults are struggling under overwhelming role demands. Something will have to give. A twenty-first-century revolution in age structure seems inevitable" (Productive Aging News, 1993, p. 8). Riley thinks that we need to break down the current "age-differentiated structure" of work and move to a lifelong view of work. "Altered institutions and norms may well allow people at all ages to move in and out of education, to change jobs or start new careers, and to intersperse leisure with other activities throughout life."

In this regard, Bass and Caro (1996) state that "over the last decade in the United States, there has been a growing interest in involving older people in significant economic and social roles" (p. 262). Bass and Caro call it "elder engagement." Thus, Bass, Caro, Butler, Riley, and others give a lot of attention to the barriers that prevent that from happening—age discrimination, lack of training opportunities, punitive pension provisions (like the Social Security retirement test), and more opportunities for part-day work in industry.*

A Reflective Old Age

Bass, Caro, and Chen (1993), in their excellent overview of the concept of productive aging, state that the goal of people using this concept is "to expand the ways in which both the general public and the scientific community approach the discussion of aging—to explore the potential of older people" (p. 5). But immediately there arises the question of how one defines "potential." In general, the common approach is to include traditional market and nonmarket economic activities that result in the production of goods and services (as in the lifelong productive aging frame discussed above). Caro, Bass, and Chen (1993) expand this view by adding activities that develop the capacity to produce goods and services to their definition of productive aging.

But most definitions of productive aging exclude "many important and

---

*For example, Rowe and Kahn (1998) propose that paid employment be organized on the basis of four-hour modules in order to increase the flexibility of work arrangements.

constructive activities undertaken by the elderly. They exclude, for example, such activities as reflection, worshiping, meditation, reminiscing, reading for pleasure, carrying on correspondence, visiting with family and friends, traveling, and so forth" (Caro, Bass, & Chen, 1993, p. 5). Given these exclusions, and others, not everyone agrees with an approach that focuses a discussion of roles in later life almost solely on older persons' economic activities and potential.

A very different approach is the one that seeks to escape from the economic paradigm and looks at the later years of life in primarily noneconomic terms. Thus, Martin Sicker writes:

> I must confess that the use of the phrase "productive aging" to convey the underlying message of its proponents causes me a good deal of discomfort. Despite the unquestionably good intentions of the advocates of "productive aging," I find the formulation anomalous, since it forces us to discuss the issues of retirement from the workplace in terms of workplace values. The phrase may even be counterproductive, given the current economic climate. (1994, p. 12)

Harry Moody (1993, p. 34) puts the matter this way:

> By insisting on the productivity of the old, we put the last stage of life at the same level as the other stages. This transposition implicitly sets up a kind of competition or struggle (who can be the most productive?) which the old are doomed to lose as frailty increases. But celebrating efficiency, productivity or power, we subordinate any more claim for the last stage of life in favor of values that ultimately depreciate with meaning of old age.*

Moody (1993) warns that while the proponents of productive aging emphasize noncoercion, options, and opportunity, "productive aging easily can become a subtle means of social control and implies a modification of the 'bureaucratized' life course, and in ways that at present remain imponderable" (p. 37).

Another commonly used term in the literature is *successful aging*, which

---

*Moody (1993, p. 35) goes on to point out that the countervailing view in favor of productive aging is that "in a social world that increasingly prizes only instrumental values, productive aging represents a vindication of the continued vitality and social contributions of older people."

also seeks to take account of and respond to the "historically negative view of aging promoted by both science and society" (Rowe & Kahn, 1998, p. xii). However, as Bass et al. point out, the emphasis in this focus is on individual physiological and physiological capacity and performance—although the recent *Successful Aging* study sponsored by the MacArthur Foundation also includes a short discussion of "productivity in old age" (Rowe & Kahn, 1998).

Moody (in my opinion) correctly points out that productive aging is more than a matter of semantics; it is a substantive answer to the question: What is later life for? He calls for a "wider vision" of late-life productivity that includes altruism, citizenship, stewardship, creativity, and the search for faith (what Moody calls the elements of "transcendence").

It is appropriate to ask the question at this point: What do people actually say about what they want to do in later life? According to the authors of the report coming out of the MacArthur Foundation study, "clearly, older people [in the United States] do not feel guilty or disapproving about increased rest and leisure in old age" (Rowe & Kahn, 1998, p. 177). However, the report immediately qualifies this conclusion by pointing out that answers to the study's various survey questions on work clearly indicated people's ambiguity about work. The majority of people agree that people should work as long as they are able, but at the same time they think that older workers should step down to let younger people take their places, and they feel that "life is not worth living if you cannot contribute to the well-being of others." Thus, we have come full circle in our discussion—back to the problem of ambiguity.

Toward the Reduction of Ambiguity

We have argued in this chapter that there is great ambiguity with regard to the economic roles of people in later life and the policies of society in general with regard to these ambiguous roles. Figure 7.1 illustrates the historical continuum of policy options that have shaped past and present behavior of employers and older workers. At the extremes are policies that, on the one hand, require people to work and, on the other hand, prohibit people from working. Policies operationalizing both extremes have existed in American history. There were, for example, the early welfare policies with work requirements patterned on the British "Poor Laws" and the recent federal welfare "reform" law "to end welfare as we know it" takes us back to many of the rules of those colonial days. There were also (at the other extreme) the mandatory retirement rules that were very common during the middle of the twentieth century (and now illegal). In addition to these extremes, there is a whole range of policies that to a greater or lesser degree either encourage or discourage work in the later years. Figure 7.1 lists only a few for illustrative purposes.

And finally, Figure 7.1 reminds us that policies determine options and influence behavior not just in the formal labor force but also in the informal sector. On the one hand, federal and state governments and foundations have financially supported programs to encourage older persons to help others in need and to provide services to the community. On the other hand, the attitudes of different segments of the population against "working for nothing" and an inhospitable neighborhood environment (particularly in the areas of transportation and crime prevention) negatively influence the mobility of older people to get out into their communities to provide services.

The ambiguity toward participation in the labor force by the elderly is not likely to be resolved—ever. As in many policy areas, it is in large part the product of conflicts in values and goals that are themselves not resolvable. But what can be accomplished is to move beyond the current simplistic practice of blaming the elderly for many of the current economic problems related to (1) slow economic growth and (2) the demographic aging of the population (government deficits, "unsustainable" pension costs, and low rates of economic growth). Putterman, Roemer, and Silvestre (1998), in their recent review of the controversy over equity versus efficiency trade-offs, argue that the welfare state and its policies transferring money to people in old age will not disappear. "The future is . . . likely to be one of increasing efforts to improve, rather than dismantle, these institutions, keeping incentive issues at the forefront of reform so as to achieve better combinations of both equity and efficiency" (Putterman, Roemer, & Silvestre, 1998, p. 874).

The welfare state and demographic aging debate has been addressed elsewhere at great length. Certainly it is not the focus of this chapter (see Schulz, Borowski, & Crown, 1991). But our focus is, in one basic sense, quite related. As the chapter discussed, the nation does not necessarily need the elderly to be productive, given its ever-growing economic potential (Schulz, 1995). It is a matter of individual and ultimately national choice as to how we want to divide up the nation's growth potential between goods and services and greater nonparticipation in the formal labor force. Thus, I think we should admit to the reality that the possibilities

Formal Labor Force

	Encourage Work			Discourage Work				
Require Work	Partial retirement options	Age Discrimination in Employment Act	Job Training Partnership Act	Social Security retirement test*	Employer age discrimination	Special early retirement programs	Mandatory retirement rules	**Prohibit Work**
"Poor Laws"								
Work	Senior Community Service Employment Program	Experience Corp	Americans with Disabilities Act	Union attitudes toward volunteerism	Inadequate public transportation	Age discrimination	No help for family caregivers	**Work**
Materialistic society discourages altruism								

Informal Labor Force

Figure 7.1   Work policies for older workers, United States

*Persons under age 65.

posed by the "reflective frame" discussed above are possible and take that frame very seriously in discussing roles in old age. This may sound strange coming from someone trained in economics, where the emphasis (among other things) is on worker incentives in the paid labor force. However, one of the common misapprehensions about economics is that it focuses entirely on profits and the consumption of goods and services (the "rational, selfish economic man"). The truth is that economics has always been about the whole range of values that people think important. It is about deciding *whose* values will determine what a society will produce and not produce in both the market and outside the market.

But more important, it is not necessary to abandon one's noneconomic values while acknowledging the usefulness of the economic paradigm. The American economists Armen Alchian and William Allen (1967) pointed out many years ago that there is no assumption in the economic paradigm's postulates that people are interested only in their own wealth or welfare:

> [It is *not* assumed] that man [sic] is greedy—meaning solely that he wants command over more rather than less goods. But a man may want control over more goods precisely in order to give some to charity to help other people. It is not assumed that he is oblivious to other people, that he is uncharitable or not solicitous of other people's welfare. Nor is he assumed to be concerned only with more wealth. . . . What is meant by "selfish" man is that he wants the right to choose among options that will affect his ensuing affairs. In short, the *right to make choices* about the future is a desired thing, an "economic good." (p. 20)

So I share the concerns of Sicker, Moody, and others who caution researchers interested in the productive aging frame. And in the policy arena, I would encourage us to clarify and pay more attention to what people (young and old) do, and say they want to do, in later life and to pay less attention to what the advocates of radical reform in old age policies say we "must" do.

REFERENCES

Alchian, A., & Allen, W. (1967). *University economics* (2nd ed.). Belmont, CA: Wadsworth.

Alpaugh, P. K., & Birren, J. E. (1967). Variables affecting creative contributions across the adult life span. *Human Development, 20,* 240–248.

American Association of Retired Persons. (1989). *Business and older workers: Current perceptions and new directions for the 1990s.* Washington, DC: Author.

Barth, M. C., McNaught, W., & Rizzi, P. (1993). Corporations and the aging workforce. In P. H. Mirvis (Ed.), *Building the competitive workforce* (pp. 156–200). New York: John Wiley & Sons.

Bass, S. A., & Caro, F. G. (1992). The new politics of productive aging. *In Depth, 2* (3).

Bass, S. A., & Caro, F. G. (1996). Theoretical perspectives on productive aging. In W. H. Crown (Ed.), *Handbook on employment and the elderly* (pp. 262–275). Westport, CT: Greenwood.

Buchanan, J. M. (1993). We should save more in our own economic interest. In L. M. Cohen (Ed.), *Justice across generations: What does it mean?* (pp. 269–282). Washington, DC: AARP.

Butler, R. N. (1989). Productive aging. In V. L. Bengtson & K. W. Schaie (Eds.), *The course of later life: Research and reflections.* New York: Springer.

Butler, R. N. (1994). Foreword. In S. A. Bass, *Productive aging and the role of older people in Japan* (pp. xiii–xvii). New York: Japan Society.

Caro, F. G., Bass, S. A., & Chen, Y.-P. (1993). Introduction. In S. A. Bass, F. G. Caro, & Y.-P. Chen (Eds.), *Achieving a productive aging society.* Westport, CT: Auburn House.

Cowgill, D. O. (1986). *Aging around the world.* Belmont, CA: Wadsworth.

Dennis, W. (1966). Creative productivity between the ages of 20 and 80 years. *Journal of Gerontology, 21,* 1–8.

Disney, R. (1996). *Can we afford to grow older?* Cambridge, MA: The MIT Press.

Donahue, W., Orbach, H. L., & Pollak, O. (1960). Retirement: The emerging social pattern. In Clark Tibbitts (Ed.), *Handbook of social gerontology* (pp. 330–406). Chicago: University of Chicago Press.

Easterlin, R. A. (1995). Implications of demographic patterns. In R. H. Binstock & L. K. George (Eds.), *Handbook of aging and the social sciences* (4th ed., pp. 73–93). San Diego: Academic.

The Economist. (1997, March 29). Education and the wealth of nations. *The Economist, 15.*

Friedmann, E. A., & Havighurst, R. J. (1954). *The meaning of work and retirement.* Chicago: University of Chicago Press.

Herzog, A. R., & Morgan, J. N. (1992). Age and gender in the value of productive activities. *Research on Aging 14* (2), 169–198.

Jacobson, D. (1988). Optional early retirement: Is it a painless alternative to involuntary layoffs? In S. Bergman, G. Naegele, & W. Tokarski (Eds.), *Early retirement: Approaches and variations: An international perspective.* Jerusalem: Brookdale Institute of Gerontology.

Kausler, D. H. (1992). *Experimental psychology, cognition, and human ageing.* New York: Springer-Verlag.

Kohli, M., Rein, M., Guillemard, A., & van Gunsteren, H. (1991). *Time for retirement: Comparative studies of early exit from the labor force.* Cambridge: Cambridge University Press.

Kreps, J. M. (1977). Age, work, and income. *Southern Economic Journal, 43,* 1423–1437.

Leone, R. C. (1997, January–February). Why boomers don't spell bust. *The American Prospect,* 68–71.

Moody, H. R. (1993). Age, productivity, and transcendence. In S. A. Bass, F. G. Caro, & Y.-P. Chen (Eds.), *Achieving a productive aging society.* Westport, CT: Auburn House.

Myles, J., & Quadagno, J. (1991). *States, labor markets, and the future of old-age policy.* Philadelphia: Temple University Press.

Okun, A. (1975). *Equality and efficiency: The big tradeoff.* Washington, DC: Brookings Institution.

O'Reilly, P., & Caro, F. G. (1994). Productive aging: An overview of the literature. *Journal of Aging and Social Policy, 6* (3), 39–71.

Pierson, P. (1994). *Dismantling the welfare state? Reagan, Thatcher, and the politics of retrenchment.* Cambridge: Cambridge University Press.

Productive Aging News. (1993, July–August). NIA expert sees a revolution in living for 21st century Americans.

Putterman, L., Roemer, J. E., & Silvestre, J. (1998). Does egalitarianism have a future? *Journal of Economic Literature, 36,* 861–902.

Quinn, J. F. (1996). *Entitlements and the federal budget: Securing our future.* Washington, DC: National Academy on Aging.

Riley, M. W., & Foner, A. (1968). *Ageing and society: An inventory of research findings.* New York: Russell Sage Foundation.

Rowe, J. W., & Kahn, R. L. (1998). *Successful aging.* New York: Pantheon.

Schön, D., & Rein, M. (1994). *Frame reflection: Toward the resolution of intractable policy controversies.* New York: Basic Books.

Schulz, J. H. (1974). The economics of mandatory retirement. *Industrial Gerontology, 1* (1), 1–10.

Schulz, J. H. (1991). Epilogue: The "buffer years": Market incentives and evolving retirement policies. In J. Myles & J. Quadagno (Eds.), *States, labor markets, and the future of old-age policy* (pp. 295–308). Philadelphia: Temple University Press.

Schulz, J. H. (1995). *The economics of ageing* (6th ed.). Westport, CT: Auburn House.

Schulz, J. H. (1999). Saving, growth, and Social Security: Fighting our children over shares of the future economic pie? In R. Butler & M. R. Oberlink (Eds.), *Life in older America* (pp. 121–150). New York: Twentieth Century Fund.

Schulz, J. H. (2000). "The Full Monty" and life-long learning in the 21st century. *Journal of Aging and Social Policy, 11*, 2/3, 71–82.

Schulz, J. H., Borowski, A., & Crown, W. (1991). *Economics of population aging: The 'greying' of Australia, Japan, and the United States.* New York: Auburn House.

Sicker, M. (1994). The paradox of productive aging. *Ageing International, 21* (2), 12–14.

Sonnenfeld, J. (1988). Continued work contributions in late career. In H. Dennis (Ed.), *Fourteen steps in managing an ageing work force* (pp. 19–211). Lexington, MA: Lexington Books.

Sterns, A. A., Sterns, H. L., & Hollis, L. A. (1996). The productivity and functional limitations of older adult workers. In W. H. Crown (Ed.), *Handbook on employment and the elderly* (pp. 276–303). Westport, CT: Greenwood.

Sterns, H. L., & McDaniel, M. A. (1994). Job performance and the older worker. In S. E. Rix (Ed.), *Older workers: How do they measure up?* (pp. 27–51). Washington, DC: AARP.

Thurow, L. C. (1996, May 19). The birth of a revolutionary class. *New York Times Magazine,* 46.

Wattenberg, B. J. (1987). *The birth dearth.* New York: Pharos Books.

III

EMERGENT THEORIES

IN GERONTOLOGY

8

PRODUCTIVE AGING
AND THE IDEOLOGY OF OLD AGE

Harry R. Moody, Ph.D.

When the railroad was introduced in the nineteenth century, it was hailed, understandably enough, as "the iron horse." Nothing is more natural than to imagine the future according to the past. So too, when confronted by a new paradigm—for that is what "productive aging" finally is—we may react with alarm or celebration. Expressions of alarm or celebration alert us that productive aging is inevitably the locus of ideological struggle, just as much as the economic ideal of free trade. What follows is a historical and critical account of this ideological struggle surrounding productive aging—a contentious idea, an arena for conceptual and political debate.

The ideological struggle around productive aging takes place in a specific historical context. Today the shape of the human life course, including the meaning of old age, is changing in dramatic ways. Moreover, we stand at the threshold of a great transition, a demographic change that comes as the proportion of the U.S. population above age 65 rises from 13 percent to 20 percent over the next two decades. Already there are many who view this prospect of population aging with profound misgiving—seen, most recently, in public debate over the future of the U.S. Social Security system. Similar fears of population aging have been heard in other societies confronting this phenomenon of population aging, in Japan and Western Europe.

It is not my purpose to argue whether such "apocalyptic demography"

(Robertson, 1997) is, or is not, justified: for the record, I think fears about an aging society are wildly exaggerated. Rather, I note that productive aging is one response to a specific recent controversy, the generational equity debate, which surfaced in the United States in the 1980s. That debate turned on the question of fairness to different generations and age groups and it has continued in different forms ever since. Proponents of generational equity raised the specter that we might not be able to afford an aging society. One response to fears of population aging is to reform aging policy systems to reflect anticipated scarcity: for example, by privatizing income redistribution or by rationing health care on grounds of age. Another, quite different response is to argue that such bleak choices would be unnecessary if only we could convert our aging population from a burden into an asset. Here is precisely the strategy of productive aging. Productive aging, then, is an optimistic response that challenges certain elements of the liberal welfare state since the New Deal, and that fact inevitably makes it ideologically contentious.

Productive aging, like its close cousin *successful aging,* embodies quintessential American values of success and productivity. With the triumph of global capitalism in the 1990s, these values are likely to prove dominant in shaping a positive image of aging in the future. However, these positive images also contain a hidden or "dark" side: what about "failure" and "unproductive" people? Productive aging and successful aging are not the only positive visions of the future. *Radical gerontology* challenges us to put the agenda of equality and social justice as the foundation for the aging welfare state, while *conscious aging* offers consciousness expansion and personal growth as the guiding principles for an aging society. How the ideological struggle among these alternatives will unfold is not predictable. Yet we know that in the next two decades, the huge baby boom generation will enter old age. For an influential segment of boomers in the 1960s political protest and consciousness expansion were prominent themes. As this cohort of boomers moves into old age, they are likely to carry these critical values along with them.

But cohort flow is only part of the story we need for the future. We need not look at historical change the way we look at a weather report: as a summary of movements beyond our control. On the contrary, in the last decade of the twentieth century, nothing was more astonishing than *unpredicted* events, like the fall of the Berlin Wall and the collapse of communism. In the face of historical complexity and population aging, what is most called for is, on the one hand, new ideas—such as productive aging—and also a critical reflexiveness that can be called ideology critique. The purpose of critical consciousness is to become aware of the assumptions and implications of alternative futures that lie before us, and, above all, to preserve our sense of an open future.

Four Ideologies of Old Age

I turn now to Table 8.1 to examine four alternative ideologies of old age. The first two, successful aging and productive aging, may be grouped together—not because they are identical but because they express a common, optimistic stance toward the scarcities and problems often antici-pated with population aging. Instead of "gloom and doom," successful aging and productive aging see old age as a time for "abundance of life" (Moody, 1988a). The third and fourth of these alternatives, radical ger-ontology and conscious aging, may also be paired together inasmuch as they express an attitude subversive with respect to the dominant values of success and productivity.

Successful Aging

The idea of successful aging is not new but has been intertwined with the history of gerontology from its earliest years (Havighurst, 1961; Neuhaus & Neuhaus, 1982). Indeed, the covert ideology of old age always oscillates between two poles: depicting, on the one hand, the "well-derly" (active, healthy, "normalized") and, on the other hand, the "ill-derly"—in Richard Kalish's memorable phrase: the "failure model." Successful aging insists that age can be a time, not of failure but of success, indeed of new creativity (Adams-Price, 1998). Successful aging can be defined across a continuum either in subjective terms (positive morale and life satisfac-tion) or in objective terms (survival and health status). Rowe and Kahn distinguish, dichotomously, between "usual" and "successful," both fall-ing within the category of "normal" aging (1987). The goal of successful aging, in their view, is to move from "usual" functional decline instead to higher levels of functioning: that is, the more health, longevity, and life satisfaction the better (1998). By contrast, Baltes and Baltes (1990) define successful aging as (pessimistically) "decrement with compensation" or (optimistically) "selective optimization with compensation."

In terms of its axial values, successful aging can be understood as some combination of survivorship and health. In some trivial sense the healthier

TABLE 8.1 Countergerontology: A Conceptual Taxonomy

	Axial Values	Key Motifs	Locus	Prominent Ideas	Caricature	Practice
SUCCESSFUL AGING	Health	Life satisfaction	Individual	Compression of morbidity	Privatism	Health promotion
	Survivor	Success	Homeostasis	J. Rowe & R. Kahn, *Successful Aging*		
PRODUCTIVE AGING	Need for achievement	Generativity	Economy	Activity theory	Busy ethic	Worklife extensions
	Worker	Productivity	Efficiency	S. Bass et al., *Achieving a Productive Aging Society*		
RADICAL GERONTOLOGY	Social justice	Diversity	Polity	Political economy	Political correctness	Radical politics
	Citizen	Protest	Equality	C. Estes, *The Aging Enterprise*		
CONSCIOUS AGING	Lifespan development	Gerotranscendence	Individual	Transpersonal	New Age philosophy	Life-review meditation
	Spiritual seeker	Self-actualization	Self-actualization	Z. Schachter, *From Age-ing to Sage-ing*		

you are, the more likely you are to survive into old age. Population aging, with an increasing proportion of each cohort living into advanced age, can be trumpeted (as it has been) as "the triumph of survivorship." But, as we know, the triumph has been marred by what we may call, following Jonathan Swift, the "Struldbrug phenomenon." Namely, like the ill-fated Struldbrugs of *Gulliver's Travels*, there are too many instances of paraplegics, stroke victims, and the demented who survive into extreme old age under conditions of severe impairment. Survivorship, obviously, is not always a triumph (Brooks, 1996).

Successful aging begins and ends as a strategy for the promotion of personal health, which is a very different approach from the rescue-oriented, high-technology approach usually associated with American health care. Others have called for a reorientation of health care in light of the geriatric imperative. For example, in the early 1980s, as the generational equity debate began to unfold, Dr. James Fries articulated a strategy he called "compression of morbidity": namely, the argument that medical science should strive to postpone, as far as possible, diseases and impairments of age until a point not long before terminal drop. Fries' strategy is closely akin to successful aging (Fries, 1989). In short, we should all be healthy and happy right up to the moment when we drop dead from a heart attack coming off the tennis court at age 95. As a pathologist's report from 1900 put it succinctly: "Went to bed healthy. Woke up dead." This old joke does have the merit of calling our attention to the fact that the successful aging strategy is a close cousin of Dr. Kevorkian. If the aim of life is to be successful, and if success is measured by life satisfaction, then when homeostasis and quality of life decline below a certain point, it's time for assisted suicide. As Erik Erikson, a prophet in his own way of successful aging, once put it: "Our lives are to be one-way streets to success—followed by sudden oblivion" (Erikson, 1950).

What is striking about the successful aging strategy is its unrelenting focus on individual responsibility: "The frailty of old age is largely reversible. . . . What does it take to turn back the aging clock? It's surprisingly simple. . . . Success is determined by good old-fashioned hard work" (Rowe & Kahn, 1998, p. 102). This language reminiscent of Horatio Alger comes perilously close to "blaming the victim." Indeed, historian Thomas Cole has shown how the ideas of health promotion and successful aging are in many ways a version of Victorian morality in a new guise (Cole, 1992). Along with assisted suicide (appropriate when other forms of self-help fail), these ideas may be just the thing to appeal to aging baby boomers, who are attracted by libertarian and individualistic motifs ("Do your own thing"). Although the strategy of successful aging may seem to be peculiarly American, it actually has proven to have broad international appeal (Gingold, 1992).

The shift toward individualism and individual responsibility for health is currently reinforced by tendencies such as the privatization of social services and health care. Managed care providers, for example, may be attracted to health promotion strategies as a way to reduce expenses. But current scientific advances, such as the Human Genome Project, also reinforce this shift toward individualism as against solidarity. As knowledge grows about genetic causes of chronic disease, individuals seek more prediction and control of their future health in later life. Poor health becomes perceived less as a matter of fate and more as a matter of individual responsibility, thus weakening norms of solidarity. Successful aging fits in well with an era of privatism in health care.

Of course, putting the matter in terms of extreme privatism is a caricature. On the positive side, health promotion and successful aging will prove to be indispensable strategies as the population grows older. Research by Kenneth Manton and others has shown, remarkably enough, that we have already made substantial gains in this direction and more is possible (Manton, Stallard, & Corder, 1997).

Successful aging as an ideological strategy involves a shift in how we think about the meaning of the last stage of life. Any definition of successful aging entails high quality of life, a measure of "life satisfaction." Few ideas in gerontology have been investigated more extensively than the notion of life satisfaction, which is more or less equivalent to a sense of personal happiness or feeling of success in life. This is not a new idea but one that originally appeared in Cicero (*De Senectute*) in terms almost identical to what contemporary writers call for. Successful aging has appeared in the popular literature of medical self-help (Rossman, 1989) and also as a measurable, empirically based agenda for research in social gerontology (Palmore, 1979). In the Duke Longitudinal Study, successful aging was investigated as an aspect of "normal aging" (Lowry, 1985). Robert Butler has been a strong proponent of both successful aging and productive aging (Butler & Brody, 1995), to which we turn now.

Productive Aging

The ideology of productive aging envisions a new image of later life as a time of personal growth and social contribution (Bass, Caro, & Chen, 1993). Instead of depicting elders as consumers of services, and thus as a burden or drain on society, productive aging sees the old as workers and lifelong contributors, either in the paid labor force or in nonmonetized roles of volunteers, caregivers, and so on. But whether as paid workers or not, the emphasis is always on achievement, on the "need to be needed," as a way of validating later life. Psychologically speaking, this motivation was hailed by John Kotre in his book *Outliving the Self,* building on Erik Erikson's idea of generativity—an idea, by the way, which Erikson himself linked to mid-life, not old age. But productive aging anchors generativity as the supreme value throughout all of life. The locus of discourse for productive aging is always on the economy—both the monetized exchange of goods and services and the nonmonetized realm of interpersonal dependency. Even beyond that, productive aging addresses a fundamental problem of the *moral economy:* namely, why should we support the elderly at all (Minkler & Cole, 1992).

Instead of answering the question in terms of past contributions, the ideology of productive aging insists that the elderly continue to give back to society, or to claim, as the Commonwealth studies do, that the elderly already are giving back and contributing in manifold ways (Bass, 1995). Like successful aging, productive aging too has international appeal among advanced industrialized societies undergoing the process of population aging (Kumashiro, 1995).

Productive aging has earlier roots in gerontology, just as the ideology of successful aging does. The early classic debate between disengagement theory and activity theory was a forerunner of productive aging, which comes down squarely on the side of activity. Keep busy, keep productive to the very end of life, and you'll feel good about yourself. This idea, of course, is easily caricatured as the "busy ethic" (Ekerdt, 1986). But productive aging is far from being just a personal "feel good" revision of old age. More broadly, it tries to persuade us that society as a whole should feel good about the elderly, knowing that they are pulling their weight and not in danger of becoming a drain on society. Fears about "apocalyptic demography" can be dismissed as fears of the Big Bad Wolf that are just an illusion.

But what about liberals and old age advocates who are fearful of productive aging itself'? Are their fears to be dismissed so easily? The answer depends partly on some distinctions in the many meanings of productive aging itself. We can appreciate this problem by looking at a central practical implication of most varieties of productive aging: namely, worklife extension. Productive aging can also be defined either as an opportunity—removing barriers to work—or as an obligation—offering incentives or penalties to insist on greater individual responsibility. For example, enforcing age discrimination laws in the workplace would not prove controversial to liberal defenders of the welfare state. However, at the other extreme, further pushing up the age of eligibility for Social Security as a work incentive would be problematic for most liberals. Finally, there are recent policy changes such as liberalizing the Social Security earnings test. These policy shifts are ideologically ambiguous: for example, is eliminating the earnings test more like opening up opportunity (a good thing for aging advocates) or a means of enriching the affluent beneficiaries and putting the Trust Fund at risk (a bad thing for aging advocates)?

The misgivings of old age advocates come down to one basic fear. Under the guise of opening up opportunity, productive aging may prove to be a new means of blaming victims and depriving the vulnerable—the poor, minorities, and older women, for example—of benefits achieved by age-based entitlements under the liberal welfare state (Holstein, 1992).

Productive aging, we have seen, is related to successful aging, and both ideologies flourish in part because of their multiple, often ambiguous meanings (O'Reilly & Caro, 1994; Robinson, 1994). For example, productive aging can be defined either externally (paid employment or nonmonetized services) or internally (reducing dependency on others). This internal definition shows how productive aging coincides with successful aging: to the extent that we remain healthy and postpone dysfunction or morbidity, we are also being indirectly "productive" by reducing our dependency on other people (Butler & Gleason, 1985).

I have argued that successful aging and productive aging are actually ideological cousins for reasons that are now clear (see Bond, Cutler, & Grams, 1995). Being active and productive, it can be argued, is a way of enhancing self-esteem and life satisfaction (successful aging). At the same time, without some degree of health and vigor, productive activity in later life becomes difficult. The challenge, then, is to translate the new biology of successful aging into a social policy for productive aging (Butler, Oberlink, & Schechter, 1990). Those who have long reflected on this problem, like Matilda Riley (Riley & Riley, 1994), see productive aging as a challenge to our age-segmented society: a point we return to in examining productive aging in relation to the postmodern life course.

Both successful aging and productive aging reflect a positive, upbeat view of later life as a time, not of burden and disability, but of healthy and productive living: a kind of extension of middle age (Krain, 1995). This spirit is apparent in popular books on aging. In the 1970s two popular books deserve note: Robert Butler's Pulitzer Prize–winning *Why Survive?* (1975) and Simone de Beauvoir's *The Coming of Age* (1973). Both convey an overwhelmingly negative view of aging and construe the condition of the aged as a matter for urgent public action. The meaning of age is understood as a social problem, an item for remedial intervention, an idea in keeping with the failure model and with Binstock's description of old age politics responsive to elders as the "deserving poor."

Both books also underscore the connection between the failure model and liberal old age advocacy. Butler's book is an example of a familiar genre of landmark works, like Michael Harrington's *The Other America,* Rachel Carson's *Silent Spring,* and Betty Friedan's *Feminine Mystique*— all books that launched significant social movements (antipoverty, environmentalism, modern feminism). Butler, who coined the term *ageism,* stands in this line of contemporary prophets and critics. The link with feminist criticism is also notable because of Simone de Beauvoir's groundbreaking *Second Sex* in the 1940s. Betty Friedan, like de Beauvoir, would also, as she herself grew old, turn her attention to aging-as-social-problem. But when she did so, in *The Fountain of Age* (1993), Friedan echoed the new ideology of both successful aging and productive aging. By the 1990s, popular books on aging signaled a shift away from the failure model toward a more positive vision of the meaning of old age.

Radical Gerontology

A third strategy for old age can be called radical gerontology (Marshall & Tindale, 1978–1979), which has perhaps the most explicit ideology of any of the four responses displayed in Table 8.1. Radical gerontology gives priority to equality rather than liberty or equal opportunity and, instead, favors the polity as opposed to the economy and the free market. The axial values of citizenship and social justice make radical gerontology closely aligned with the traditional American liberalism of age-based advocacy. Yet there are important differences. Traditional liberalism as an ideology of old age found an embodiment in the New Deal of the 1930s

(Social Security) and the Great Society of the 1960s (Medicare). During both the 1930s and the 1960s liberal advocates successfully depicted the elderly as "the worthy poor" and age-based entitlements represented a major effort to remedy their need for income and health care (Myles, 1989).

By the 1970s and 1980s it gradually came to be recognized that such entitlement programs were having two effects on the elderly as a group. First, the previously high rate of poverty among the aged (40 percent) has been reduced to a level that is, on average, not much different from other adult groups (13 percent). Second, there are still dramatic differences in the economic well-being of subgroups of the older population: for example, the poverty rate of white men over age 65 is around 6 percent while the rate for black women is close to 60 percent—10 times greater. A similar inequality in health care distribution has also been apparent. Thus, whatever benefits age-based entitlement programs were having, the problem of inequality among vulnerable subgroups was not fully remedied by policies of the liberal welfare state. In old age, as across life, hierarchies linked to class, race, and gender serve to support systems of privilege and disadvantage (Stoller & Gibson, 1997).

At the same time, during the 1980s and 1990s, there were major policy initiatives to roll back some of the liberal welfare measures on behalf of the poor and the elderly. With the collapse of communism in Eastern Europe after 1989, the triumph of capitalism as an ideology on the world stage seemed assured. After the generational equity debate of the 1980s, the aged themselves were no longer so easily portrayed as a uniformly needy or vulnerable constituency. True, despite loose talk about "greedy geezers," the aged were never successfully depicted in the negative terms of, say, welfare recipients. But in the 1990s, an atmosphere of fiscal crisis and budget cutting did create an environment far different from the 1960s or 1970s. Aging policy was increasingly on the defensive. The fit between liberal politics and age-based advocacy is no longer as perfect as it once was (Hudson, 1996).

This new complexity of the aging policy environment has been the background for the ideology of radical gerontology and for methods of analysis known as the political economy of aging, a framework that owes much to Marxism (Olson, 1982; Estes et al., 1984). On this view, the status of old age itself can be seen as a "construction" of capitalism (Phillipson, 1982). The early, and still classic, statement of radical gerontology is found in Carroll Estes' *The Aging Enterprise* (1979), which departed from mainstream liberalism by depicting the liberal social service establishment as a form of domination. Her theme would be elaborated in succeeding works exploring the political economy of aging (Estes et al., 1984; Minkler & Estes, 1984). Her ideological critique of hegemony would find echoes in other writers such as Katz (1996), who draws on thinkers like Foucault and Althusser.

After the 1980s radical gerontology also came to mirror the conventional liberal celebration of diversity with its tendency toward identity politics and advocacy on behalf of specific subgroups such as women, minorities, and gays. Naturally, this tendency easily lends itself to caricature as "political correctness." But whatever the validity of such a label for disciplines like literary criticism or sociology, there is little ideological adherence to radical ideas within gerontology as a field. On the contrary, radical gerontology is still a perspective with limited appeal, very much in opposition to the dominant interest-group liberalism of the aging network. The aging service network remains closely aligned with a perspective of value-free social science tied to the geriatric professions of health care and social service.

It was Robert Butler who once described gerontology itself as the union of science with advocacy. One can hardly offer a better description of ideology—indeed, what I have called the "overt ideology" of gerontology (Moody, 1988b). But, as with other ideological mixtures of this kind, advocacy can mean many different things and the balance between science and advocacy will always be a bone of contention. For radical gerontology, at least, advocacy and social justice remain in the forefront. As in other forms of radical ideology, there is always a suspicion that what is called science is actually a masquerade for vested interests of the power elite (Aronowitz, 1988). Following in that spirit, radical gerontology has had its own ideology critique as an important part of its agenda (Bornat, Phillipson, & Ward, 1985).

In view of these origins and sympathies, radical gerontology cannot be expected to accept productive aging without grave doubts and hostility. It is certainly going too far to see productive aging as an extension of capitalist ideology. Yet the economistic origins of the primary category—productivity—cannot be denied (Herzog & House, 1991). And proponents of productive aging themselves acknowledge that advancing the agenda of productive aging will entail serious debate—for example, about how to promote late-life productivity while protecting the interests of the least advantaged. As long as the environment is characterized by fiscal crisis and conservatism, on the one hand, and population aging, on the other, we can expect that the encounter between radical gerontology and productive aging will continue to be an arena for ideological conflict.

Conscious Aging

The final ideological response to be considered here is conscious aging, a term apparently first used at a national conference under that name convened by the Omega Institute in 1992. Where other ideological strategies see the older person as a worker or a citizen, conscious aging depicts elders as spiritual seekers: in short, as individuals aspiring to a higher stage of fulfillment, toward what Maslow termed "self-actualization." Freud described the goals of human life as *lieben und arbeiten* (to love and to work). In those words he invoked a purely secular ideal, akin to generativity through family and career. Late life could indeed be seen as a period for "more of the same": namely, a time when the motives of Eros and Achievement continue to guide our lives. By contrast, conscious aging sees the last stage of life as a time for going beyond the roles and purposes of mid-life. Conscious aging draws its inspiration from religion, art, and other forms of self-transcendence, as described, for instance, in the growing field of transpersonal psychology (Wilber, 1996).

One of the most accessible popular books on conscious aging is Schachter and Miller's *From Age-ing to Sage-ing* (1995). Schachter writes from the Jewish mystical tradition, but Christian writers also depict later life as a time of "spiritual journey" (Bianchi, 1982). Robert Atchley (1993) has drawn on the Vedantic or Hindu mystical perspective to offer his own description of the wisdom attainable in the last stage of life. Not all varieties of conscious aging take their point of departure from religion. Rosenmayr (1981) depicts the wide range of personal growth and creativity in later life that fall under the category he calls "the late freedom." Hazan (1996) describes the practice of such freedom through older adult education in the University of the Third Age in Britain, a phenomenon that has its parallel in the American Elderhostel experience. Hazan emphasizes the importance of community and social networks in late-life freedom. Drawing on this theme, Drew Leder (1996) has also emphasized the importance of spiritual community for conscious aging.

The diversity of all these varieties of "consciousness"—education, art, meditation, and so on—raises a question. What *is* conscious aging and why should it be categorized as an ideological response to population aging? One answer can be given in terms of the idea of psychological development. Tornstam (1997) has posited a need for what he calls "gero-transcendence" in later life: namely, a movement beyond self-actualization or ego-integrity toward the contemplative dimension of life, where "being" rather "doing" is the purpose of existence. His account finds echoes among those who have looked at cognitive development in terms of "postformal operations" (Pascual-Leone, 1990; Sinnott, 1996), where late-life wisdom becomes tantamount to mysticism (Moody, 1995; Atchley, 1997).

The strategy of conscious aging is easily caricatured as just another variety of New Age philosophy for seniors (Heelas, 1996). Yet ideas of healing and meaning are increasingly part of both popular culture and academic discourse. For example, there is an important scientific literature documenting the importance of spirituality and the search for meaning in later life (Koenig, 1994). Popular self-help books, like *The Road Less Traveled* and *Care of the Soul,* find their parallel in the spiritual psychology of later life (Moody, 1997). Activities like meditation and life-review have already shown that conscious aging can make an important practical contribution to enhancing the quality of life in old age. In sum, what conscious aging does is to insist that healthy survivorship or productivity or equal access to services in later life is not enough. The personal search for meaning and spiritual growth must be part of any overarching ideology of old age to provide a positive vision of the future.

The Emergence of Productive Aging

Having considered four different ideological responses to old age, we now must turn back to the question posed at the outset of this inquiry: Why did the idea of productive aging emerge in the 1990s? and What conditions are likely to favor productive aging in the early decades of the twenty-first century? The answers to these two questions are both social-structural and ideological.

Structural Forces. Among the structural forces that favor the emergence of productive aging are the following trends:

- Pressures toward cost-containment in health care spending (e.g., Medicare budgets)

- Improving health status of the young-old
- Increasing heterogeneity of the aging population (due to immigration and cultural diversity)
- Rising level of education of successive cohorts of older people
- Impending population aging and aging of baby boomers
- Anticipated labor shortage (due to declining number of younger workers)
- Retreat from defined benefit retirement plans
- Rise of a part-time "contingent" workforce
- Information technologies permitting decentralized labor (e.g., employment by homebound disabled)

These historical trends are evident enough as we look back at the decade of the 1990s. Some reflect predictable demographic shifts (e.g., ethnic diversity, aging baby boomers); others reflect new technology (e.g., the Internet); others reflect benefits of earlier social investments (improved health status of the young-old, rising levels of education). Still other trends represent the evolution of retirement and the erosion of age-based benefits (e.g., the spread of managed care and defined contribution pension plans). The structural trends enumerated here are likely to continue through the first decade of the twenty-first century and in that sense seem relatively predictable.

Ideological Trends. Less definitely predictable but still clearly in evidence are the following tendencies that influence the ideological climate in which the idea of productive aging is received:

- Aftermath of the generational equity debate (e.g., "Can we afford an aging society?")
- Privatization as a generic policy strategy (in health care, school vouchers, prisons, etc.)
- Social Security pessimism (especially among elites and younger cohorts)
- Individualism and libertarianism among younger age cohorts
- Decline of solidarity and the rise of identity politics
- Waning influence of traditional (New Deal) liberalism
- Postmodernism in the cultural sphere

Several of these tendencies have already been discussed in analyzing the four categorical ideological responses. What is noteworthy is the persistence of these trends throughout the decade of the 1990s. For example, public opinion surveys repeatedly show that all age groups tend to support Social Security. Yet surveys also show lack of confidence in the future integrity of Social Security. The younger the respondent, the less the confidence. The waning influence of traditional New Deal liberalism has been much commented on; the trend seems likely to continue in the future as the World War II generation dies out. At the same time, younger cohorts (Generation X) appear to exhibit less traditional forms of loyalty toward employers, spouses, political parties, and so on. Other forms of liberalism increasingly focus on differences and claims of subgroups, thus reinforcing a decline in solidarity (to use the European phrase for consensus values underlying welfare state politics.)

Another trend worth noting is an erosion of consensus about the shape of the human life course: the so-called deinstitutionalization of the life course (Phillipson, 1982). It would appear that the adult life course is becoming less and less predictable in the timing of key life events such as marriage, birth of children, retirement, and higher education. The modernized life course can be said to be the product of bureaucratic interventions that increasingly segmented life into the "three boxes" of education, work, and retirement with predictable age-based transitions: kindergarten at age 5, retirement at age 65, and so on. A new "postmodern" life course can be defined objectively as a loss of predictability in the timing of life transitions in favor of a more fragmented, discontinuous, and individual course of life. In ideological terms, the postmodern life course entails a loss of normative consensus on age-appropriate roles.

The fate of productive aging will depend not only on structural forces or the timing of life events but on elite and mass opinion, including ideas of moral economy and the self-identity of the old themselves (Minkler & Estes, 1998). In that respect, ideology is not merely an epiphenomenon reflecting deeper forces but a crucial variable in political mobilization. In this respect, a point deserving attention is the rise of a broad cultural tendency known as "postmodernism," by which I mean ironic distancing (hence a loss of belief) toward traditional forms of culture. Postmodernism is an attitude that takes for granted that all practices and beliefs are socially constructed by human initiative, rather than reflecting enduring natural or objective norms. Consider, for instance, Erik Erikson's view that the human life course has a sequence of stages, culminating in old age with its distinctive virtue of "ego-integrity." Instead of seeing any such pattern as natural or universal, the postmodern reading of the life course would emphasize contingency, relativity, and the multiplicity of ideas about old age.

It is not clear what "development" would mean according to such a postmodern reading of the life course (Young, 1998). What is clear is that all public images of aging need to be progressively "deconstructed" (Featherstone & Wernick, 1995), just as the discourse we use to talk about aging is to be unmasked (Green, 1993) in the spirit of Nietzsche or Foucault. A postmodern reading of the life course might lead us to view today's version of old age as merely a "mask" (Featherstone & Hepworth, 1991) and an arena for "cultural combat" (Gullette, 1997) in the ongoing "cultural politics of selfunderstanding" (Rosenwald & Ochberg, 1992). Postmodernism, at least in the academic world, has prompted many commentators to see race, like gender, not as "natural" but as socially constructed. That skeptical attitude has had influence far beyond academia. For example, the rise of the Internet and of self-publishing leads ever larger numbers of people to view writing and publication, even knowledge itself, as construction inherently open to anyone (therefore indefinitely revisable). This polycentric universe of postmodernism is available on the World Wide Web and can now be a matter of daily experience.

Finally, two points deserve attention in this (all too brief) characterization of postmodernism and aging. The first is that the rise of postmodern sensibility fosters an attitude of suspicion or doubt toward any of the "givens" about age that might have been accepted in earlier epochs: for example, the idea of a natural life course or of age-appropriate behavior. As a result, all claims to knowledge (including those in gerontology) become political claims and enter into an arena of ideological dispute. For that reason alone, the coming of a postmodern sensibility must mean greater attention to the ideology of old age—especially, for example, women and aging (Ray, 1996; Kunneman, 1997). Productive aging comes to center stage at the historical moment when this ideological shift toward postmodernism attains wide public influence, in part because of a pervasive influence of media in our society (Gabler, 1998).

The second point is the very notion of a "postmodern life course" itself entails certain political consequences unfavorable to traditional liberalism and age-based entitlements. Age-based entitlements like Social Security and Medicare, after all, are publicly legitimated because of shared political norms that people above a certain age deserve special benefits of income or health care. If we were to move toward a society where age is less and less a predictor or basis for anything at all—as Matilda Riley, for example, wants to do (Riley, Kahn, & Foner, 1994)—then it is not hard to imagine that the consensus supporting age-based entitlements will be weakened. Thus, on the one hand, postmodernism intensifies an atmosphere of ideological struggle surrounding all claims of knowledge or social action; and, on the other hand, postmodernism weakens a traditional view of the life course that might see old age as a legitimate period of retirement (i.e., nonproductivity). Whatever its future, the postmodern life course has huge implications for the ideology of old age and for productive aging.

Critical Gerontology and the Ideology of Old Age

It has been the argument of this chapter that ideological constructions of aging must be judged in a historical context—namely, the emergence of the postmodern life course, and within a specific framework of ideology critique: what has come to be called critical gerontology. The aim of historical and philosophical criticism is to promote consciousness about assumptions and alternatives and a more self-reflexive approach to research, education, and advocacy in gerontology.

Critical gerontology involves a clear alternative to the "value-free" empiricist orientation prevailing in mainstream gerontology (Moody, 1992). Critical gerontology need not entail a rejection of objective truth but it does demand attention to the normative questions, human interests, and covert ideological agenda of gerontology itself. Like postmodernism critical gerontology insists that old age is not merely an empirical "given" but that it is always itself socially constituted (Baars, 1991). The problem for mainstream gerontology is that an exclusively scientific paradigm of gerontology contains concealed values and disguised human interests (Tornstam, 1992).

By contrast, the agenda for critical gerontology has often included cultural dimensions (Luborsky & Sankar, 1993) and the role of the humanities in gerontology (Moody, 1988b). But the label *critical gerontology* cannot be limited to either political critique (as in radical gerontology) nor to the creation of culturally alternative visions of age. Drawing on the critical theory of Jürgen Habermas, critical gerontology would emphasize the primacy of communicative action (such as discourse and public images of old age and the moral dimension of the social sciences). In keeping with radical gerontology, critical theory would expose the connection between ideology and human interests, whether in professionalized gerontology or in what Habermas termed "colonization of the life-world" in manifestations such as the medical-industrial complex, the "Gray Market" for commodified aging services, and so on. In place of this colonization and commodification, critical gerontology would insist on the primacy of emancipatory interests and even, on the example of Ernst Bloch, on behalf of utopian ideals. Such utopianism would include both social justice (the example of Maggie Kuhn) and cultural productivity (universities of the third age). It would include the "Eden Alternative" for nursing homes along with "Spiritual Eldering" and intergenerational solidarity in local communities. In summary, a genuinely critical perspective would not be pie in the sky utopianism but the celebration of concrete experiments that create role models for a positive vision of aging in the future.

From all that has been said, it should be clear that the four alternative ideologies described here need not be understood as mutually exclusive. On the contrary, successful aging and productive aging depend on each other in crucial ways. Similarly, radical gerontology would presumably not wish to limit older people to a role as being passive consumers of services but would also insist on wider opportunities to contribute to the common good. And conscious aging has its own contribution to make toward healthy aging and continued productivity where contributive roles are defined in the widest possible terms. If there is one theme that unites all four alternative ideologies, it is just this widening of the sense of possibilities for the later part of life. If the struggle to understand and advance an agenda for productive aging opens us all and keeps us alive to these possibilities, it will have made an immeasurable contribution to our vision of an aging society in years to come.

REFERENCES

Adams-Price, C. E. (Ed.). (1998). *Creativity and successful aging: Theoretical and empirical approaches*. New York: Springer.

Aronowitz, S. (1988). *The power of science: Discourse and ideology in modern society*. Minneapolis: University of Minnesota Press.

Atchley, R. C. (1993). Spiritual development and wisdom: A Vedantic perspective. In R. Kastenbaum (Ed.), *Encyclopedia of adult development*. Phoenix, AZ: Oryx.

Atchley, R. C. (1997). Everyday mysticism: Spiritual development in later adulthood. *Journal of Adult Development, 4* (2), 123–134.

Baars, J. (1991). The challenge of critical gerontology: The problem of social constitution. *Journal of Aging Studies, 5*, 219–243.

Baltes, P. B., & Baltes, M. M. (Eds.). (1990). *Successful aging: Perspectives from the behavioral sciences.* Cambridge: Cambridge University Press.

Bass, S. A. (Ed.). (1995). *Older and active: How Americans over 55 are contributing to society.* New Haven: Yale University Press.

Bass, S. A., Caro, F. G., & Chen, Y.-P. (Eds.). (1993). *Achieving a productive aging society.* Westport, CT: Auburn House.

Bianchi, E. C. (1982). *Aging as a spiritual journey.* New York: Crossroads.

Bond, L. A., Cutler, S. J., & Grams, A. (Eds.). (1995). *Promoting successful and productive aging.* Thousand Oaks, CA: Sage.

Bornat, J., Phillipson, C., & Ward, S. (1985). *Manifesto for old age.* London: Pluto.

Brooks, J. D. (1996). Living longer and improving health: An obtainable goal in promoting aging well? *American Behavioral Scientist, 39* (3), 272–287.

Butler, R. N. (1975). *Why survive? Being old in America.* New York: Harper & Row.

Butler, R., & Brody, J. A. (Eds.). (1995). *Strategies to delay dysfunction in later life,* New York: Springer.

Butler, R. N., & Gleason, H. P. (Eds.). (1985). *Productive aging: Enhancing vitality in later life.* New York: Springer.

Butler, R. N., Oberlink, M. R., & Schechter, M. (Eds.). (1990). *Promise of productive aging: From biology to social policy.* New York: Springer.

Cole, T. (1992). *The journey of life: A cultural history of aging in America.* New York: Cambridge University Press.

de Beauvoir, S. (1973). *Coming of age.* New York: G. P. Putnam's Sons.

Ekerdt, D. J. (1986). Busy ethic: Moral continuity between work and retirement. *The Gerontologist, 26* (3), 239–244.

Erikson, E. (1950). *Childhood and society.* New York: Norton.

Estes, C. L. (1979). *The aging enterprise: A critical examination of social policies and services for the aged,* San Francisco, CA: Jossey-Bass.

Estes, C. L., Gerard, L. E., Sprague-Zones, J., & Swan, J. H. (1984). *Political economy, health, and aging.* Boston: Little, Brown.

Featherstone, M., & Hepworth, M. (1991). The mask of ageing and the postmodern life course. In M. Featherstone, M. Hepworth, & B. Turner (Eds.), *The body: Social process and cultural theory* (pp. 370–389). London: Sage.

Featherstone, M., & Wemick, A. (1995). *Images of aging: Cultural representations of later life.* London and New York: Routledge.

Friedan, B. (1993). *The fountain of age.* New York: Simon & Schuster.

Fries, J. F. (1989). *Aging well: A guide for successful seniors.* Reading, MA: Addison-Wesley.

Gabler, N. (1998). *Life the movie.* New York: Knopf.

Gingold, R. (1992). *Successful ageing.* New York: Oxford University Press.

Green, B. (1993). *Gerontology and the construction of old age: A study in discourse analysis.* Hawthorne, NY: Gruyter.

Gullette, M. M. (1997). *Declining to decline: Cultural combat and the politics of the midlife.* Charlottesville: University of Virginia Press.

Havighurst, R. J. (1961). Successful aging. *The Gerontologist, 1,* 4–7.

Hazan, H. (1996). *From first principles: An experiment in ageing.* Westport, CT: Bergin & Garvey.

Heelas, P. (1996). *The new age movement.* Oxford: Blackwell.

Herzog, A. R., & House, J. S. (1991). Productive activities and aging well. *Generations, 15* (1), 49–54.

Holstein, M. (1992). Productive aging: A feminist critique. *Journal of Aging and Social Policy, 4* (3–4), 17–34.

Hudson, R. B. (1996). Changing face of aging politics. *The Gerontologist, 36* (1), 33–35.

Katz, S. (1996). *Disciplining old age: The formation of gerontological knowledge.* Charlottesville: University Press of Virginia.

Koenig, H. G. (1994). *Aging and God.* New York: Haworth.

Krain, M. A. (1995). Policy implications for a society aging well: Employment, retirement, education, and leisure policies for the 21st century. *American Behavioral Scientist, 39* (2), 131–151.

Kumashiro, M. (Ed.). (1995). *Paths to productive aging.* London: Taylor & Francis.

Kunneman, H. (1997). Relevance of postmodern and feminist philosophy for the study of aging. *Journal of Aging Studies, 11* (4), 273–282.

Leder, D. (1996). Spiritual community in later life: A modest proposal. *Journal of Aging Studies, 10* (2), 103–116.

Levin, J. S. (1993). Age differences in mystical experience. *The Gerontologist, 33* (4), 507–513.

Lowry, J. H. (1985). Predictors of successful aging in retirement. In E. Palmore, E. Busse, G. L. Maddox, & I. C. Siegler (Eds.), *Normal aging III: Report from the Duke Longitudinal Studies, 1975–1984* (pp. 394–404). Durham, NC: Duke University Press.

Luborsky, M. R., & Sankar, A. (1993). Extending the critical gerontology perspective: Cultural dimensions. *The Gerontologist, 33,* 440–454.

Manton, K. G., Stallard, E., & Corder, L. (1997). Education-specific estimates of life expectancy and age-specific disability in the U.S. elderly population. *Journal of Aging and Health, 9* (4), 419–450.

Marshall V. W., & Tindale, J. A. (1978–1979). Notes for a radical gerontology. *International Journal of Aging and Human Development, 9* (2), 163–175.

Minkler, M., & Cole, T. R. (1992). Political and moral economy of aging: Not such strange bedfellows. *International Journal of Health Services, 22* (1), 113–124.

Minkler, M., & Estes, C. L. (Eds.). (1984). *Readings in the political economy of aging.* Farmingdale, NY: Baywood.

Minkler, M., & Estes, C. L. (Eds.). (1998). *Critical gerontology: Perspectives from political and moral economy of growing old.* Amityville, NY: Baywood.

Moody, H. R. (1988a). *Abundance of life: Human development policies for an aging society.* New York: Columbia University Press.

Moody, H. R. (1988b). Toward a critical gerontology: The role of the humanities to theories of aging. In J. Birren & V. Bengtson (Eds.), *Emergent theories of aging: Psychological and social perspectives on time, self, and society.* New York: Springer.

Moody, H. R. (1992). What is critical gerontology and why does it matter? In T. R. Cole (Ed.), *Voices and visions: Toward a critical gerontology.* New York: Springer.

Moody, H. R. (1995). Mysticism and aging. In M. A. Kimble, S. H. McFadden, J. W. Ellor, & J. J. Seeber (Eds.), *Aging, spirituality, and religion: A handbook.* Minneapolis: Fortress.

Moody, H. R. (1997). *The five stages of the soul: Charting the spiritual passages that shape our lives.* New York: Doubleday Anchor Books.

Myles, J. (1989). *Old age in the welfare state: The political economy of public pensions* (rev. ed.). Lawrence: University Press of Kansas.

Neuhaus, R. H., & Neuhaus, R. H. (1982). *Successful aging.* New York: John Wiley & Sons.

Olson, L. K. (1982). *The political economy of aging.* New York: Columbia University Press.

O'Reilly, P., & Caro, F. G. (1994). Productive aging: An overview of the literature. *Journal of Aging and Social Policy, 6* (3), 39–71.

Palmore, E. (1979). Predictors of successful aging. *The Gerontologist, 19,* 427–431.

Pascual-Leone, J. (1990). Reflections on life-span intelligence, consciousness, and ego development. In C. N. Alexander & E. Langer (Eds.), *Higher stages of human development.* New York: Oxford University Press.

Phillipson, C. (1982). *Capitalism and the construction of old age.* London: Macmillan.

Ray, R. E. (1996). Postmodern perspective on feminist gerontology. *The Gerontologist, 36* (5), 674–680.

Riley, M., Kahn, R., & Foner, A. (Eds.). (1994). *Age and structural lag: Society's failure to provide meaningful opportunities in work, family and leisure.* New York: Wiley-Interscience.

Riley, J. W., Jr., & Riley, M. W. (1994). Beyond productive aging: Changing lives and social structure. *Ageing International, 21* (2), 15–19.

Robertson, A. (1997). Beyond apocalyptic demography: Towards a moral economy of interdependence. *Ageing and Society, 17* (4), 425–446.

Robinson, B. (1994). In search of productive aging: A little something for everyone. *Ageing International, 21* (4), 33–36.

Rosenmayr, L. (1981). *Die späte Freiheit* (The late freedom). Vienna: Severin & Siedler.

Rosenwald, G. C., & Ochberg, R. L. (1992). *Storied lives: The cultural politics of self- understanding.* New Haven: Yale University Press.

Rossman, I. (1989). *Looking forward: Complete medical guide to successful aging.* New York: E. P. Dutton.

Rowe, J., & Kahn, R. (1987). Human aging: Usual and successful. *Science, 237* (4811), 143–149.

Rowe, J., & Kahn, R. (1998). *Successful aging.* New York: Pantheon.

Schachter, Z., & Miller, R. S. (1995). *From age-ing to sage-ing: A profound new vision of growing older.* New York: Warner Books.

Sinnott, Jan. (1996). Postformal thought and mysticism: How might the mind know the unknowable? *Aging and Spirituality, 8,* 7–8.

Stoller, E. P., & Gibson, R. C. (1997). *Worlds of difference: Inequality in the aging experience* (2nd ed.). Thousand Oaks, CA: Pine Forge.

Tornstam, L. (1992). The quo vadis of gerontology: On the scientific paradigm of gerontology. *The Gerontologist, 32,* 318–326.

Tornstam, L. (1997). Gerotranscendence: The contemplative dimension of aging. *Journal of Aging Studies, 11* (2), 143–154.

Wilber, K. (1996). *Eye to eye: The quest for a new paradigm* (3rd ed.). Boston: Shambala.

Young, G. (1998). *Adult development, therapy and culture: A postmodern synthesis.* New York: Plenum.

9

THE POLITICAL ECONOMY
OF PRODUCTIVE AGING

Carroll L. Estes, Ph.D., and Jane L. Mahakian, Ph.D.

This chapter incorporates the moral economy perspective as we examine the assumptions and values behind the concept of productivity as applied to the aging process. We attempt to show how we believe this application of productivity to old age will generally affect the elderly (i.e., creates new problems) and resource allocations to them (i.e., holds them in place with continuing race, class, and gender inequity). A moral economy perspective looks "beyond the appearance of things—at the underlying foundational assumptions, facts, loyalties, and values that undergird the superstructure of public policy" (Minkler & Estes, 1999, p. 2).

Social Context and Antecedents of Productive Aging

During the 1960s and 1970s and continuing into the 1980s, social movements emerged around civil rights, consumer rights, holistic health, fitness, self-care, feminism, and ageism. These popular movements grew out of and fostered a new emphasis on individual rights and the role of society. The 1980s, under the leadership of President Reagan in the United States and Margaret Thatcher in the United Kingdom, saw a resurgence of the market ideology and the responsibility of the individual, which has been vigorously promoted by private-sector business and institutionalized through laws that have begun to challenge the "rights" of entitlement to welfare and to an array of other welfare state benefits (Estes, 1998). Mainstream political and economic systems of Western industrialized nations have variously experimented with changes in their retirement and health systems (Esping-Andersen, 1996).

A Broader Conceptual Framework:
The Social Determinants of Health

The 1970s marked a watershed in understanding the importance of social, environmental, and behavioral determinants of health status (Estes, Fox, & Mahoney, 1986). Dubos (1979), McKeown (1978/1997), and Belloc and Breslow (1972) contributed to an increased understanding of the social determinants of health, particularly the environment, social class and other social factors, and lifestyle as major determinants of individual health status. Dubos's (1970) pioneering work addressed individual adaptation to the social and physical environment. McKeown (1978/1997) demonstrated the role of improved nutrition, changing personal habits, and sanitation in achieving the marked improvements in health status during the past 150 years, calling into question the strong belief that improved medical care and technology have been the major source of health gains. Belloc and Breslow (1972) demonstrated an association between lifestyle habits and physical health status, supporting the promotion of individual behavior change as part of preventive health principles. Physical health was measured in terms of disability, chronic conditions, impairments, symptoms, and energy level. Positive behaviors for health were sleeping seven or eight hours each night, maintaining normal weight, engaging in physical exercise, not smoking cigarettes, and drinking a certain number of drinks.

More recently, McKinlay and McKinlay (1977, p. 425) pushed this point further, showing that "at most 3.5% of the total decline in mortality since 1900 could be ascribed to medical measures" for the eight infectious diseases they studied. They found, instead, that social factors, including a rise in income, better sanitation, and nutrition, were more significant in improving the health of the U.S. population than medical interventions, including both prevention and treatment.

During this same period, two reports spoke to the elderly. The 1977 report of the President's Council on Physical Fitness and Sports states that older persons (1) believe their need for exercise diminishes and eventually disappears with age; (2) exaggerate the risks involved in regular exercise beyond middle age; (3) overrate the benefits of light, irregular exercise;

and (4) underrate their own capabilities and abilities to participate in fitness activities. The 1979 Surgeon General's Report on Health Promotion and Disease Prevention set specific quantifiable national health status goals for the first time for the health of older adults: "by 1990, to reduce the average annual number of days of restricted activity due to chronic and acute conditions by 2004 to fewer than thirty days per year for people aged 65 and older" (U.S. Department of Health, Education, and Welfare, 1979, p. 71). This document laid out a conceptual framework for national health promotion activities, focusing on individual behavior and lifestyle as a major determinant of health and illness.

In 1980, Minkler and Fullarton noted the exclusion of the elderly from health promotion programs as due to the following characteristics: (1) focus on life extension, while the elderly are perceived as not having a future; (2) focus on reducing risk factors associated with premature mortality and morbidity, whereas many of the elderly have already lived beyond risk of premature death; (3) advocacy of youthfulness and the prevention of signs of aging; therefore "old folks" are unwelcome; and (4) focus on absence and avoidance of chronic disease, which is an irrelevant goal for most elderly who already have one or more chronic conditions that may or may not limit their functioning.

Simultaneously, in 1980, Fries observed the increase in the incidence of chronic disease, as people are more likely to survive illnesses that used to strike early in life. Because chronic disease is now the major cause of death, the major emphasis of health care, he argued, must shift from the treatment of acute illness toward the removal of risk factors associated with chronic illness. Because lifestyle is a major risk factor associated with the onset of chronic illness and resulting functional disability, Fries postulated that modification of lifestyle and behavior to promote health can alter the process of aging; improve the physical, mental, and social functioning of the elderly; reduce disability normally associated with aging; and extend a vigorous life up to the end of what they describe as the natural biological life span.

The 1981 White House Conference on Aging recommended increased governmental, voluntary, and private-sector activity in health promotion and fitness for the elderly (U.S. Department of Health and Human Services, 1982). During the 1980s the rising interest in health promotion provided a hopeful sign that public health policy would shift (or at least somewhat rebalance priorities) from the dominant biomedical definition and model of health and disease toward a broader bio-psycho-social view that encompassed the social and physical environment, as well as individual lifestyle and behavior (McKeown, 1978/1997, pp. 79–90). Toward such an aim, the Kaiser Family Foundation supported several major initiatives, including (1) Green's (1980) work on a model of health promotion that combined health education with related organizational and politico-economic interventions designed to facilitate behavioral and environmental adaptations to improve or protect health, and (2) a project on the links between health and community (Amick et al., 1995; Haan et al., 1989).

The Biomedicalization of Aging

In spite of the accumulating research evidence documenting the import of social as opposed to medical factors in health and aging, as well as fledgling health promotion efforts, the hegemony of the medical model in health and aging policy in the United States persists. We have written about the pitfalls of the "biomedicalization of aging" (Estes & Binney, 1989) in which society has constructed old age as a disease and aging as a medical problem requiring more and more medical services. This biomedicalization has contributed to the acute care bias of Medicare and the failure of health policy to provide long-term care and the rehabilitative and social supportive services needed by the chronically ill. More important, it diverts our resources and attention from other factors that are more important in determining the experience and quality of life of older persons—an adequate income and a safe and secure physical environment, among others. And finally, the biomedicalization of aging has contributed substantially to the expansion of multiple highly profitable medical industries and professions that provide acute and high-tech care to the elderly.

Former Assistant Secretary for Health, Dr. Philip Lee, cites three problems with U.S. health policy for the elderly that impede its ability to promote successful or productive aging: (1) the continuing dominance of the biomedical paradigm; (2) the acute care model when a long-term care paradigm is more appropriate; and (3) the priorities in health promotion and disease prevention that concentrate on children and leave the problems of the elderly unaddressed (Lee, 1998).

Major health care policies for the aging reflect the biomedical definition of health in which health is seen as the absence of disease, disease as a deviation from a biological norm of a young and "healthy" society, and aging as a biologically determined process of inevitable decline. Health maintenance is thus focused on treating these processes of disease and decline. More recently, a perceptible yet subtle shift has been to treating the risk factors for these processes of disease and decline.

To sum up, although knowledge of the determinants of health in the aging has grown and health promotion and disease prevention programs also have grown in visibility in Congress, in federal agencies, and at state and local levels of government, policies that build on this knowledge and perspective remain frustratingly illusive to the American people. The Surgeon General's recent report, *Healthy People 2010,* and recent Medicare legislation (the 1997 Balanced Budget Act) contain new coverage of a number of preventive benefits (e.g., the full cost of mammograms, prostate cancer screening). These efforts have been aided by many groups outside government, including the Institute of Medicine of the National Academy of Sciences and a growing number of university and business interests. Private-sector groups actively advocating for health promotion include voluntary professional health organizations, health and life insurance companies, fitness and health food industries, and some employers. Nevertheless, health policy that actually promotes health (rather than simply be bounded by a sickness model) receives limited support or funding, in large part because of the difficulty of cracking the already medically committed and potentially volatile financing of the big categorical health programs such as Medicare and Medicaid. Current policy, thus, represents a formidable obstacle to the advancement of health and aging policy that would truly challenge the medical model with health goals that would maximize the likelihood of successful or productive aging.

Gerontology Embraces Successful Aging: Modifiable and Reversible

Advances in gerontological theorizing and research are consistent with the efforts of health promotion advocates to improve individual outcomes as they increase individual choices and personal control. The 1980s saw an energizing of gerontology with the notion of the plasticity (even the potential reversibility) of aging, the differentiation of "usual" aging from "successful aging" (Rowe & Kahn, 1987), and the idea of the modifiability of previously considered inevitable biological, behavioral, and social processes. The well-received optimism about aging continues with the MacArthur Foundation Network on Successful Aging (Rowe & Kahn, 1998) and the findings of Manton, Corder, and Stallard (1997) regarding the decline in the prevalence of chronic disability among the elderly, from 24.9 percent to 21.3 percent between 1982 and 1994. Nevertheless, amid predictions concerning changing morbidity and its "compression," there is both controversy and certainty that there will be enormous increases in the number of very old elderly that will still require serious attention in terms of economic, health, and long-term care issues.

In the case of successful aging, the positive new framework points to the identification of individual risk factors for unsuccessful aging and the choices for successful health-promoting behaviors. The work theoretically holds out hope of challenging the biomedical paradigm, while giving a nod to the importance of social and environmental factors in making successful aging a possibility. These social and environmental factors, however, remain underexplicated, undertheorized, and underresearched in the work on successful aging, as they have in the work on health promotion more broadly.

Riley (1998, p. 151) describes the shortcoming well:

> Rowe and Kahn's . . . 1997 article, "Successful Aging" is a signal contribution to gerontology. . . . . However, . . . their model remains seriously incomplete. Although it elaborates the potentials for individual success, it fails to develop adequately the social structural opportunities necessary for realizing success. . . . Changes in lives and changes in social structures are fundamentally interdependent (Riley & Riley, 1994). Thus successful aging involves the interplay between lives and the complementary dynamic of structural change.

Social class is, from our viewpoint, the most important structural element that must be considered in shaping whatever may be possible in aging, for social class is the single most consistent structural factor that is empirically related to virtually every measure of health and illness. Race, ethnicity, and gender each weigh in very heavily as well. Dramatically reduced incomes, decreased power and social standing, the threat of economic and social dependency, chronic illness, and the loss of social support systems, as well as individual lifestyle, are all powerful determinants of the well-being of the elderly in our society.

From "Successful" to "Productive" Aging

Gerontologists have recently engaged in serious attempts to reconstruct the reality of aging—first from what is "usual" to what is "successful" and, now, from aging as a negative value (i.e., as "unproductive") to something valued (i.e., as "productive"). Both efforts speak broadly to the social, environmental, behavioral, and other factors involved, yet each underplays the profoundly difficult task of truly conceptualizing what it would take in the form of altered policy and social (to wit, economic) arrangements (and redistribution) to achieve the measure of their promise. In a capitalist society where the market is king and its primary (perhaps only) value is what is monetized and its economic value, there are formidable political, economic, and social barriers to the proposed reevaluation of what elders "do," under the productive aging banner.

Productive Aging: Definitions

The focus of productive aging is primarily on social and economic production of goods and services that creates value (paid for or not) or develops the capacity to produce them (paid for or not) (Caro, Bass, & Chen, 1993). With productive aging, it is said that there is (or will be) a sense of achievement and life engagement and a view of older adult as a major and valuable resource (Caro, Bass, & Chen, 1993).

According to Herzog (1989), productive aging is any activity that produces goods or services, whether paid for or not, including activities such as housework, child care, volunteer work, and help to family and friends. Morgan (1988) defines productivity as activities that produce goods and services that otherwise would have to be paid for and that reduce the demand on goods and services produced by others.

Butler and Schechter (1995) define productive aging as the capacity for an individual or a population to serve in the paid workforce, to serve in volunteer activities, to assist in the family, and to maintain as independent an existence as possible. The aging are viewed individually and collectively as a resource to meet their own and society's needs.

A Critique

Well-intentioned and developed by leading scholars in the field of gerontology, the concept of productive aging seeks a positive recognition of the resources of old age. In a major sense, the concept of productive aging seeks a redemption of old age itself.

We agree with Holstein that it aims to show that old people are already productive (seeking to reverse the "decline and loss" paradigm) and that it seeks to counteract the greedy geezer stereotypes by showing that old people are contributors to society—not just selfish consumers (Holstein, 1992, p. 359). And, as Holstein observes, it "affirms a cultural ideal— that it is good to elevate productivity as a ruling metaphor for a good old age" (Holstein, 1992, p. 359).

This is where the problems begin. Economic status has a profound impact on the older adult's ability to experience a meaningful and pro- ductive aging experience. So does race, ethnicity, and gender.

Crucial questions raised by ourselves and others as well:

Who exactly defines productive aging?
Who is productive aging for?
What is the role of and who will benefit from productive aging?

To these questions, we would add the following:

What does productive aging mean in the face of:
    –increasing inequality in society?
    –increasing inequality within the aging population?
    –the potential "end of work" and changes in the meaning of work?
    –challenges to the meaning of retirement?

Productive aging, in one sense, may be seen as the perfect extension of market logic (and potentially the market discipline) to old age. Market logic is defined as placing the individual in complete authority over the produc- tion of goods and services. The market rationale is imposed on individual aging through the concept of productivity in what may be described as a different but nonetheless judgmental and normative view of aging.

Trying to get aging defined as productive is an unnecessary capitula- tion to the power of the market, rendering up all human experience (and living) to (and subject to) controls of the market and as "work" (and at any price). What disappears is any notion of value or meaning that is detached from economic worth and defined according to capitalist logic. Also what disappears is any legitimacy for the notion of social need or deservingness based on the human condition.

The use of the concept obfuscates what is a macro problem—a society that stigmatizes and "throws away" a particular age segment (and more) of its people—and redefines it as a micro problem of individuals who are aging. Productive aging obliterates all other values than the economic metric. This approach threatens to redefine every stage of the life course as being required to meet productivity standards (imposed norms of production).

A Political Economy Perspective on Productive Aging

The political economy perspective brings a critical lens to a concept such as productive aging and its uses and implications. Such a concept can be understood only in the context of the social structures and the power relations within which individual persons in the society age. The political economy perspective looks at social structural factors that affect aging, both as individual and as societal processes and structural phenomena of global proportions and consequences. Political economy is not an individual theory of aging but is concerned with both the existing structural arrangements and resource distributions that vitally affect the individual experience of old age, and older persons and the aging as a collectivity and as subgroups (Estes, 1979, 1999).

A central assumption of the political economy perspective is that aging and old age are directly related to the nature and historical moment of the society in which they are situated and, therefore, cannot be considered or analyzed in isolation from other societal forces and characteristics, including the wider power structures in society and global politics and economics.

The power of the state (government), of business, and of workers and the role of the economy are all central in determining the life chances of older persons in society, and these life chances are seen as highly differentiated by race, class, and gender. Explicitly recognized in this framework are the structural influences on the aging experience and the role of societal institutions and social relations in understanding how aging and old age are defined and treated in society. The major problems facing the elderly such as dependency are understood as socially constructed as a result of societal conceptions of aging and the aged (Estes, 1979).

The political economy perspective calls attention to five areas, each of which is discussed below. These are: (1) the social and structural production of aging; (2) the role of ideology; (3) the types of social interventions that are called for by dominant perspectives; (4) the role of the aging enterprise and medical-industrial complex; and (5) social policy.

1. A political economy perspective calls attention to the socially and structurally produced nature of aging and the lived experience of old age as these vary by gender, social class, race, ethnicity, and generation.

The concept of productive aging portrays aging as a problem of individuals. It is subject to interpretations that begin and end on the individual level, with the individual seen (and blamed) as productive or unproductive. The measures of evaluation are also at the individual level. Matilda White-Riley (1998) spoke to this problem with the work of Rowe and Kahn (1998) on successful aging and noted the vital importance of thinking and working on societal and institutional levels (e.g., of schools, employers, churches, government) as well as on the individual level.

The linking or confounding of the view of positive aging with productivity is likely to have unintended but discriminatory effects against older people as well as others who live outside a well-defined normative mainstream, and particularly those on the margins—those who are "not normal," perhaps disabled, the oldest-old, and those without resources.

Directly or indirectly, the productivity movement in aging is entirely consistent with the larger political economic context in which the market is seen as the best (or only) way to meet social needs. The "giving away" of the public sphere and public responsibility for the aging is an incalculably high cost indeed.

There are formidable social, structural, and institutional impediments to making it as a "productive ager." The concept of productive aging tends to gloss over the gender, race, and ethnic inequalities from birth on and the different life chances and opportunities afforded under these different circumstances and explicit social policy—for example, policy that results in the highest poverty levels for older women in the United States of any in the Western industrial world and even higher poverty levels for older women of color.

Holstein argues, persuasively, that the call for a productive aging society will truncate, rather than expand, older women's chances to construct a meaningful last chapter of life. Further, she argues, the definition perpetuates a perception of perceived personal and social needs that is especially damaging to women (Holstein, 1992).

There are competing constructions of reality regarding what is positive aging. The consequences of these competing definitions, labels, and constructions have to be considered. Who has the power to define the problem (i.e., "the reality") of productivity? Productivity is owned by the field as a problem, in the terms of the market and on its own terms. And with what implications for those who are defined as productive or unproductive?

Holstein (1992) identified its negative effect, especially for people who suffer from chronic health problems or major disabilities. Moody alluded to the inescapable semantic significance of the term (Moody, 1993) and to the problem of the narrow standards we use to define a productive life. Productive aging is not the only imaginable ideal for what the last stage of life might mean.

We may be socially adopting a negative concept of people who are failures. This is so, as the concept implicitly accords normative value to aging that is equated with success. Lack of productive aging equals failure—failure to produce goods or services, whether paid or unpaid—and potentially the *obligation* to produce more, particularly more of the "free" labor of elder caregiving that women already provide in large quantities (Estes, 1998). The concept of productive aging lulls us into believing that there are no losers—that productive aging is a positive goal synonymous with apple pie and motherhood (Estes, 1998).

Labels or social constructions of reality are crucial in defining "the problem" and the policy solutions attendant to the problem. The importance of the labels that we apply to the elderly has been documented elsewhere (Estes, 1979). Labels that are applied to others contribute significantly to the process by which we define ourselves, our worth, and our self-esteem (an illustration of the "Looking Glass Self" and the contributions of labeling theory; see Thomas, 1967). Much has been written about the fact that the elderly are particularly vulnerable to such labels and definitions as worthless or unproductive, given the cumulating losses occurring in old age and our societal vacuum in dealing with aging in a holistic or respectful way. The productivity label (being so or not so) is likely to contribute to the already worrisome construction of aging as a burden. It is consonant with the constructions of aging as a demographic and fiscal crisis—as a burden that the nation (i.e., especially the government) cannot bear.

2. From a political economy perspective, ideology is a central element in the processing of the old and old age in society and its implications by gender, race, and social class.

The concept of productive aging is consistent with, if not an extension of, the ideology of the market into the aging process. This ideology limits a vision of the possible as well as options and actions to what is imaginable. The onus is on the individual, not our society or the state.

The ideology of individualism is at the heart of the resurgence of the market, in which preference for the market far outweighs considerations of the growing inequality being produced in U.S. society.

3. The political economy perspective examines the types of social interventions that are legitimated by the dominant construction of aging and the role of the (nation) state therein.

The use of the productivity notion to determine what the best of aging "is" may transfer the risk from the state to the individual, and from the community to the older person. Such a transfer of responsibility is consistent with efforts to convert or privatize Social Security and Medicare.

The movement to enhance elder productivity, which inevitably confounds successful aging with productivity, provides the necessary cognitive framework for the retreat of the state and for cuts in Medicare and Social Security. In this way, the concept of productive aging may be useful in advancing the interests of those who wish to contain and roll back the welfare state.

Productive aging paves the way for the extension of the market mentality (and its purportedly politically neutral "invisible hand" or inexorable laws of competition) into judgments about doing housework, caring for others, and, by extension, even when we walk, what we eat, and our personal health behaviors.

We find ourselves left largely with the concept of responsibility at the individual level—consistent with the individualization of risk, apart from all of the social forces and social factors (race, class, and gender) that our scientific research demonstrates to significantly determine the differential exposure to risk (health risks and other types of risks) and how that risk is individually experienced (as well as with what economic and political weapons to combat it).

It is here, also, that there is an important link between productive aging and the field of health promotion and disease prevention. It is here that there has been a persistent decoupling of what we know about the social determinants of health and aging and what our health policy supports.

We know the importance of socioeconomic status (SES) in every measure of health at every stage of life and aging (House, Kessler, & Herzog, 1990). The social and the behavioral factors in determining health risks are well documented (McKinlay & McKinlay, 1986; Amick et al., 1995) and seen by many as increasingly important with age.

Yet, as a nation, we persist in policies that pay for medical care (Medicare) while we do almost nothing in support of policies that would truly promote health. There are a few examples in the area of prevention (mammograms, influenza and vaccines, prostate and colon cancer screening, and Pap smears) that have been recently added to Medicare benefits. Nevertheless, 99 percent of Medicare dollars are for acute care, provided within a biomedical paradigm—in spite of the well-documented needs of elders for chronic and long-term care, supportive services, and policies to support healthy and safe communities, adequate income, and housing to promote and support healthy lifestyles. There are assorted federal and state initiatives, many of them disease-specific, on hypertension, diabetes, and heart disease. Work on healthy communities involves more local initiatives, although the "safe streets" initiatives will affect the environment in which persons might be encouraged to walk.

If we are to promote productive aging, there is a need for enlarged public- and private-sector responsibility. Community and social institutional responsibility (including policy changes and resource commitments) are essential elements of any program to promote productive aging in order to permit and promote positive individual and societal outcomes. Otherwise, the certain outcome will be the continuous reproduction of inequalities of race, class, and gender. We need to explore perceptions of the public and how they define productive aging, productivity, and older adults' contributions.

A problem, in our view, is that the most tangible focus remains on the individual to make changes to his or her lifestyle by being energized and motivated to work (paid or unpaid) and to exercise and improve one's nutrition, control stress, reduce one's use of alcohol and drugs, and quit smoking—independent of real and meaningful changes in the larger structural arrangements.

4. From a political economy perspective, the aging enterprise and the medical-industrial complex are treated as influences in and potential beneficiaries of the definition and treatment of aging.

Attention to aging at the individual level is consistent with the individualized notion of aging from a biomedical perspective. With the aging of the population, the highly profitable biomedically oriented medical-industrial complex remains intact and unchallenged (Estes, Harrington, & Davis, 1992). Insofar as health-promoting and lifestyle behaviors converge or are defined synonymously with (or antecedent to) productive aging, a vast new array of private-sector product lines and industries to promote dietary, exercise, and other behavioral changes—again primarily aimed at the individual level—are legitimated by aging experts. The economic and social resources to avail oneself of these are likely to continue to be determined on the basis of the market or the ability to pay for them privately, rather than as a right to health or well-being in old age.

5. A political economy approach examines the nature and consequences of social policy with attention to its effects on older persons, and particularly in accord with their gender, social class, and racial and ethnic status.

On the policy level, the concept of productive aging does little to challenge the status quo. If anything, it holds everything in place. There are no accompanying or requisite economic or health policies to address problems of market failure or of unequal access to whatever is defined as productive aging. (Unequal access is a problem that Butler and Schecter [1995] say should be addressed.) Without compensatory strategies, public policy will remain class-based, racialized, and gendered in its outcomes (Estes, 1998). Indeed, without explicit policy to the contrary, social class, racial, and gender inequalities will surely deepen.

To be aging successfully or productively, elders may be expected to take on more work (paid or unpaid) and to expect less from the state (government and the public sector). The redefined productivity of unpaid labor, for example, in the form of long-term caregiving (one-third of which is provided by the elderly, most of them women) is also seen as good because it is productive (this, irrespective of the costs to the caregiver). This redefinition of aging, however, comes at a price since support for the application of the norm of productivity to what the elderly do leaves intact other critical elements of the situation—the substantial problems of gender (in)justice, racial and ethnic (in)justice, and class (in)justice that characterize the everyday lives of older persons (and all Americans for that matter).

Significantly, productive aging, in itself, necessitates no policy prescription to provide the material resources to compensate (or even provide disability coverage) for unpaid work such as long-term caregiving. Instead it only blesses and encourages such work. In the extreme, the aged may find themselves dogged by market judgments to the end of life, and in ways that become troubling new sources of stigma and social control.

References

Amick, B. C., Levine, S., Tarlov, A. R., & Walsh, D. C. (1995). Introduction. In B. C. Amick, S. Levine, A. R. Tarlov, & D. C. Walsh (Eds.), *Society and health* (pp. 3–17). New York: Oxford University Press.

Belloc, N. B., & Breslow, L. (1972). Relationship of physical health status and health practices. *Preventative Medicine, 1,* 409–421.

Butler, R. N., & Schechter, M. (1995). Productive aging. In G. L. Maddox (Ed.), *The encyclopedia of aging.* New York: Springer.

Caro, F., Bass, S., & Chen, Y.-P. (1993). Introduction. In S. Bass, F. Caro, & Y.-P. Chen (Eds.), *Achieving a productive aging society.* Westport, CT: Greenwood.

Dubos, R. J. (1970). *So human an animal.* New York: Scribner.

Dubos, R. (1979). *Mirage of health.* New York: Harper & Row.

Esping-Anderson, G. (Ed.). (1996). *Welfare states in transition.* Thousand Oaks, CA: Sage.

Estes, C. L. (1979). *The aging enterprise.* San Francisco: Jossey Bass.

Estes, C. L. (1998). Crisis, the welfare state and aging. Paper presented at the meeting of the American Sociological Association, San Francisco.

Estes, C. L. (1999). Critical gerontology and the new political economy of aging. In M. Minkler & C. L. Estes (Eds.), *Critical gerontology: Perspectives from political and moral economy* (pp. 17–35). Amityville, NY: Baywood.

Estes, C. L., & Binney, E. A. (1989). The biomedicalization of aging: Dangers and dilemmas. *The Gerontologist, 29* (5), 587–596.

Estes, C. L., Fox, S., & Mahoney, C. W. (1986). Health care and social policy: Health promotion for the elderly. In K. Dychtwald (Ed.), *Wellness and health promotion for the elderly* (pp. 55–69). Rockville, MD: Aspen.

Estes, C. L., Harrington, C., & Davis, S. (1992). The medical industrial complex. In E. F. Borgatta & M. L. Borgatta (Eds.). *The encyclopedia of sociology* (Vol. 3, pp. 1243–1254). New York: Macmillan.

Fries, J. F. (1980). Aging, natural death and the compression of morbidity. *New England Journal of Medicine, 303,* 130–135.

Green, L. W. (1980). *Health education planning: A diagnostic approach.* Palo Alto: Mayfield.

Haan, M., Kaplan, G., & Syme, S. (1989). Old observations and new thoughts. In J. Bunker, D. Gomby, & B. Kehrer (Eds.), *Pathways to health: The role of social factors* (pp. 76–117). Menlo Park, CA: The Henry J. Kaiser Family Foundation.

Herzog, A. R. (1989). Age differences in productive activity. *Journal of Gerontology: Social Sciences, 44* (B), S129–S138.

Holstein, M. (1992). Productive aging: A feminist critique. *Journal of Aging and Social Policy, 4* (3–4), 17–33.

House, J. R., Kessler, C., & Herzog, A. R. (1990). Age, socioeconomic status, and health. *Milbank Quarterly, 68,* 383–411.

Lee, P. R. (1998). Personal communication.

Manton, K., Corder, L., & Stallard, E. (1997). Chronic disability trends in elderly U.S. populations: 1982–1994. *Proceedings of the National Academy of Sciences, 94,* 2593–2598.

McKeown, T. (1997). Determinants of health. *Human Nature Magazine* (April, 1978). Reprinted in P. R. Lee & C. L. Estes (Eds.), *The nation's health* (5th ed., pp. 9–17). Sudbury, MA: Jones & Barlett.

McKinlay, J. B., & McKinlay, S. M. (1977). The questionable contribution of medical measures to the decline of mortality in the U.S. in the twentieth century. *Milbank Memorial Fund Quarterly/ Health and Sociology, 55* (3), 405–428.

McKinlay, S. M., & McKinlay, J. B. (1986). Aging in a healthy population. *Social Science Medicine, 23* (5), 531–535.

Minkler, M., & Estes, C. L. (Eds.). (1999). *Critical gerontology: Perspectives from political and moral economy.* Amityville, NY: Baywood.

Minkler, M., & Fullarton, J. E. (1980). *Health promotion, health maintenance, and disease prevention for the elderly.* Background paper for the 1981 White House Conference on Aging (pp. 1–2).

Moody, H. R. (1993). Age, productivity, and transcendence. In S. Bass, F. Caro, & Y.-P. Chen (Eds.), *Achieving a productive aging society* (pp. 28–40). Westport, CT: Greenwood.

Morgan, J. (1988). The relationship of housing and living arrangements to the productivity of older people. In Committee on an Aging Society, *The social and built environment in an older society* (pp. 250–280). Washington, DC: National Academy Press.

President's Council on Physical Fitness and Sports. (1977). *Exercise and aging.* Washington, DC: U.S. Government Printing Office.

Riley, M. W., & Riley, J. W. (1994). Structural lag: Past and future. In M. W. Riley, R. Kahn, & A. Foner (Eds.), *Age and structural lag* (pp. 15–36). New York: John Wiley & Sons.

Riley, M. W., & Riley, J. W. (1998). Letters to the Editor. *The Gerontologist, 38* (2), 151.

Rowe J. W., & Kahn, R. L. (1987). Usual and successful aging. *Science, 237,* 143–149.

Rowe J. W., & Kahn, R. L. (1997). Successful aging. *The Gerontologist, 37* (4), 433–440.

Rowe J. W., & Kahn, R. L. (1998). *Successful aging.* New York: Pantheon.

Syme, L., & Berkman, L. (1976). Social class, susceptibility, and sickness. *American Journal of Epidemiology, 104,* 1–8.

Thomas, W. I. (1967). *The unadjusted girl, with cases and standpoint for behavioral analysis.* New York: Harper & Row.

U.S. Department of Health, Education, and Welfare. (1979). *Healthy people: The Surgeon General's report on health promotion and disease prevention, 1979.* Washington, DC: U.S. Government Printing Office.

U.S. Department of Health, Education, and Welfare. (1982). *White House Conference on Aging, 1981. Final Report.* Washington, DC: U.S. Government Printing Office.

U.S. Department of Health and Human Services. (1998). *Healthy people: The Surgeon General's report on health promotion and disease prevention, 2010.* Washington, DC: U.S. Government Printing Office.

10

CHANGES OVER THE LIFE COURSE
IN PRODUCTIVE ACTIVITIES
Comparison of Black and White Populations

James S. Jackson, Ph.D.

The most common definitions have viewed activities to be "productive" if they generate valued goods and services (Herzog et al., 1989) and contribute in some meaningful way to society (e.g., Bass, 1995; Bass & Caro, 1992; O'Reilly & Caro, 1994). In prior work we proposed that individual and social characteristics, responsiveness of the opportunity structure, and economic necessity combine to affect patterns of productive participation in "economic networks" (Jackson, 1996; Jackson, Antonucci, & Gibson, 1993). These networks form the environmental, social, and psychological contexts for the choice and expression of productive activities over the individual life course, resulting in what we term "aging productively" (Jackson, 1996; Jackson, Antonucci, & Gibson, 1993; Butler, 1989; Butler & Gleason, 1985). Productive activities conducted within these different networks have been shown to be qualitatively and perhaps quantitatively distinct.

Productive activities can be assessed by at least three indicators. The first is the traditional count of hours of participation or imputed values of these hours (Morgan, 1986; Herzog & Morgan, 1992). The second indicator is the psychological process benefits that derive from participation in these hours of activities (Juster, 1985). These include subjective judgments of enjoyment and satisfaction of the activities and attributions of benefits to self. The final indicator is the attribution of potential benefits to others (altruistic or obligatory motives), including family, friends, or more generalized social identity groups. In prior work we examined whether the antecedents and consequences of productive activities within the three different networks, assessed by the three different indicators, are influenced by gender, socioeconomic status, and ethnic (racial) influences.

We also hypothesized (Jackson, 1996; Jackson, Antonucci, & Gibson, 1993) that differential participation in economic networks and involvement in formal and primary social networks over time are reciprocally related. Productive activities within these economic and formal and primary social networks are hypothesized to affect individual and group material, social, and psychological well-being. In prior work in a national U.S. sample of adults, we examined how engagement in productive activities in different types of economic networks influence social, psychological, and health outcomes. We also showed that these outcomes may be different at different points in the life course (Jackson, 1996; Glass et al., 1995).

The theoretical model of productive activities in this chapter builds on a long history of work in social gerontology. Particularly important is the past and current research on age stratification (Riley, 1985; Riley & Riley, 1992; Streib, 1985), well-being and adjustment (George & Bearon, 1980), voluntary associations (Cutler, 1976), activity theory (Neugarten, 1976), health (Satariano & Syme, 1981), and social support systems (Antonucci, 1990; Lowenthal & Robinson, 1976). Recent authors point to the needs of the future elderly, growth of an aging U.S. society (Committee on an Aging Society et al., 1986; Friedland & Summer, 1999; Siegel & Taeuber, 1986; Manton & Soldo, 1985), and the need for more integrative theory and research on aging and the life course, especially work on successful aging (Baltes & Baltes, 1990; Bass & Caro, 1996; Morgan, 1981; Riley, 1987).

Succinctly, this chapter has several purposes. The first is to present a description of a life course, network model of productive economic activities. In prior work (e.g., Jackson, 1996) we provided empirical support for the existence of the three economic networks and their observable indicators, and showed that the antecedents of participation differ by type of economic network and by significant demographic subgroups of the American population, notably age, gender, and racial group membership. We also provided empirical support for how the different indicators of productive involvement (behavioral, psychological, and social) influence individual social and psychological consequences within the contexts of the three different types of economic networks. In the present chapter I provide a descriptive examination of changes over the period 1989 to 1994, using three waves of panel data from a national longitudinal study of the American adult population, Americans' Changing Lives (House et al., 1994). My purpose is to compare and contrast by race, gender, age, and education how patterns of productive activities within and between these different economic networks change over this near-decade period.

Economic Network Framework

As we discussed in prior work (e.g., Jackson, 1996), the general assumption of the network model is that blocked opportunities and economic necessity motivate differential participation by individuals and families over the life course in three distinct but interrelated economic networks. The first is the regular economy network. This is the one most frequently engaged in and is characterized by exchanges of labor for pay and an efficient government accounting and taxation system (Pencavel, 1986; Rendall & Speare, 1993, 1994). The second network also involves pay but does not include government oversight and regulation as in the regular economy. This one has been called the underground, illegal, or irregular economy (Ferman, Henry, & Hoyman, 1987; Glutmann, 1977; Henry, 1982; Henry & Brown, 1990; Smith, 1982; Witte & Simon, 1983).

The final one, the social economy network, is based on a barter system that does not include exchanges for money (Lowenthal, 1975, 1981). In this case economic exchanges, largely among family and friends, are made without the explicit transfer of money. These three networks are interrelated and may be tightly interwoven. Participation in the three networks is also hypothesized to be integrally related to involvement in traditional familial and friend, social, and emotional support networks (Glanz, 1994).

Evidence for the Three Distinct Economic Networks

Briefly, overall, the results of prior exploratory and confirmatory factor analyses support our theorizing about the existence of definable and meaningful networks of economic activities that can be empirically examined (Jackson, 1996). These measurement models suggest that individual assessments of activities generally considered productive by traditional yardsticks form three distinct and independent latent factors, as predicted by our theoretical framework.

Prior work demonstrated the efficacy of expanding the definition of productivity to include hours measured among a greater number of activities (Antonucci et al., 1994; Herzog et al., 1989; Herzog & Morgan, 1992; Jackson, 1996; Jackson, Antonucci, & Gibson, 1993; Robinson, 1994). For example, another set of analyses reveals that when this expanded set of activities is considered, blacks and whites differ little in the number of overall productive hours engaged in over a period of a year, and, if anything, blacks may be slightly more engaged than whites in midlife, tapering off in older ages. Thus, our prior analyses suggest that we need to: (1) consider a broader range of possible productive activities; (2) include the economic context in which these activities transpire as well as hours of participation in each; and (3) attend to the psychological and social process benefits that accrue from hours of participation in activities within each economic context (Juster, Courant, & Dow, 1981; Juster, 1985; Juster & Stafford, 1985).

Predictors and Consequences of Participation in Different Networks

To quickly summarize prior research (Jackson, 1996), what is important about our findings is that while the extent of working in a particular network may have positive, negative, or no effects on a particular outcome, the psychological and social process benefits derived from those behaviors (measured in hours) may have different effects. For example, among younger individuals increased regular work hours increase depressive symptoms. But the psychological process benefits derived from these hours lower depressive symptoms and the social process benefits (others better off) have no influence on depressive symptoms. However, among the older age group, behavior (hours of participation) has no direct influence on depressive symptoms but the psychological process benefits derived from this behavior decrease depressive symptoms, whereas the social process benefits have no effects. The results of prior analyses suggest that individuals do indeed conceptualize and perhaps engage in different (by network) economic activities that have important differential contextual meanings for the individual, families, and other social relations (Mannel & Dupuis, 1994). The results of the predictors of traditional and nontraditional measures of productivity suggest that race, gender, and social and economic statuses have different influences on the amount of productive involvement. Individual well-being and health do not show simple relationships to productive activities, but instead are differentially affected by different factors within different economic networks (Jackson, 1996).

Life Course Approach

This chapter takes a life course perspective, stressing the importance of early experiences with the labor force and the environment as influencing later opportunities and types and levels of productive activities (Committee on an Aging Society et al., 1986; Jackson, 1996; Jackson & Gibson, 1985; Jackson, Antonucci, & Gibson, 1993; Sicker, 1994). A life course framework is needed to explore how environmental stressors influence and interact with group and personal resources to both impede and facilitate the quality of life of successive cohorts over the group life course and the nature of individual human development and aging experiences (Baltes, 1987; Riley & Riley, 1992). It is the premise of a life course perspective that already-born and aging cohorts are being currently exposed to the foundations for their social, health, and psychological statuses as they reach older ages in the years and decades to come (Jackson, 1996; Baltes, 1987; Barresi, 1987).

Central to the proposed process of economic network involvement is the fact that because of economic necessity individuals, perhaps largely but not solely, participate in a variety of different types of economic networks for individual and family survival (Hill, 1981). Socioeconomic position may play an important role in the qualitative and quantitative aspects of participation in the three economic networks (Cantor & Little, 1985). Other sociocultural distinctions, however, may also contribute to important differences between social groups (e.g. race) in the rate, frequency, and type of participation. Differences between blacks and whites have been reported for such things as attachment to the labor force (Anderson & Cottingham, 1981); level of involvement in subjective experiences in regular economic participation (Ferman, Berndt, & Selo, 1978); and rates and types of participation in social or barter economies (Stack, 1974). Other data indicate differential sets of relationships and participation in primary social support group activities (Cantor, 1981; Taylor & Chatters, 1986; Taylor, Chatters, & Jackson, 1993). This suggests that more than socioeconomic factors may contribute to observed differences among social groups in productive activities (Ferman, Berndt, & Selo, 1978).

We proposed (Jackson, 1996; Jackson, Antonucci, & Gibson, 1993) that the involvement in productive activities begins early in preadult life in the irregular and social economic networks. This early participation may be dictated by a variety of motivating factors, but the overriding condition is that of economic necessity. We further suggested that this participation strengthens over the years. By mid-adulthood and old age, participation has become well entrenched and the individual has perhaps played a variety of key roles in the operation of the irregular economy and the social economy networks. We expect that similar types of parallel activities have also transpired in the regular market economy, although for many disadvantaged Americans this is not necessarily the case (Hamilton, 1975; Headen, 1992; Kalleberg & Sorenson, 1979; Montagna, 1977).

For many ethnic and racial minority groups, for example, participation in the regular economy is less than satisfactory, particularly in terms of economic subsistence, as well as the noneconomic incentives and rewards gained from market employment (Hill, 1983; Montagna, 1977). Thus, there are clear economic and noneconomic reasons for participating in these other economic networks (Ferman, Berndt, & Selo, 1978; Lowenthal, 1975, 1981; Myers, Manton, & Bacellar, 1986).

Among the important noneconomic factors may be religious values and church participation; family attachment and intergenerational relationships; perceptions and experiences with the opportunity structure; social identity and group consciousness; and differences in basic values regarding the role and importance of individual versus family and group achievement. We expect that these factors will contribute to participation in the economic networks and both influence and are influenced by primary group affiliations, resulting in subsequent differences in behaviors as well as other social, psychological, and health outcomes. We proposed (Jackson, Antonucci, & Gibson, 1993; Jackson, 1996) that the major, but not sole, motivating factor for entry into any of these networks is economic necessity. This motivation, however, may be tempered by several important factors. Personal characteristics may play an important role in regulating entry into economic networks. For example, because of differences in family responsibilities, young people may not have the same level of economic motivation as adults. Similarly, economic necessity may be conditioned by the nature of the social environment (situation). The neighborhood where an individual is raised, as well as family structure, may affect the extent to which economic necessity functions as a motivator of behavior.

Economic necessity is predicted to have the strongest influence on involvement in irregular and social economic network activity. For example, economic necessity may be stronger in low-income groups (e.g., blacks), more so than among whites, and thus overall these low-income groups should show greater involvement in the social and irregular economy networks than whites. It is predicted that socioeconomic status variables, such as education and occupation, will reduce the relationship between race and participation in social and irregular network economies.

Participation patterns within the social, irregular, and regular economy networks are viewed as interrelated. A person may participate in all three simultaneously, two, or only one. Similarly, participation may be sequential or periodic. For example, a person with an episodic formal employment history may maintain an adequate level of individual productivity by moving between the regular and irregular economy networks as a function of general economic conditions, but consistently maintaining relationships and position within the social economy network. As indicated earlier, however, the nature and interpretation of participation in these economic networks may affect and be affected by the primary group relationships in which the individual is enmeshed (Moen, Kain, & Elder, 1983). We are especially concerned with the effects of participation within these economic networks on primary group relationships and how these relationships may affect productive activities, and in turn, social, psychological, and health outcomes (Herzog et al., 1996).

Some productive behaviors will be more or less likely to occur as a function of the type of networks in which an individual participates. Thus, if an individual's network relationships are in the regular economy, the productive activity of prime importance is likely to be paid work. The person may also be engaged, however, in the full range of other activities. Whether these other activities are related to the regular economy network or not may be a function of the degree of connection to the irregular economy and social economy networks.

One of the major outcomes in conceptualizing productive behaviors as occurring within the context of these three different types of networks is the fact that the same productive behavior performed within different networks may differ qualitatively and quantitatively. For example, paid employment within the regular economic network may be important for securing a salary to help meet monthly bills and provide for a basic standard of living. Engaging in the same activities within the irregular network, even for less pay, perhaps may be viewed as more enjoyable and self-satisfying because it occurs within a milieu of friends, neighbors, and kin.

We also propose that one set of the major outcomes of productive activities will be at the individual level. Some of the outcomes that we envision occurring in the elderly as a function of participating in these activities will be in the areas of formal and informal social integration, self-esteem, psychological health, and general well-being (Ferman, Berndt, & Selo, 1978). Further, we feel that positive outcomes derived from engaging in these productive activities will positively affect noneconomic incentives for further participating in these networks. One of the most common observations has been the fact that involvement in the social, irregular, or even the regular economy network is dictated by noneconomic considerations (Stack, 1974; Ferman, Berndt, & Selo, 1978; Lowenthal, 1975, 1981; Sarason, 1977). While we propose that economic necessity is the overriding consideration for participation in these networks, at least initially (Oppenheimer, 1981), we believe that other incentives (e.g., altruism, religious motivation, group identity, etc.) may gain importance over time as a function of these individual outcomes.

Participation in the social economy network and, to some extent, the irregular economy network, is pervasive in some communities. In addition, this involvement may have direct beneficial effects on the community itself by providing work and income (Morris & Caro, 1995). Several authors have reported on the importance of networks in maintaining the viability and integrity of the community (Ferman, Berndt, & Selo, 1978; Headen, 1992; Lowenthal, 1975; Stack, 1974).

Generally, we predicted that different social groups may diverge significantly in their involvement and participation in different economy networks. More advantaged groups may be more likely to participate solely in the regular economy network, while less advantaged groups may participate more in the social and irregular economy networks. As indicated earlier, these are only working hypotheses. Not much empirical research has been conducted on these networks (Ferman, Henry, & Hoyman, 1987; Ferman, Berndt, & Selo, 1978), but we expect participation and productive activities to show continuity for less advantaged groups within the irregular and social economy networks and more sporadic and perhaps entry later in life for more advantaged members of society. The opposite is predicted for the regular economy network. These predictions suggest a different set of relationships over time among major network indicators as well as the types of activities engaged in within the networks.

Changes in status within the regular economic network should have less impact on the total productivity scores, defined as the total hours of participation across all three economic networks, of disadvantaged group members than it will for others. This prediction is predicated on the belief that the former groups are much more likely to be involved in the other two networks and that more of their individual productivity returns are derived from these networks. We predict that the total productivity score for all social groups should be reduced over time with changes in regular economy network participation. This reduction should be greater and more debilitating for advantaged groups because of the disproportionate contribution of regular economic network participation to total productivity scores in comparison to less advantaged groups. Thus, loss of jobs, retirement, or disability should have the effect of disproportionately reducing individual productivity scores in advantaged groups, subsequently leading to greater reductions in well-being and health outcomes than for less advantaged groups.

We further suggested that the viability and integration of communities have some direct relationship to the well-being of the larger society. Obviously, activities within the regular economy network have direct and measurable effects on the society through estimates of national income and the gross national product (Ferman, Berndt, & Selo, 1978; Leichter, 1984; National Research Council, 1979; Committee on an Aging Society et al., 1986; Rosen, 1984). The contributions of productive behaviors in other economic networks, however, have gone largely unrecognized in terms of their implications for individual well-being, and community survival and viability, which in turn have direct effects on the larger society.

To reiterate, the purpose of this chapter is to explore similarities and differences across race, age, gender, and education in the involvement in productive activities in the different economic networks over a nearly decade-long period. We predicted that blacks would show less regular work involvement and perhaps higher involvement in the other two networks. Similar effects were expected by gender, education, and age (Holstein, 1992). Similarly, we explored differences in the patterns of participation over the three waves of data collection for this period. Although we did not have firm hypotheses about the patterning of engagement by network, we did predict declines in participation over time in regular economic involvement and steady involvement in the other two networks.

Empirical Support

Data

Data from an original 1986 sample of 3,617 black and white respondents age 25 to 96 from the Americans' Changing Lives Study (ACL) (Herzog et al., 1989; House et al., 1994) and follow-ups on the same individuals in 1989 and 1994 were analyzed (see Table 10.1). The 1986 first wave was a multistage, stratified probability sample of individuals 25 years of age and older. Respondents were interviewed in their homes by interviewers from the Survey Research Center at the University of Michigan's Institute for Social Research. Blacks and persons over age 60 were sampled at twice the rate of whites under 60 to facilitate age and race comparisons. This sampling approach resulted in complex design effects (Herzog et al., 1989). Subsequent data collections were based largely on telephone surveys of the original respondents.

Measures

Following a standard approach, productivity was measured by hours spent in the activity during the past year (Herzog & Morgan, 1992). Questions ascertaining reported hours of participation were asked in the following manner:

Regular economy network. Respondents were asked if they were doing any work for pay at the present time; and if so, how many hours per week they worked.

Irregular economy network. Respondents were asked if they were paid to do work or chores that were not part of a regular job; and how many hours per year they spent doing such work in the past 12 months.

Social economy network. In order to keep this measure commensurate with those in the prior two networks, and because they reflect a prototypical assessment of our conceptualization of the social network, a combination of two items was used. (1) Respondents were asked how many hours they spent doing volunteer work for organizations such as religious institutions, schools, or political groups. (2) Respondents were asked about hours spent in giving help to friends, neighbors, or relatives who did not live with the respondent. These were tasks such as transportation, shopping, errands, car or house upkeep.

Findings

Participation

Table 10.2 shows the differences by race for each year. As expected, blacks show a greater decline in regular work participation over the period, a total of 20 percentage points (Honig, 1998). Whites show a similar but somewhat lesser decline. There are actually few differences between blacks and whites in terms of irregular work or social economic participation and little decline over the years for blacks or whites. Whites show a slight tendency to be involved in more activities in all three networks than blacks at all three points in time. Table 10.3 shows these effects disaggregated by gender. Generally, for both blacks and whites, males participate in both regular and irregular work more than females. These differences are more pronounced for whites than blacks, although by 1994, black males showed appreciably more irregular work participation. There are few gender differences in social network participation for either blacks or whites over the three waves.

Table 10.4 shows broad age differences by race over the three time points. As expected older black and whites show similar declines in regular economic participation as they age. These findings are similar in irregular networks and not present at all in social network participation. As expected, Table 10.5 reveals that having more education is related to greater regular work participation for both blacks and whites at all three waves. To a slight degree for whites, but to an even larger extent for blacks, this is also true for social network participation. Higher education among blacks is associated with increased participation in irregular work. Unlike among blacks, there is a tendency among whites for lower education to be associated with higher proportions of participation in irregular activities. Thus, these results suggest that, among blacks, education at each wave of measurement provides opportunities not only for regular work, but also for irregular and social network activities as well. This is also true among whites in regular work and social network participation, but not true for irregular work.

Patterns of Participation

Table 10.6 shows the patterns of participation over the three waves of measurement. As done in Tables 10.2–10.5, I examined the ways in which race, age, gender, and education influenced these patterns. As shown in Table 10.6, slightly more whites (57 percent) than blacks (53 percent) participate in regular work over all three periods. In fact, nearly 20 percent of both blacks and whites do not participate in any regular work activities over this period. What is interesting about Table 10.6 is that whites (80 percent) much more so than blacks (67 percent) participate in social network activities over all three periods and blacks (75 percent) are more likely than whites (68 percent) to not participate in irregular activities over the period. Although not shown, these same racial patterns are found by gender. While both black and white males are much more likely than females to engage in regular and irregular activities, males and females of both race groups participate just about evenly in social network activities. Similarly, younger blacks and whites are more likely than their comparable counterparts to be engaged in regular and irregular work over all three periods; this is more true for whites than blacks. Finally, higher education is linked to more consistent participation in regular and social activities over the three periods for both blacks and whites; blacks show low but similar consistent patterns for irregular work.

Patterns of Network Participation

Next, we turn to an examination of the nature of participation in the three networks over time by race, and race by gender, age, and education (see Table 10.7). Although not shown here, we find that whites are slightly more likely than blacks to participate in all three networks over the three periods of measurement. Blacks are more likely than whites to show more erratic patterns of participation over the same period. If the data are disaggregated by gender, we find that white males (in comparison to black males) are more likely than their female counterparts to engage in all three activities at similar levels during each period of measurement. Both black and white females are less likely than males to be involved in all three networks at each wave of measurement, but these differences are larger for whites than blacks. As we might expect, we find that younger as, compared to older, respondents, regardless of race, are more likely to be active in all three networks over the three periods.

Finally, we find that more educated respondents are more likely to be involved in all three networks at each wave of measurement, and less likely to have no involvement than are their less educated counterparts. This effect is much more pronounced for blacks in comparison to whites.

In sum, these results suggest differences over this small part of the life course in the percentage of activities engaged in by race, gender, education, and age. Similarly, the results indicate differences in the patterns of participation in activities by the same factors and, in fact, differences in whether individuals participate consistently in the three networks. The findings are somewhat surprising, since they suggest a racial, social, gender, and resource advantage that favors those who are already materially and socially advantaged. Unlike our overall hypothesis that participation in nonregular networks (irregular and social) might offset lack of involvement, actually whites, males, more highly educated, and younger respondents enjoy the benefits of participating in all three networks. While this is less true for social economic activities, for the most part, few differences are found for gender, age, education, and race, contributing to the overall findings of greater participation in all networks by whites, males, highly educated individuals, and younger respondents.

Conclusions and Implications

Two compelling factors provide a rationale for the proposed economic network framework. First, previous work on productive activities has not developed a theoretically meaningful definition of productive activities at the individual level. The proposed conceptualization of individual productivity and productive aging (Rosen, 1984) includes the traditional behavioral productivity measure of hours engaged or actual or imputed monetary value (Herzog & Morgan, 1989; Herzog & Morgan, 1992) but also attempts to assess the role of ancillary processes, notably psychological and social process benefits, as possible mediators of traditional productivity indicators (Jackson, 1996). As summarized in this chapter, the model also provides independent assessments of productive activities separate from their predicted effects on individual social and psychological functioning (Jackson, 1996; Moss, 1979).

Second, by placing the relationship of individual productivity and well-being within an economic network context, differential predictions are possible regarding the same behaviors across settings and situations that may differ both qualitatively and quantitatively. We believe that the proposed life course / productive activity framework will facilitate a nontraditional approach to the study of gender, socioeconomic, race, ethnicity, and cultural factors related to aging productively. It has been proposed (Hamilton, 1975; Ferman, Berndt, & Selo, 1978; McAdoo, 1981) that these networks gain particular value for elderly disadvantaged groups by providing an avenue for engaging in activities that are of value to the community and also to the groups themselves (Noelker & Zarit, 1983).

The framework presented in this chapter provides a conceptual and theoretical life course approach to the empirical study of racial, ethnic, and cultural influences on the relationships of opportunity-structure factors to processes and behaviors related to aging productively (Jackson, 1996; Noekler & Zarit, 1983). The results of our analyses suggest that over the life course individuals systematically view different activities as clustering in three distinct and theoretically meaningful networks. This framework provides a potentially useful conceptual approach to the empirical study of the relationships among the opportunity structure, social and cultural factors, productive activities, formal and primary group affiliations, and health, well-being, and effective functioning across the individual life course.

The proposed framework should contribute to the study of productive behaviors over the individual life course. The model emphasizes the importance of these networks for productive behaviors at all life stages (Herzog et al., 1989). As McAdoo (1981) and others (Ferman, Berndt, & Selo, 1978; Ferman & Berndt, 1981; Hamilton, 1975) have indicated, however, these networks are of particular value for disadvantaged groups in providing an avenue for engaging in activities that are of value to the community and also to themselves.

Although Ferman, Berndt, and Selo (1978) did not do extensive analyses by race, they reported that blacks were slightly more likely to indicate using the irregular economy for services. Life for poor people, African Americans, and members of many other racial and ethnic groups, at every income level and at every stage of the life course, is often a struggle, both physically and psychologically (Jackson, 1993). For example, in examining the social economy network, several researchers commented on the importance of this network for poor and black elderly (Stack, 1974; Lowenthal, 1975; Cantor, 1979). While it may be true that black and other minority elders receive assistance from family and friends with no observable reciprocity, this may be in keeping with a lifetime of involvement with the social economy network and an extensive history of providing goods and services to other members of the community.

In conclusion, then, definitions of what activities we construe as productive need expansion. These definitions should at least include measures of reported behaviors, for example, hours (or imputed values), psychological process benefits (enjoyment, satisfaction, benefits to self), and social process benefits (benefits for others) (Juster, 1985).

The range and context of what constitutes economic exchanges and productive activities need expansion. The contexts of regular, irregular, and social economic work may be a useful conceptualization of what constitutes the universe of important productive activity contexts. A life course framework is necessary to understand how the mix of productive activity and the involvement in economic networks may change over the individual life span. And finally, the influence of gender, ethnic, and social- and economic-related processes on differences in productive involvement must be considered in addition to their influence on the consequences of such activities on social, psychological, and health outcomes.

The very nature of what is considered to be productive behaviors may show significant shifts with advancing age (Glass et al., 1995). While declining physical abilities may severely limit some forms of productive behaviors, others may become more prominent (Harlow, Swindell, & Turner, 1991). For example, counseling and advice for younger family members and friends may assume greater importance as productive activities among older, rather than younger, adults (Freedman, 1997; Herzog et al., 1989).

Surprisingly, the results of the descriptive analyses on this longitudinal panel suggest that whites actually report participating more than blacks in these nontraditional networks and that this participation may be more consistent over time. These relationships suggest that our early theorizing about economic necessity motivating involvement in different economic contexts may be correct, but in a different way than originally hypothesized. It may be the case that such motivation leads to involvements in all networks, which, in turn, provide greater economic and noneconomic rewards.

We have assumed that these hypothesized economic networks are of particular value for elderly disadvantaged groups by providing an avenue for engaging in activities that produce material resources for the community and also for themselves (Noekler & Zarit, 1983). The framework and analyses presented in this chapter provide a basis for a conceptual and theoretical life course approach to the empirical study of the economic, behavioral, social, psychological, ethnic, and cultural influences on the relationships of opportunity-structure factors to processes and behaviors related to aging productively. Somewhat surprisingly, it may turn out that such involvement supports material and social advantages over the life course that may be of more benefit to groups in society that begin their lives in more favored positions.

Tables 10.1 to 10.7 follow on pages 230–34.

TABLE 10.1   Sample Description,
Americans' Changing Lives Survey, 1986–1994

	Wave 1 1986	Wave 2 1989	Wave 3 1994	
			Nonproxy	w/Proxy
Sample size	3,617	2,867	2,398	2,562
All waves	2,348	2,348	2,223	2,348
All waves, black/white	2,285	2,285	2,161	2,285
Response rate #1*	67.0%	83.1%	76.4%	81.7%
Response rate #2**			87.1%	92.0%
Number of deaths		166	314	
Average age, all waves	53.6	55.6	57.7	59.0
Average age of blacks and whites only, all waves	50.5	53.1	58.1	59.2
Males	37.5%	36.2%	36.7%	36.1%
Females	62.5%	63.8%	63.3%	63.9%
Blacks	64.2%	66.5%	68.7%	68.4%
Whites	32.5%	30.5%	28.5%	28.8%
Other	3.3%	3.0%	2.8%	2.8%
High school or less	59.9%	N/A	N/A	N/A
High school or more	40.1%	N/A	N/A	N/A
South	40.0%	N/A	N/A	N/A
Non-South	60.0%	N/A	N/A	N/A

*Response rate #1 for wave 3 was calculated based on the wave 1 sample since the wave 3 sample includes 214 original not interviewed at wave 2.

**Response rate #2 for wave 3 was calculated based on the wave 2 sample and excludes the 214 nonpanel cases.

TABLE 10.2   Changes in Participation in Productive Activities by Race (%)

	Wave 1 1986		Wave 2 1989		Wave 3 1994	
	Black	White	Black	White	Black	White
Regular work	69	67	66	63	49	53
Irregular work	13	14	13	15	11	13
Social network	86	90	85	93	84	87

NOTE: Percentages are adjusted for region (North, South).

TABLE 10.3   Changes in Participation in Productive Activities by Gender (%)

Black						
	Wave 1 1986		Wave 2 1989		Wave 3 1994	
	Male	Female	Male	Female	Male	Female
Regular work	79	59	74	58	53	45
Irregular work	14	12	15	10	15	7
Social network	88	83	88	82	84	85

White						
	Wave 1 1986		Wave 2 1989		Wave 3 1994	
	Male	Female	Male	Female	Male	Female
Regular work	76	58	70	56	57	48
Irregular work	18	10	19	10	18	8
Social network	89	90	93	93	87	88

TABLE 10.4   Changes in Participation in Productive Activities by Age (%)

	Black					
	Wave 1 1986		Wave 2 1989		Wave 3 1994	
	25–54	55+	25–54	55+	25–54	55+
Regular work	83	55	85	46	78	19
Irregular work	16	10	15	11	16	6
Social network	89	82	89	80	87	82
	White					
	Wave 1 1986		Wave 2 1989		Wave 3 1994	
	25–54	55+	25–54	55+	25–54	55+
Regular work	85	49	87	39	85	21
Irregular work	23	5	19	10	17	9
Social network	93	86	94	91	93	82

TABLE 10.5   Changes in Participation in Productive Activities
by Education (%)

	Black					
	Wave 1 1986		Wave 2 1989		Wave 3 1994	
	≤HS	>HS	≤HS	>HS	≤HS	>HS
Regular work	58	80	54	77	40	57
Irregular work	9	17	10	16	10	12
Social network	77	94	76	93	75	93
	White					
	Wave 1 1986		Wave 2 1989		Wave 3 1994	
	≤HS	>HS	≤HS	>HS	≤HS	>HS
Regular work	65	70	61	65	49	56
Irregular work	16	12	15	14	14	12
Social network	88	92	90	95	83	92

NOTE: HS = high school.

TABLE 10.6   Patterns of Productive Activities over Time by Race (%)

Waves		Regular Work		Irregular Work		Social Network	
1 2 3		Black	White	Black	White	Black	White
X X X		53	57	2	4	67	80
X X O		11	9	2	4	8	6
X O X		3	3	2	2	6	3
O X X		4	4	3	2	6	5
X O O		4	5	6	8	3	2
O X O		4	2	4	5	3	1
O O X		2	2	5	6	3	1
O O O		20	19	75	68	5	2

NOTE: Wave 1 = 1986, Wave 2 = 1989, Wave 3 = 1994. X = active, O = not active.

TABLE 10.7   Pattern of Productive Activities across Networks (%)

			Wave 1		Wave 2		Wave 3	
Reg	Irr	Soc	Black	White	Black	White	Black	White
X	X	X	10	14	10	13	9	11
X	X	O	***	1	***	***	***	***
X	O	X	53	53	55	54	48	51
O	X	X	2	3	2	3	2	3
X	O	O	8	5	7	4	4	4
O	X	O	***	***	***	***	1	***
O	O	X	19	20	17	22	22	25
O	O	O	9	4	9	3	14	7

NOTE: Wave 1 = 1986, Wave 2 = 1989, Wave 3 = 1994. Reg = regular work, Irr = irregular work, Soc = social network. X = active, O = not active.

*** = no data or less than one percent.

References

This chapter is based on a presentation to the conference, "Perspectives on Productive Aging: Toward a Knowledge-building Agenda," George Warren School of Social Work, Washington University, St. Louis, Missouri, December 3–4, 1998. I would like to thank Myriam Torres and Jeremy Salvatori for their statistical and organizational help. Partial support for this research and writing was provided by grants from the National Institute of Mental Health (grant # 1 POL MH58565-01) and the National Institute on Aging (grant # 1-P30-AG15281-02).

Anderson, B. E., & Cottingham, D. H. (1981). The elusive quest for economic equality. *Daedalus, 110,* 257–274.

Antonucci, T. C. (1990). Social supports and social relationships. In R. H. Binstock & L. K. George (Eds.), *The handbook of aging and the social sciences* (3rd ed., pp. 205–226). Orlando, FL: Academic.

Antonucci, T. C., Jackson, J. S., Gibson, R. C., & Herzog, A. R. (1994). Sex differences in age and racial influences on involvement in productive activities. In M. Stevenson (Ed.), *Gender roles through the life-span* (pp. 259–282). Muncie, IN: Ball State University.

Baltes, P. B. (1987). Theoretical propositions of life-span developmental psychology: On the dynamics between growth and decline. *Developmental Psychology, 23,* 611–626.

Baltes, P. B., & Baltes, M. M. (1990). Psychological perspectives on successful aging: A model of selective optimization with compensation. In P. B. Baltes & M. M. Baltes (Eds.), *Successful aging: Perspectives from the behavioral sciences* (pp. 1–34). New York: Cambridge University Press.

Barresi, C. M. (1987). Ethnic aging and the life course. In D. E. Gelfand & C. M. Barresi (Eds.), *Ethnic dimensions of aging* (pp. 18–34). New York: Springer.

Bass, S. A. (Ed.). (1995). *Older and active: How Americans over 55 are contributing to society.* New Haven: Yale University Press.

Bass, S. A., & Caro, F. G. (1992). The new politics of productive aging. *In Depth, 2* (3), 59–79.

Bass, S. A., & Caro, F. G. (1996). Theoretical perspectives on productive aging. In W. H. Crown (Ed.), *Handbook of employment of the elderly.* Westport, CT: Greenwood.

Butler, R. N. (1989). Productive aging. In V. L. Bengtson & K. W. Schaie (Eds.), *The course of later life: Research and reflections* (pp. 55–64). New York: Springer.

Butler, R. N., & Gleason, H. P. (Eds.). (1985). *Productive aging: Enhancing vitality in later life.* New York: Springer.

Cantor, M. H. (1979). The informal support system of New York's inner city elderly: Is ethnicity a factor? In D. E. Gelfand & A. J. Kutzik (Eds.), *Ethnicity and aging: Theory, research and policy.* New York: Springer.

Cantor, M. H. (1981, November). *Factors associated with strain among families, friends, and neighbors, and neighbors caring for the frail elderly.* The 34th Annual Scientific Meetings of the Gerontological Society of America, Toronto, Canada.

Cantor, M. H., & Little, J. K. (1985). Aging and social services. In E. Shanas & R. H. Binstock (Eds.), *Handbook of aging and the social sciences* (2nd ed.). New York: Van Nostrand Reinhold.

Committee on an Aging Society (U.S.) / Institute of Medicine / National Research Council. (1986). *Productive roles in an older society.* Washington, DC: National Academy Press.

Cutler, S. J. (1976). Age profiles of membership in sixteen types of voluntary organizations. *Journal of Gerontology, 31,* 462–470.

Ferman, L. A., & Berndt, L. E. (1981). The irregular economy. In S. Henry (Ed.), *Can I have it in cash?* London: Astragal Books.

Ferman, L. A., Berndt, L. E., & Selo, E. (1978). *Analysis of the irregular economy: Cash flow in the informal sector.* A report to the Bureau of Employment and Training, Michigan Department of Labor, Institute of Labor and Industrial Relations, University of Michigan–Wayne State University.

Ferman, L. A., Henry, S., & Hoyman, M. (1987). Issues and prospects for the study of informal economies: Concepts, research strategies, and policy. *The Annals, 493,* 154–172.

Freedman, M. (1997, September–October). Golden years, indeed: Senior citizens are our greatest repository of untapped civic capital. *The New Democrat,* 24–26.

Friedland, R., & Summer, L. (1999, November). *Demography is not destiny.* Paper presented at the Annual Meeting of the Gerontological Society of America, Washington, DC.

George, L. K., & Bearon, L. B. (1980). *Quality of life in older persons: Meaning and measurement.* New York: Human Sciences.

Glanz, D. (1994). Older volunteers and productive aging: What do we know? *The Gerontologist, 34* (2), 276–278.

Glass, T. A., Seeman, T. E., Herzog, A. R., Kahn, R., & Berkman, L. F. (1995). Change in productive activity in late adulthood: Macarthur Studies of Successful Aging. *Journal of Gerontology: Social Sciences, 50B* (2), S65–S76.

Glutmann, P. M. (1977). The subterranean economy. *Financial Analysts Journal, 34,* 26–27.

Hamilton, R. N. (1975). *Employment needs and programs for older workers: Especially blacks.* Washington, DC: National Center on the Black Aged.

Harlow, K. S., Swindell, D., & Turner, M. J. (1991). Productivity in late life: Does contribution continue? *Agedata: Special Issues Report #16,* Heartland Center on Aging, Disability, and Long Term Care.

Headen, A. E. (1992). Time, costs and informal social support as determinants of differences between black and white families in the provision of long-term care. *Inquiry, 29,* 440–450.

Henry, S. (1982). The working unemployed: Perspectives on the informal economy and unemployment. *The Sociological Review, 30,* 460–467.

Henry, S., & Brown, J. (1990). Something for nothing: The informal economy outcomes of free market economics. In I. Taylor (Ed.), *The social effects of free market policies.* New York: Harvester.

Herzog, A. R., Franks, M. M., Markus, H. R., & Holmberg, D. (1996). Productive activities and agency in older age. In M. Baltes & L. Montada (Eds.), *Produktives leben in Alter Conference* (pp. 323–343). Hamburg, Germany: Campus.

Herzog, A. R., Kahn, R. L., Morgan, J. N., Jackson, J. S., & Antonucci, T. C. (1989). Age differences in productive activities. *Journals of Gerontology, 44* (4), S129–S138.

Herzog, A. R., & Morgan, J. (1992). Age and gender differences in the value of productive activities. *Research on Aging, 14* (2), 169–198.

Hill, M. (1983). Trends in the economic situation of U.S. families and children: 1970–1980. In R. R. Nelson & F. Skidmore (Eds.), *American families and the economy.* Washington, DC: National Academy Press.

Hill, R. B. (1981). *Economic policies and black progress: Myth and realities.* New York: National Urban League.

Holstein, M. A. (1992). Productive aging: A feminist critique. *Journal of Aging and Social Policy, 4* (3–4), 17–34.

Honig, M. (1998). *Minorities face retirement: Worklife disparities repeated?* Paper presented at the Economics of Aging Symposium at the Annual Meetings of the Gerontological Society of America, Philadelphia, PA.

House, J. S., Lepkowski, J. M., Kinney, A. M., Mero, R. P., Kessler, R. C., & Herzog, A. R. (1994). The social stratification of aging and health. *Journal of Health and Social Behavior, 35,* 213–234.

Jackson, J. S. (1993). Racial influences on adult development and aging. In R. Kastenaum (Ed.), *The encyclopedia of adult development* (pp. 18–26). Phoenix, AZ: Oryx.

Jackson, J. S. (1996). Aging productively: An economic network model. In M. Baltes & L. Montada (Eds.), *Produktives leben in Alter Conference* (pp. 211–238). Hamburg, Germany: Campus.

Jackson, J. S., Antonucci, T. C., & Gibson, R. C. (1993). Cultural and ethnic contexts of aging productively over the life-course: An economic network framework. In S. A. Bass, F. G. Caro, & Y.-P. Chen (Eds.), *Achieving a productive aging society* (pp. 249–268). Westport, CT: Auburn House.

Jackson, J. S., & Gibson, R. C. (1985). Work and retirement among black elderly. In Z. Blau (Ed.), *Current perspectives on aging and the life cycle* (pp. 193–222). Greenwich, CT: JAI.

Jackson, J. S., Lockery, S. M., & Juster, F. T. (1996). Introduction: Health and retirement among ethnic and racial minority groups, *The Gerontologist, 36* (3), 282–284.

Juster, F. T. (1985). Preferences for work and leisure. In F. T. Juster & F. P. Stafford (Eds.), *Time, goods and well-being.* Ann Arbor, MI: Institute for Social Research.

Juster, F. T., Courant, P. N., & Dow, G. K. (1981). The theory and measurement of well-being: A suggested framework for accounting and analysis. In F. T. Juster & K. C. Land (Eds.), *Social accounting systems.* New York: Academic.

Juster, F. T., & Stafford, F. P. (Eds.). (1985). *Time, goods and well-being.* Ann Arbor, MI: Institute for Social Research.

Kalleberg, A. L., & Sorenson, A. B. (1979). The sociology of labor markets. *Annual Review of Sociology, 5,* 351–379.

Leichter, H. M. (1984). National productivity: A comparative perspective. In M. Holzer & S. S. Nagel (Eds.), *Productivity and public policy.* Beverly Hills, CA: Sage.

Lowenthal, M. (1975). The social economy in urban-working class communities. In G. Gappert & H. M. Rose (Eds.), *The social economy of cities.* Beverly Hills, CA: Sage.

Lowenthal, M. (1981). Non-market transactions in an urban community. In S. Henry (Ed.), *Can I have it in cash?* London: Astragal Books.

Lowenthal, M. F., & Robinson, B. (1976). Social networks and isolation. In R. H. Binstock & E. Shanas (Eds.), *Handbook of aging and the social sciences.* New York: Van Nostrand Reinhold.

Mannell, R. C., & Dupuis, S. L. (1994). Leisure and productive activity. In M. P. Lawton & J. A. Teresi (Vol. Eds.), *Annual review of gerontology and geriatrics* (Vol. 14, pp. 125–141). New York: Springer.

Manton, K. G., & Soldo, B. J. (1985). Dynamics of health changes in the oldest old: New perspectives and evidence. *Milbank Memorial Fund Quarterly, 63,* 206–285.

McAdoo, H. P. (1981). *Black families*. Beverly Hills, CA: Sage.

Moen, P., Kain, E. L., & Elder, G. H., Jr. (1983). Economic conditions and family life: Contemporary and historical perspectives. In R. R. Nelson & F. Skidmore (Eds.), *American families and the economy*. Washington, DC: National Academy Press.

Montagna, P. D. (1977). *Occupations and society: Toward a sociology of the labor market*. New York: John Wiley & Sons.

Morgan, J. N. (1981). Behavioral and social science research and the future elderly. In S. B. Kiesler, J. N. Morgan, & V. K. Oppenheimer (Eds.), *Aging: Social change*. New York: Academic.

Morgan, J. N. (1986). Unpaid productive activity over the life course. In Committee on an Aging Society (U.S.) / Institute of Medicine / National Research Council (Ed.), *Productive roles in an older society* (pp. 250–280). Washington, DC: National Academy Press.

Morris, R., & Caro, F. G. (1995). The young-old, productive aging, and public policy. *Generations, 19* (3), 32–37.

Moss, M. (1979). Welfare dimensions of productivity measurement. In National Research Council (Ed.), *Measurement and interpretation of productivity*. Washington, DC: National Academy Press.

Myers, G. C., Manton, K. G., & Bacellar, H. (1986). Sociodemographic aspects of future unpaid productive roles. In . In Committee on an Aging Society (U.S.) / Institute of Medicine / National Research Council (Ed.), *Productive roles in an older society*. Washington, DC: National Academy Press.

National Research Council (Ed.). (1979). *Measurement and interpretation of productivity*. Washington, DC: National Academy Press.

Neugarten, B. L. (1976). Personality and aging. In J. E. Birren & K. W. Schaie (Eds.), *Handbook of the psychology of aging*. New York: Van Nostrand Reinhold.

Noelker, L., & Harell, Z. (1983). The integration of environment and network theories in explaining the aged's functioning and well-being. *The Gerontologist, 17*, 84–95.

Oppenheimer, V. K. (1981). The changing nature of life-cycle squeezes: Implications for the socioeconomic position of the elderly. In R. W. Fogel, E. Hatfield, S. B. Kiesler, & E. Shanas (Eds.), *Aging: Stability and change in the family*. New York: Academic.

O'Reilly, P. O., & Caro, F. G. (1994). Productive aging: An overview of the literature. *Journal of Aging and Social Policy, 6* (3), 39–70.

Pencavel, J. (1986). Labor supply of men: A survey. In O. Ashenfelter & R. Layard

(Vol. Eds.), *Handbook of labor economics* (Vol. 1, pp. 17–28). North-Holland: Elsevier Science.

Rendall, M. S., & Speare, A. (1993). Comparing economic well-being among elderly Americans. *Review of Income and Wealth, 39* (1), 1–21.

Rendall, M. S., & Speare, A., Jr. (1994). United States elderly poverty alleviation through household extending and work. *Life Course Institute Working Paper Series,* College of Human Ecology, Cornell University.

Riley, M. W. (1985). Age strata in social systems. In R. H. Binstock & E. Shanas (Eds.), *Handbook of aging and social science* (2nd ed). New York: Van Nostrand Reinhold.

Riley, M. W. (1987). On the significance of age in sociology. *American Sociological Review, 52,* 1–14.

Riley, M. W., & Riley, J. W. (1992). Individual and social potentials of older people. In P. B. Baltes & J. Mittelstrass (Eds.), *Zukunft des Alterns und gesellschaftliche Entwicklung.* Berlin: Walter de Gruyter.

Robinson, B. (1994). In search of productive aging: A little something for everyone. *Ageing International, 21* (4), 33–36.

Rosen, E. D. (1984). Productivity: Concepts and measurement. In M. Holzer & S. S. Nagel (Eds.), *Productivity and public policy.* Beverly Hills, CA: Sage.

Sarason, S. B. (1977). *Work, aging and social change: Professionals and the one life–one career imperative.* New York: The Free Press.

Satariano, W. A., & Syme, S. L. (1981). Life changes and disease in elderly populations: Coping with change. In J. L. McGaugh & S. B. Kiesler (Eds.), *Aging: Biology and behavior.* New York: Academic.

Sicker, M. (1994). The paradox of productive aging. *Ageing International, 21* (2), 12–14.

Siegel, J. S., & Taeuber, C. M. (1986). Demographic perspectives on the long-lived society. *Daedalus, 115,* 77–118.

Smith, J. D. (1982). *The measurement of selected income flows in informal markets.* Final report to the Internal Revenue Service (Contract No. TIR 81-28). Ann Arbor, MI: Institute for Social Research.

Stack, C. B. (1974). *All our kin: Strategies for survival in the black community.* New York: Harper & Row.

Streib, G. F. (1985). Social stratification and aging. In R. H. Binstock & E. Shanas (Eds.), *Handbook of aging and the social sciences* (2nd ed.). New York: Van Nostrand Reinhold.

Taylor, R. J., & Chatters, L. M. (1986). Church based informal support among elderly blacks. *The Gerontologist, 26,* 637–642.

Taylor, R. J., Chatters, L. M., & Jackson, J. S. (1993). A profile of familial relations among three-generation black families. *Family Relations, 42,* 332–341.

Witte, A. D., & Simon, C. D. (1983). The impact of unrecorded economic activity on American families. In R. R. Nelson & F. Skidmore (Eds.), *American families and the economy.* Washington, DC: National Academy Press.

IV

FUTURE DIRECTIONS

IN PRACTICE, THEORY,

AND RESEARCH

11

STRUCTURAL LEAD

Building New Institutions
for an Aging America

Marc Freedman, M.B.A.

According to a recent *New York Times* (Noble, 1998) headline, "The Elderly Are Becoming More Active, and Activity Is Improving Their Lives." The photo accompanying the *Times* article depicts a grimacing septuagenarian wearing tennis whites and delivering an especially ferocious serve.

The article was a reminder of how much progress we have made in the past four decades trading in the rocking chair for "a new active way of life," as the Del Webb company used to say in its Sun City marketing brochures. However, as we are declaring victory on this front, it is time to ask whether we can't do better than all this activity—so much of it self-indulgent.

In this context, productive aging marks a significant step forward. In arguing that older adults can not only keep themselves busy but be contributing members of society, it challenges so much that is distressing about the activity obsession and its implicit suggestion that older adults are superfluous—jogging in place on the sidelines as society goes about its important business.

However, productive aging too could stand to face the content test. All productivity is not created equal, and some forms hold much greater promise as a vehicle not only for enriching individual lives but also for helping to meet the pressing needs of society.

Thinking about Productive Aging

I was reminded of this basic truth recently on a visit to Minneapolis to spend time with a volunteer in the Senior Companion Program. For a week, I shadowed Yakov Gritchener, a 65-year-old immigrant from Moldavia. The retired mathematics teacher now spends his Wednesdays with Harry Dychal, a disabled postman who is Yakov's age and legally blind. Theirs is a reciprocal relationship—each partner is convinced that he is the helper and the other is the recipient of his altruism. Harry helps Yakov with his English, correcting grammatical errors, while Yakov helps with some of the basic functions that would make independent living impossible for Harry. Mostly this assistance is with simple things, such as going to the store.

On one day I was visiting they took me to lunch at their favorite destination: Burger King. (Burger King is particularly generous with discount coupons, and Yakov and Harry clip them assiduously.) Once in the restaurant we were waited on by Dave, a tall, gray-haired man who looked to be Yakov and Harry's age, wearing an orange and blue polyester outfit and a Burger King beanie, punching in icons of shakes and fries alongside giggling 15-year-olds acquiring their first job experience.

The juxtaposition between Yakov and Dave was unsettling. While Dave surely makes twice as much money as Yakov, I can't imagine the Senior Companion swapping his $9 daily stipend for the minimum wage at Burger King. It would come at a great price in dignity and sense of purpose. It would also be a loss to the community—both in terms of the social fabric and in the actual expense of prematurely institutionalizing individuals like Harry.

I take the trouble to recount this story because I don't think the choice represented by Yakov's and Dave's situations is farfetched. As we proceed further into the postindustrial society there is likely to be growing demand for service sector jobs like Dave's, and it is no secret that the fast food companies are hot on the trail of older recruits. At the same time there is urgent need for the kind of "relationship work" Yakov is engaged in, not only within the older population, but between adult generations and young people—so many of whom are growing up starved for guidance and support (Freedman, 1999a).

Yet much of what I read of the literature on productive aging fails to distinguish between various kinds of productivity and their relative merits. In fact, there seems to be an implicit valuing of private-sector employment over work in communities—unpaid, stipended, even salaried.

In fact, this imbalance is not always implicit. Consider syndicated columnist Robert Samuelson's essay, "Off Golden Pond," which appeared in *The New Republic* in April 1999. According to Samuelson, we "need to reject the platitudes that the elderly can contribute to society by volunteering or offering 'wisdom'," adding, "this may be true, but it is a tiny truth." How might older adults use their skills? "The main way that older Americans can contribute," he concludes, "is by doing the same thing that other adults do: that is, by working, and not becoming a premature social burden."

In Samuelson's reasoning, the leisure ethic gets replaced with more work in the labor market. Rather than a second childhood of unrelenting leisure, we are offered instead a part-time, warmed over version of mid-life. Lost is any sense that later life might be a season with its own particular advantages and definition of success.

Most of all the Samuelson perspective fails to recognize that what really matters is not the form of the work (we need to encourage a wide variety of forms, paid and unpaid, part-time and full-time), but the content. We must cultivate and encourage particularly those kinds of contributions that promise to provide the greatest payoff for individuals and society—in other words, the biggest win-win situations for both sides (Samuelson, 1999).

The Aging Opportunity

There is reason to believe that the great opportunity of the aging society may be in roles that enable older Americans to play a much more substantial part in civil society and the public-purpose sector, where a human resource crisis of staggering proportions currently exists. Voluntarism is down a full 5 points, PTA membership has fallen through the floor, and we face a teacher shortage of nearly 220,000 over the coming decade. Meanwhile, Americans in the middle generation struggle under the weight of simultaneously trying to work long hours and raise their children (Putnam, 1995).

Changes in the role of women are surely a significant piece of this overall crisis. For a century, American women have been the glue in civil society, performing an array of undervalued, often utterly unnoticed tasks that have held our communities together. Today, a great many of those women are working, and we should waste little time hoping that history will suddenly begin running backwards (Hochschild, 1989, 1997).

Besides, there is no need to be nostalgic. America's burgeoning older population could come to succeed women as the new trustees of civic life in this country, provided we create the kinds of institutions and opportunities that could enable them to make a genuine contribution while benefiting themselves in the process. This country now possesses not only the largest, but also the healthiest, best-educated, and most vigorous population of older adults in our history. And this group has what the middle-aged population so desperately lacks: time (Freedman, 1996).

Despite all these assets, a raft of surveys suggesting that older Americans want to be more involved in civic life, and a body of research linking productive engagement and strong social networks to prolonged physical and mental health, the older population serves less than any other group in society—even those overwhelmed adults in the middle generation (Peter D. Hart Research Associates, 1999; Independent Sector, 1996).

Is it that older adults just don't care? Their stellar voting record suggests otherwise. One common explanation is that we need to ask, and there can be no doubt that we ask too little of the older generation. But my research over the past decade suggests that the real culprit is at the institutional level, in the dearth of compelling opportunities for people to serve. Even projects like Yakov's Senior Companion Program are restricted to individuals living below 125 percent of the poverty line. All too many individuals who want to give back to society and who have little or no financial needs and terrific resumes to recommend them run persistently into brick walls while trying to make a contribution. They might be characterized as "all dressed up with no place to go" (Freedman, 1999b).

The New Wave of Social Entrepreneurs

How will we remedy the growing gap between the potential and actual contributions of older Americans to society, and do so in time for the arrival of the boomers to later life—in an era of quiescence in public policy initiatives to promote this activity?

The good news is that there is currently a vigorous but little appreciated upsurge in social entrepreneurship in this area, much of it coming from older adults themselves, who are taking matters into their own hands and providing a glimpse of what some of the new institutions for an aging society might look like.

One example is Jack McConnell, a retired pediatrician living in a gated retirement community in Hilton Head, South Carolina, who created the

Volunteers in Medicine program five years ago. McConnell's story is by now somewhat familiar (Congressman John Kasich from Ohio devoted an entire chapter to him in his recent book, *Courage Is Contagious*). Nevertheless, it remains a compelling tale. In retiring to Hilton Head he was planning on a sheltered life of golf, relaxation, and dining; however, after a year the peripatetic McConnell was feeling the lack of purpose. He was also aware of the juxtaposition of wealth and poverty in Hilton Head that never found its way into the Chamber of Commerce brochures. This was particularly evident when driving out the rear exit of his guard-gate community. At times McConnell would offer rides to workers from the resort, and he discovered that these individuals rarely had any health coverage. Meanwhile he was golfing all day with retired doctors, dentists, and other health care professionals who he could tell were adrift, without the opportunity to be useful (McConnell, 1998).

In the classic spirit of American efficiency, McConnell transformed this untapped resource and unmet need into a clinic that serves upward of 1,000 people a month using hundreds of retired volunteer physicians, dentists, nurses, and lay volunteers whose job is primarily to create a caring atmosphere at the clinic. McConnell managed to convince everybody from the Robert Wood Johnson Foundation through the local mayor (who donated the land for the facility) into supporting his dream. He also drove a bill through the South Carolina legislature enabling these retirees to serve using a special volunteer medical license, provided a practicing, licensed physician supervises all charts. At the same time he convinced the major insurance underwriter in the state to provide liability coverage with a 20-year tail at a total of $5,000 a year.

Before actually visiting the clinic, I worried about whether the quality of care would be up to speed. This concern was quickly dissipated. In fact, the standard of care provided is clearly higher than that which most Americans receive at their HMOs. The doctors are top flight. Most are refugees from the commercialization of medicine, who absolutely thrive in an environment where they can spend an hour with a patient, not have to think about paperwork, profits, or malpractice insurance, and be part of a community of other physicians who all "want to be there" (a phrase I heard repeatedly).

Just as significant, while McConnell himself was critical in establishing the institution, he plays very little role in it anymore. In other words, it does not require a charismatic leader to make it run. Equally important, it is not limited to a retirement Mecca for the affluent like Hilton Head (although it is interesting to note that local real estate agents now use the presence of the clinic as a selling point in trying to convince retiring doctors to settle there as opposed to other upscale retirement destinations).

In some ways, an even more compelling example than Volunteers in Medicine exists in San Mateo, California. The Samaritan House Medical Clinic is not an example of the grand entrepreneurship of Jack McConnell, but rather a much more incremental incarnation. Almost a decade ago, John Kelley, a former priest and the director of the nonprofit community group Samaritan House, placed an ad in the county medical bulletin requesting a volunteer physician to provide care to some of the low-income individuals who come to Samaritan House for food, clothing, and shelter. A few local physicians responded.

One night a week Dr. Bill Schwartz, then in the last year of practicing internal medicine as a paid physician, started seeing patients in the Samaritan House conference room. Today, the Samaritan House clinic has its own building on "Doctors Row" in town and sees 500 patients a month—almost all Latino men and women who are working poor. There is no charge and the backbone of the effort is 40 retired local physicians. The drab brown building is a quarter the size of the Volunteers in Medicine palatial facility in Hilton Head, but other than that there is no difference in care.

Bill Schwartz continues to serve as clinical professor of medicine at UCSF. Most of the other doctors are recently retired UCSF and Stanford Medical School attending physicians and faculty. There is also a strong multigenerational dimension to Samaritan House Clinic: two full-time practicing physicians, both women in their 30s and both fully bilingual, serve as medical director and clinic director. In addition, there are dozens of volunteer translators. And the clinic is currently a rotation for fourth-year UCSF medical students.

Just as the retired physicians at Samaritan House have the time required to provide in-depth care to the patients—and to build relationships with them and to educate them on prevention issues—they have time to spend with the medical students. The mentoring relationships that form are unhurried and substantial, and the students talk excitedly about the clinic being the one place where they learn "the art of medicine."

Will Samaritan House or Volunteers in Medicine serve as a solution to the more than 40 million Americans who have no health insurance? Not a chance. However, the broader significance likely resides elsewhere. These clinics offer a compelling glimpse of what medicine can be, when there is enough time "to do things right," as one retired doctor observes. It is also a glimpse of what later life can be, when highly skilled individuals get to ply their trade not for monetary reward or status, but for the intrinsic joy of practicing something they are good at and love. In the process they pass their passion on to younger generations, showing them that there are other possibilities than what they are experiencing through the managed care system.

Although I have concentrated on retired physicians, one might just as easily have described Brenda Eheart, creator of Hope Meadows, a foster care village that has been created on the grounds of a downsized military base near the University of Illinois. At Hope Meadows older adults are offered reduced rent in apartments interspersed among foster families in return for serving six hours a week as tutors and crossing-guards. However, the real benefit is in all the informal contact that occurs between the generations. Hope Meadows is a powerful example of how age-integrated housing can stimulate intergenerational support (Johnson, 1996). Another compelling example is the Troops to Teachers project, started by the late Washington University history professor Jack Hexter at age 81. Troops to Teachers retrains military retirees for teaching science and math in the inner cities. The project has been an extraordinarily successful vehicle for recruiting African American men into teaching, and the retention rates in the program are five times the national average. Hexter's creation is an important reminder that civic work can take many forms, including second careers in the public interest—particularly in areas like teaching, where there is a massive shortage of individuals willing to work in our inner cities (Feinsilber, 1994).

Launching Experience Corps

Another example is in the realm of national service—an enterprise we have come to associate with young people in President Clinton's AmeriCorps program. In 1995, I was involved directly in the development of a new national service program focused on mobilizing older Americans around urban elementary schools. This project, the Experience Corps, was underwritten with funds from Congress to the National Senior Service Corps of the Corporation for National Service, the group that currently operates the Foster Grandparent, Senior Companion, and RSVP programs. This appropriation was a first: never before had Congress allocated money to innovate within the context of these three Senior Corps programs (Freedman & Fried, 1999).

Drawing on practices emerging from some of the most innovative Senior Corps projects, lessons from youth service programs, and research about the kinds of features that might attract the boomers in retirement, the Experience Corps model is built around the following features:

- *The name.* The Experience Corps name (coined by former HEW secretary John Gardner, who chaired the advisory board for the project) was designed to purge the words *senior citizen, elderly, retired,* or *aged.* We wanted to get away from these loaded terms, and from the notion of chronological age, to an identity focusing on the asset older adults were bringing: experience. We also were wary of anything too grandiose—wisdom, elder, and so on. The Experience Corps name also turned out to have a wonderful double meaning: the volunteers referred to it in talking about "all the experiences they were having!"

- *Critical mass.* The focus in Experience Corps was on making a difference. It was made clear from the outset that this project was not going to be about envelope stuffing or about giving the old folks something to keep them busy. The emphasis was on helping to support urban public schools under tremendous stress. Thus, we placed approximately 15 individuals in each school being served, so that the project would constitute a central presence in the institution.

- *Flexibility.* The Experience Corps provided four different commitment options for the volunteers: stipended full-time and half-time positions (the half-timers received between $100 and $150 a month to cover costs associated with making such a big commitment to service, while the full-timers were made VISTA volunteers), as well as unstipended part-time (four to six hours per week) and episodic (some-time) slots. The end result was something resembling "one-stop service," where individuals in a wide variety of situations could find a way of plugging in. And we discovered that these men and women over time moved in and out of various options as their changing life circumstances dictated.

- *Leadership.* Although some volunteers worked directly one on one with children tutoring and mentoring them, others used their experience and interests to generate new projects filling gaps in the schools, involving more parents, and building community support for the institution. For example, a woman in the South Bronx who had started, with her husband, the first tap dance school in that part of New York, created an after-school tap program that also functioned as an African American heritage class. A retired mailman in Philadelphia hauled a mailbox into the school and started a creative writing program in which students wrote letters to each other. Each week he would don his postman's uniform and deliver the letters to the students. There are many other examples, but all these projects underscore the wide variety of ways the Experience Corps members draw on their work and personal experience to enhance the schools.

Two other central elements of the project are the *team concept* and an emphasis on *learning* on the part of volunteers. Experience Corps forged a strong sense of social affiliation through the project, particularly through building teams that enable the volunteers to provide mutual support, reflect on their experiences in the school, and have access to new opportunities to enhance their social networks. Part of the emphasis on learning and growth was realized through training sessions both before and during service. However, another important aspect was the provision of free Community Service Awards from Elderhostel—entitling the full- and part-time volunteers to take any domestic Elderhostel course free as a reward for their contribution to the community. The awards proved to be a wonderful way of reinforcing the message the volunteers were imparting to the students—that learning is important.

Originally, the Experience Corps was piloted in five cities: Philadelphia, New York, Minneapolis, Port Arthur (Texas), and Portland (Oregon). Three years later it is either in operation or development in over 30 locations. The Corporation for National Service has added Cleveland, Boston, Kansas City, and Lake County, Florida, to the original roster of sites. Civic Ventures, the organization I direct, is creating new elementary-school focused projects in California, Indiana, North Carolina, and Arizona, and adapting the model in four additional cities to work with Y's, Boys and Girls Clubs, and neighborhood libraries. The State of Ohio in 1998 started eight city literacy-focused versions of Experience Corps. And a year later, AARP and the Corporation for National Service launched a six-city Experience Corps for Independent Living, aimed at helping frail elders remain in their homes.

Structural Lead

These efforts are part of the growing ferment of entrepreneurial efforts that are blending public and private financing and creating new roles for Americans in the last third of life. In short, they constitute, in the words of Cornell University sociologist Phyllis Moen, a kind of structural lead, an antidote to the lag that has long prevailed.

Before concluding, there is an additional institutional idea that holds promise and is worth describing briefly. This notion is built on the possibilities that exist for taking a combination of service and learning to a new level, and in the process to create a new kind of community center that might supersede the senior centers of today. For example, such an effort might start by combining an Experience Corps and an adaptation of the Elderhostel Institute for Learning in Retirement (ILR) model in the same location, say an urban YMCA. This entity would encourage cross-fertilization between the two components, so that participants in Experience Corps would be rewarded with free courses in the ILR, and the ILR would help develop learning opportunities for Experience Corps members. The center might also sponsor lectures on topics related to the service Experience Corps members are undertaking. ILR participants would also be eligible for episodic service assignments within Experience Corps.

Over time this entity might take on additional functions, like helping individuals make the transition to second careers in the public interest (teaching, environmental work, etc.), performing both a career counseling and retraining function. There would also be a purely social function—that coffee pot to stand around. And then there could be seminars for individuals on the brink of the third age, to help them plan for a retirement that involves giving back. Altogether these opportunities would stand in sharp relief to the traditional focus of senior centers on ministering to the needs of older adults and providing activity for activity's sake—and might attract individuals who wouldn't get caught dead at the senior center. The theme here would be renewal: combining personal renewal with community renewal.

A related idea is working with a community to help them become established as a place that is oriented toward a new kind of retirement, one blending individual and community renewal. One might, over a period of time, seek to establish a *critical mass* of these centers. Such a community might become an alternative destination for people who don't want to retire to a self-indulgent, Sun City–esque environment. Even more likely, these opportunities would encourage older adults to remain in their community, rather than taking off for the Sun Belt.

A Key Role for Policy

Obviously, social programs alone will not transform the aging of America into a new era of individual and social renewal; however, they can help set the tone, give people a glimpse of what is possible, and enable many, many more people to step into opportunities that they would have great difficulty inventing themselves.

In thinking of the power of institutions to produce wider change one need only consider the example of Elderhostel. Twenty years ago the notion of learning in later life was exotic. Today it is commonplace, almost expected. Elderhostel had a lot to do with spawning the wider industry of late-life learning and producing shifts in the culture. Now we need to do for community contribution what Elderhostel has helped do for learning.

Fortunately, we won't have to start from scratch. There are a growing number of compelling models out there, waiting to be expanded, adapted, and imitated. Policy can play a critical role in this process, and the examples described above point at some of the ways:

- The Experience Corps receives funding from the federal Corporation for National Service, states like Ohio, and local school districts.
- Volunteers in Medicine received the clinic lot from the city of Hilton Head for a dollar a year, and South Carolina granted a special volunteer license enabling out-of-state physicians to practice.
- The Department of Defense has put $65 million into Troops to Teachers.
- The State of Illinois provided Hope Meadows with $1 million to retrofit housing at the closed air force base, and provides half a million dollars annually from child welfare funds to cover operating expenses (Ronald McDonald House charities has also just provided $8 million for replication of the model).

While many creative opportunities in this area exist at all levels of government, federal policy remains critical. There are numerous ways that these policies need to be overhauled, both to become less of an obstacle to the contribution of older adults, but also to help stimulate more substantial involvement. We can reform our tax policies so that individuals are not discouraged from working part-time in retirement (especially in public service careers), and so that we can more easily use creative measures like nontaxable stipends as an incentive for greater involvement in high-commitment, high-priority community projects. We might provide Medicare coverage to individuals between 55 and 65 who are involved in half- to full-time service. Additionally, there are many ways in which the federal government could be involved in reforming the existing program efforts it sponsors—such as the National Senior Service Corps and the Senior Community Service Employment Program (Title V of the Older Americans Act)—which have some strengths but are often woefully outdated (Freedman, 1994).

Specific measures such as these would undoubtedly be helpful, but a more appropriate response, I believe, is to develop a policy initiative in keeping with the magnitude of the demographic revolution. This calls for more than fine tuning or piecemeal action. And it calls for more than state and local responses. Indeed in searching for appropriate policy analogy, the example that comes most quickly to mind is none other than the Servicemen's Readjustment Act of 1944, also known as the GI Bill.

The GI Bill was devised to help assimilate in a constructive and mutually beneficial way millions of World War II veterans who would need to make a transition back into society after their service overseas. The potential consequences of these individuals being poorly reintegrated were significant, including the prospect of a very large segment of the population that was disappointed and disaffected, not to mention a great loss of human resources to the economy and the country. As a result of the magnitude of the situation and the stakes involved, the GI Bill was both large and comprehensive, including dollars not only for education and training, but also for home, farm, and business loans.

Without attempting to overstate the analogy, we would today do well to consider an ambitious, national, multifaceted policy initiative aimed at enabling the transition and integration of millions of individuals who are not crossing a geographic divide, or one from military service to private citizenship, but rather traversing a divide along the lines of age and social roles. Like the soldiers of World War II, these aging boomers must be well integrated in society, or the consequences will be dire. Having a dislocated class numbering nearly a quarter of the population, with little or no role in the life of the nation and no connection to the central institutions of society, is a recipe for a sour, gloomy, conflict-ridden nation. Alternatively, the vital involvement of this group might mean something resembling a new golden age.

We need to consider generating a new policy initiative inspired by the GI Bill—a Third Age Bill, or 3A Bill aimed at enabling the successful transition of vast numbers of aging boomers into new roles strengthening communities and revitalizing civil society. The specifics of such a measure would, of course, need to be debated and developed at much greater length, but the rough contours might include the following:

- A massive new national corps, potentially based on existing pilots like Experience Corps, aimed at involving between 5 and 10 percent of the over 55 population over the next decade in areas of highest priority to the society. This effort should include administrative grants for operating local projects, with the requirement of a 50 percent local match as well as vouchers that individuals serving half- to full-time could use to provide a nontaxable stipend along with health and prescription benefits.
- A fund for R&D, stimulating the creation of new approaches to involving third agers (such as the work of the social entrepreneurs), and providing resources, technical assistance, and evaluation designed to help identify and expand successful projects.
- A program to promote training at both institutions of higher education and nonprofit organizations aimed at enabling third agers to make the transition to second careers in high-priority service areas.
- A research initiative designed to identify key niches in the society where efforts to tap the human resources of third agers might be targeted, that is, where there is a good match between the talents of older adults and human resource needs of the society, as well as examination of potential costs and barriers.
- A national report card, issued every three years, to determine how effectively America is making use of the resources in the older population, built around a national conference that explores lessons learned, showcases new approaches for involving third agers more effectively, and charts mid-course corrections and promising new directions.
- A set of major awards, given out annually and patterned on the Presidential Medal of Freedom (perhaps a much expanded version of the Legacy Awards), highlighting Americans who either themselves are role models for a new kind of third age or who are making

it easier for others to contribute to the well-being of society in this new stage of life.

The issue of administering such a 3A Bill raises important questions. Could or should it be overseen by the Administration on Aging, or the Corporation for National Service? Or might it become part of an entirely new federal agency, a U.S. Department of Aging, that might incorporate through its various parts our efforts both to meet the needs and tap the talents of the vast and burgeoning aging population, an entity that would serve as the central impetus for national efforts as America enters into the aging century?

Whatever the ultimate nature of such a bill or its administration, the most important priority is to begin discussing national policy responses that are of a scale, scope, and potential impact in accordance with the social transformation at hand, one that might be able to enable the silver lining that is present in the graying of America (Freedman, 1999b).

A Social Windfall

The potential payoff from all of this could be enormous. Despite much hand wringing about entitlements, the aging of America is every bit as much an opportunity to be seized as a problem to be solved. And nowhere is the opportunity greater than in the realms of civil society and public purpose. If we play our cards right, the graying of America could come to be a social windfall for communities, as we usher in a new definition of success in later life that urges people to lead lives that matter.

William James observed that "the great use of life is to spend it for something that will outlast us." There could be no clearer articulation of why older Americans need the very engagement in our communities that we need of them.

REFERENCES

Feinsilber, M. (1994, May 15). Retiree helps turn drill instructors into teachers. *The Los Angeles Times.*

Freedman, M. (1994). *Seniors in national and community service.* Philadelphia: Public/Private Ventures.

Freedman, M. (1996, November–December). The aging opportunity. *The American prospect, 7* (29).

Freedman, M. (1999a). *The kindness of strangers: Adult mentors, urban youth, and the new voluntarism.* New York: Cambridge University Press.

Freedman, M. (1999b). *Prime time: How baby boomers will revolutionize retirement and transform America.* New York: Perseus Books / PublicAffairs.

Freedman, M., & Fried, L. P. (1999). *Launching experience corps.* San Francisco: Civic Ventures.

Hochschild, A. (1989). *The second shift: Working parents and the revolution at home.* New York: Avon Books.

Hochschild, A. (1997). *The time bind: When work becomes home and home becomes work.* New York: Henry Holt / Metropolitan Books.

Independent Sector. (1996). *Giving and volunteering in the United States.* Washington, DC: Independent Sector.

Johnson, D. (1996, April 1). Program creates community for foster care. *New York Times,* 1.

McConnell, J. B. (1998). *Circle of caring.* Englewood, CO: The Estes Park Institute.

Noble, H. B. (1998, October 20). A secret of health in old age: Muscles. *New York Times,* F8, 1.

Peter D. Hart Research Associates. (1999). *The changing face of retirement: Older Americans, civic engagement, and the longevity revolution.* Washington, DC: Author.

Putnam, R. D. (1995). Bowling alone: America's declining social capital. *Journal of Democracy, 6* (1), 65–78.

Samuelson, R. (1999, April 12). Off golden pond: The aging of America and the reinvention of retirement. *The New Republic,* 36–43.

12

PRODUCTIVE AGING

Theoretical Choices and Directions

Michael Sherraden, Ph.D., Nancy Morrow-Howell, Ph.D.,
James Hinterlong, M.S.W., and Philip Rozario, M.S.W.

In this chapter we identify some of the key theoretical contributions in preceding chapters, discuss theoretical issues and choices, and offer some thoughts and suggested directions on theory building in productive aging. As noted at the beginning, productive aging, like most other emergent policy concepts, has been characterized by advocacy and empirical work more than by theoretical development. As the concept matures academically, theory will increasingly be brought to bear and tested, and in doing so a knowledge base will be built. Hopefully this chapter is a small step in that direction.*

---

*This chapter is based on summary theoretical comments of Michael Sherraden at the conference on Perspectives in Productive Aging, with contributions from Nancy Morrow-Howell and James Hinterlong to this written chapter. Following the first day of the conference, Sherraden met with doctoral student observers to discuss their insights, and later that night sat down and prepared key observations used in the summary the next day. Much of this chapter is structured by this summary presentation, somewhat revised, with additional clarification and comments added. This allows us to put more into this chapter than might ordinarily be possible, although it may have the downside of moving rather quickly from point to point. We thank the doctoral students who attended the conference and provided insightful observations that contributed to this chapter: Lisa Byers, Hye-Ji Choi, David Hodge, Violet Horvath, Amanda Moore, Muriel Mosley, Chaie-Won Rhee, Philip Rozario, Patricia

Conceptual and Theoretical Contributions

Scott Bass and Frank Caro have made large contributions to conceptual development in productive aging. They offer a definition of productive aging as any activity by an older individual that contributes to producing goods or services or develops the capacity to produce them. Bass and Caro include certain activities and exclude others; for example, education or training that strengthens ability to be effective in paid work, volunteering for organizations, or informal productive family or community activities are included, but education for personal growth is excluded. If accepted, these distinctions enable researchers to quantify productive aging more reliably and treat it as a dependent or independent variable more discretely. Bass and Caro (1996) were the first to offer a conceptual framework regarding productive engagement in later life, and in this volume, they expand this thinking. They contribute a framework in which four sectors—environmental, situational, individual, and social policy—relate to participation in productive activities. They argue that conceptualizations about productive aging should go beyond social forces and examine interrelationships among policies, norms, cohort effects, the economy, individual personality, and individual behavior. Their framework highlights the complexity of the phenomenon as well as interdisciplinary efforts that will be needed to advance knowledge about the influence of multiple factors. Additionally, Bass and Caro point to three theoretical perspectives to explain current levels of participation in work and volunteer positions: affluence/leisure preference, intergenerational conflict, and cultural lag. Finally, they express their judgment as applied researchers in suggesting that we focus on macro-level policy to explain productive engagement and influence change.

Alvar Svanborg, a physician and biomedical researcher, reminds us that functional capacity is affected by exogenous factors over which we have some control; other factors are age-related, largely out of our control, and ultimately related to functional decline. Certain important biomedical functions can be retained or revitalized through lifestyle and medical intervention, while others are destined to decline with aging. Both processes occur within a given organ or organ system. Svanborg contributes an im-

Stoddard, Catherine Striley, Shannon Collier-Tenison, Trina Williams, and Hong-Sik Yoon. And we owe additional thanks to Philip Rozario, who looked up references and made substantive and editorial suggestions for the chapter.

portant concept to the discussion of maintaining functioning in later life, *reactivation*. Reactivation is recovery of function to premorbid levels after an acute illness or injury. Reactivation is important not only because it relates to resuming previous activities but also because it relates to preventing future illnesses or postponing age-related declines. Indeed, Svanborg points to the challenge of better understanding the relationship between meaningful activity and the postponement of functional decline. He offers a new and very useful insight when he suggests that a justification for late-life productivity may be the postponement of functional decline.

James Birren, a psychologist, extends the definition of productivity in ways that are new to the productive aging discussion. He points out that we consider a worker productive even if, for example, he is in a sedentary occupation, consumes a lot of alcohol and nicotine, and ends up being more of a "sink" than a "source" to society due to health care costs during retirement. Birren also points out that we have no way to quantify the value of an idea, which can lead to tremendous productivity gains in a society, and we have no way to measure the value of cognitive and affective exchanges across generations—what Erik Erikson (1950) referred to as the generative function of healthy older adults in bringing along the generations behind them. In multiple ways, Birren focuses our attention on diverse forms of productivity and difficulties in ensuring the validity of measurement. He suggests that productivity of the individual depends as much on the balance of physical effort, cognitive load, and social network as on the economic value of the output. He proposes that certain "life portfolios"—certain mixes of investment of time, energy, and concerns—may maximize productivity, claiming that more educated older adults are more productive due to better decision making and generation of information. Overall, Birren invites a much more complicated conceptualization of productivity in general, with particular applications in later life.

Two sociologists, Brent Taylor and Vern Bengtson, contribute a review of sociological theories with applications to the concept of productive aging, affirming the importance of past theoretical contributions to future development of productive aging as a concept. They note that, as with gerontology in general, most scholarship on productive aging has neglected theory. They also warn us to keep micro- and macro-level analyses distinct. At the micro level, they recommend social exchange theory as a useful lens for studying productive aging. At the macro level, they suggest that the political economy perspective and the age stratification model might be most fruitful. As an overall contribution, Taylor and Bengtson's work may encourage scholars to consider extensions of established social science theories to advance knowledge of productive aging.

Economists have long held sway over the concept of productivity in general, but they are relative newcomers to discussions on productive aging, and their theoretical perspectives will be very important to this topic. As an initial step, James Schulz identifies four "frames" that may clarify options for future economic policies addressing the elderly and population aging as a demographic trend. The four frames are: (1) the aged as a buffer, meaning that retirement policy is used as a labor market adjustment; (2) economic growth *über Alles,* referring to a focus on how retirement policy interacts with savings and labor market participation; (3) lifelong productive aging, meaning a view of productivity throughout the life course; and (4) a reflective old age, indicating that economic productivity may not be the best way to think about the older years. Schulz offers an economist's opinion that our nation, given its ever-growing economic potential, does not necessarily need older adults to be productive in the workplace, and therefore choice should be a strong value. He recommends that we take the reflective old age frame seriously, with its emphasis on choice among an array of personally meaningful activities. We should clarify, by examining both actions and stated preferences, what people want to do in later life.

Harry Moody, a major contributor to the critical gerontology perspective, points out that productive aging embodies the quintessential American values of success and productivity. Placing this in perspective, he identifies four alternative ideologies of old age: productive aging, successful aging, radical gerontology, and conscious aging. He points out that all four ideologies broaden the possibilities for the later part of life and expresses enthusiasm for concrete experiments that create new roles in later life. Also, Moody notes an erosion of consensus regarding fixed stages in the life course, and he sees new possibilities in postmodern conceptualizations of the life course. Productive aging anchors generativity as the supreme value throughout all of life. Moody celebrates this trend and the possibilities it offers, but he also notes that the purpose of critical consciousness is to become aware of the assumptions and implications of alternative futures that lie before us. In this regard, he remains cautious about expecting and prescribing active engagement for older adults, because of potentially coercive applications of this ideology. For Moody, opportunity and choice are central values. He asks perceptively: What brings about the movement toward productive aging? Why now?

Carroll Estes has been a major contributor to the political economy perspective on aging (e.g., Estes, 1991). She and Jane Mahakian express concern that productive aging advocates underestimate the difficult task of defining what it would take in the form of altered policy and social arrangements to achieve a productive aging society. They note that productive aging may support the conceptualization of aging as a problem of individuals, with measures and evaluation at the individual level and not at the institutional or societal level. Estes and Mahakian note the dominance of social class, race/ethnicity, and gender in shaping possibilities in later life, and they express concern that disadvantaged elders might be more disadvantaged under the banner of productive aging. They assert that social and environmental factors have been and may continue to be underexplicated, undertheorized, and underresearched.

Approach to Theory and Its Use

As applied social scientists, we have some particular viewpoints and probably some blinders, and it might be helpful to identify these, to the extent that we are aware of them. In particular, our observations on theory in productive aging will be shaped by our inclinations toward positivism, deduction, and application. In these matters our viewpoints are quite traditional, but in this time of widespread questioning of epistemologies in social inquiry, a few words of clarification may be useful.

Regarding *positivism,* this is the way we build knowledge in a scientific sense. It is only a tool, one way of knowing, but it has proven to be an extraordinarily useful and productive tool. The current fad of claiming that positivism is dead in the postmodern era is in all likelihood overstated, and may not be wise. While many ways of knowing are welcome, there is likely to be a distinct and continuing role for social science, and in any case, that is the method of inquiry we practice.

Regarding *deduction,* the essence of knowing in a scientific framework is to be able to specify what one thinks is happening, gather evidence, and ascertain to what extent one is right or wrong. Deduction is required for this, although it seems to be a bit underrated these days. So many social science researchers fail to specify their questions as testable propositions. As Taylor and Bengtson say in this volume, researchers too often "disown theory." Many who in fact have some idea of what they are looking for claim instead that they are only being exploratory or are building theory. Of course, there is always an important role for induction in science; many important observations and discoveries are made inductively and we should always be open to new insights. However, deduction will always be the essence of the scientific method. With few exceptions, we should strive to say what we think may be happening and ask of the social reality if indeed it is happening. This requires specifying theory and stating hypotheses so that they are testable.

Regarding *application*, this is simply our practical bias, and in this regard we are not so different from most scholars who study productive aging. We try to do work that has both intellectual content and potential impact in the world. We would assert, however, that the only way to do applied work so that it contributes to a body of knowledge is to be theoretical. As social-psychologist Kurt Lewin (1951) famously observed, "There is nothing so practical as a good theory." The notion that applied social science can or should be atheoretical is unfortunately somewhat common, but it leads nowhere. A recent example is Thyer (1999), who proposes that "outcomes" research need not be based on theory. But what good is an "outcome" if one doesn't know what it is or what caused it? As a research tool, a theory simply means a carefully thought out and specified idea. In this regard, the challenges of applied work are no less than for basic social science. Indeed, the bar for applied work is much higher: to be theoretically sound, empirically verified, and in addition, useful in application.

Toward a Definition of Productive Aging

Productive aging is almost by definition an applied concept. It has very little abstract intellectual purpose or appeal. None of us would be interested in this concept if not for the assumption that productivity in later years might be a good idea, and that changing policies, programs, institutions, and interpersonal relations, as well as individual thinking, motivation, and behavior, is possible. In brief, the primary goal of this academic agenda is that, to the extent warranted by societal values, empirical evidence, and political support, productive aging might be promoted and enhanced. Although none of the chapters in this volume makes a concerted effort to document that the elderly are marginalized in the present social and economic order, this is in fact the editors' motivation in organizing this discussion. (Of course, Estes and Mahakian in this volume and others warn that the elderly, particularly the disadvantaged elderly, might be in even worse circumstances when faced with "productive aging.")

Turning to definition and measurement, productivity is, in a strict sense, about action and positive return. In an economic sense this would mean a return on investment measurable in dollars. But economic value is not the only metric that can be used to define productivity. Many would prefer to conceptualize productive aging in a broader way, to include social and psychological dimensions, and perhaps a spiritual dimension as well. In all of these dimensions, however, the notions of action and positive return are fundamental. Where possible, efforts can and should be made to monetize investments and returns, as in a cost-benefit analysis. Putting all factors in dollar terms allows assessment across diverse constructs and a clear conclusion regarding whether an action or behavior was productive in an economic sense. This is useful in application, especially in policy and program decisions. Where this is not possible, less precise assessments of productivity might be used, as in a cost-effectiveness analysis. Beyond this, noneconomic methods of many types might be used, both quantitative and qualitative. Regarding the latter, for example, it would not be an unreasonable research method simply to ask an older person if he or she believed that a given activity was worthwhile and in what sense. Likewise, we might ask these questions of those who have benefited from the activity, such as the frail man who receives care from his spouse (see Herzog & Morgan, 1992).

Thus, a major definitional challenge is to identify all of conceptual components that may or may not be included in a definition of productive aging. In this volume, a range of definitions and examples is offered—from economic, to social/civic, to personal. Major categories of productive actions might include the following: (1) market-based economic activities, (2) nonmarket activities with economic value, (3) formal social/civic contributions, (4) informal social assistance, (5) social relationships and activities, and (6) self-improvement: learning, fulfillment, enlightenment.

This is not the only possible list, and it is not necessarily the right list, but it covers the range that is discussed in this volume. We do not insist on a specific definition of productive aging. As Moody says, we should "keep open" the definition. Our inclinations, similar to most authors in this volume, are for a broad definition. (In the next chapter, we offer a definition that includes the first four categories above, but not the last two.) All of the authors in this volume see productive aging as multidimensional. No one is advocating a narrow definition based only on paid labor. In their particular discussions or studies, scholars should say what they are including and what they are excluding in their definition of productive aging. It is not necessary that everyone agrees, but it will be helpful if each scholar is explicit. Such explicitness is important because only in comporting our definitions to that criterion will it be possible to build systematic knowledge.

Having said all this, it seems that the authors in this volume agree that older people should have greater choices of meaningful activities and roles, among these a range of productive aging activities listed above. Also, everyone seems to agree that older people should not be coerced into doing something, or stigmatized for choosing not to be active or productive. Therefore, there may be more fundamental agreement on what we are aiming at than discussions of productive aging sometimes indicate. And all of this leads us to suggest that perhaps theory and policy in productive aging should be oriented toward identifying and achieving of a greater range of choices. This would appear to be a central theme in theoretical work in this area.

Cautions

Coercion and Choice

As noted above, Estes and Mahakians's chapter warns that productive aging is a concept that carries baggage. In particular it may carry the assumption that older people *should* be productive, and this assumption may lead to pressures on them to be engaged in activities that they would prefer not to undertake. Possibly it may lead to outright coercion and exploitation of older people. Why, ask Estes and Mahakian, should society strong-arm older people to be engaged in something when the economy really doesn't need the extra workers? Why should older people be asked to bend under a yoke of productivity at a stage in their lives when they might prefer to rest and reflect?

To be sure, this warning serves an important cautionary purpose in this debate, but it is probably overstated. In our view, a greater oppression is already occurring in the lack of opportunities for older people to be engaged and make contributions. In the current scheme of things, many people retire without good choices for staying involved. Many feel disconnected and would like to make some kind of contribution but cannot find a way to do so (Bass, 1995; Peter D. Hart Associates, 1999). Nor do we think that productive aging policy would have to be coercive. As indicated above, the goal should be to offer a greater range of choices. This view is consistent with all the chapters in this volume, and it is perhaps alarmist to conclude that productive aging would become coercive. Indeed, nothing in the history of American social policy points toward increasing coercion on older adults—in fact, just the opposite, the long-term policy direction is to be more generous with the elderly. Productive aging does not have to be, and is not likely to be, any more coercive than options for adolescents to join athletic teams or to sign up for AmeriCorps.

The only major exception that we can think of is the possibility of raising the age at which people are entitled to retirement benefits, public or private. This could indeed happen (we are not quite as sure as James Schulz that older people will no longer be needed in the economy), but if it does the major reason would be the further extension of life expectancy and accompanying financial strain on retirement systems rather than changing societal values to force older people to work longer. No advocate of productive aging that we know of has suggested raising the retirement age just because he or she thinks that older people ought to be working (although others have made this argument on one side of the generational equity debate).

Values

Values are implicit in any proposal for productive aging. Values can range from economic, to social/civic, to personal. Perhaps the major value inherent in productive aging is the contributions that older people can make to the economy, that is, the potential of a vast, underutilized resource. On the other hand, critical gerontologists have warned that the concept and/or its application might be economically exploitative (e.g., Estes and Mahakian, this volume; Holstein, 1992). In the social/civic sphere, productive aging suggests a positive role for elders to participate and contribute to social bonds and political affairs. On the negative side, this could potentially lead to excessive influence of the elderly, possibly a gerontocracy in the political arena. For example, critics of the substantial political influence of AARP might raise this kind of concern, but it seems an unlikely outcome of productive aging. In the personal arena, the values of productive aging are for personal satisfaction and growth. A possible negative side would be for individuals to become harried and worn by the added obligations of being "productive," or to conclude that meaning can only be achieved through production, but again these seem to be small threats. Each proposal for productive aging should be looked at through all of these and other value lenses, both positive and negative. The reality, of course, will be of multiple and competing values. There are no easy answers to value choices of this nature; judgments are required; people will differ in their views. The best strategy at this early stage is, insofar as possible, to make value choices explicit and to engage in the debate.

Political Agendas

Like every social construct with applied implications, there will be political dimensions to the concept and definitions of productive aging. As applied social scientists, it is incumbent on us to be aware of these. Some useful questions raised in this volume include: Why are we thinking about this? What is the need? What is the opportunity? Whose agenda is it? Who will decide on the definition? Productive aging for whom? Who will decide on the policies and programs? If action is taken, how will resources be allocated? Who will benefit? Who will pay? These and other political questions must be on the mind of any good applied social scientist. However, social scientists cannot and should not attempt to be politicians. Our contributions are to define and document good policy and programs. For the most part, the political process is not in our control, and for academics to try to become political actors is usually a mistake because being political risks our most precious asset: intellectual independence and objectivity. There may be added value in attempting to theorize about political agendas and the political process in productive aging, although we cannot say what the particular lens of productive aging would bring to such theorizing, and it is beyond our present purpose.

Race/Ethnicity, Gender, Class, and Cultural Differences

Carroll Estes raises fundamental questions about the underlying values, political agendas, and effects on different populations, particularly women (e.g., Estes, 1991). And James Jackson has contributed to this discussion with his inquiries into racial and ethnic differences in aging (e.g., Jackson, Antonucci, & Gibson, 1990). An important theme in this volume, especially in the chapters of Estes and Mahakian and Jackson, is that meanings, options, and outcomes for productive aging are quite likely to vary among different populations. This is so true and meaningful that it would be intellectually and practically foolish to ignore such differences. As prior work indicates, we should anticipate differences across subgroups and test for these differences. The best theorizing will attempt to integrate and explain such differences, in effect, to listen to the voices of those on the margins. There are two basic theoretical/methodological options for handling subgroups: the first is to include subgroups as constructs in the theory, and the second is to test a theory separately with each subgroup of interest. Each approach has advantages and disadvantages. In this chapter we take the first approach. What we gain is a direct test of the variables of interest (e.g., whether race/ethnicity matters). What we give up is the construction of unique theories by subgroup that might be more explanatory (e.g., different theories for whites versus blacks). There is no singularly correct answer and, if indicated, both approaches can be taken.

Pretheoretical Tensions

Some conceptual work is pretheoretical, that is, it is a general way of thinking that is not yet specified in testable terms. Economist Joseph Schumpeter referred to these general orientations as preanalytical. Historian of science Thomas Kuhn (1970) used the word *paradigm* to describe entirely new ways of understanding an area of scientific knowledge. Unfortunately, the word has become much overused of late, spilling over into popular culture, but Kuhn's understanding of how shifts in science occur is one of the great intellectual contributions of our era. In brief, he points out that a major change in scientific theory does not come by accretion of new empirical information, but by a new way of understanding that is more fully explanatory, with fewer anomalies, than the old way. We would not assert that productive aging qualifies as a new paradigm, but it is a new way of envisioning the role of older people in the economy and society. As such, it is pretheoretical at the present stage.

Below we briefly summarize some of the large ideas and conceptual tensions that may underlie theory construction as it proceeds. We select three of these that seem to carry a lot of conceptual weight, and from which much of the discussion in this volume seemed to draw (for still others, see the four "frames" in Schulz's chapter in this volume).

Biology: Natural Limits versus Extension of Limits

The biology of aging leaves heavy footprints on this discussion. Unfortunately, those footprints are going in opposite directions, which sometimes leaves discussants a bit confused. The first direction, so fundamental to existence, is that the life span has a natural limit, and functioning declines approaching that limit. The practical conclusion is that we cannot be productive indefinitely. One of the important contributions of Svanborg's chapter is to remind us of this limit and that decline and eventual death are natural. At the same time, Svanborg's data remind us that we can make strides in improving functioning during later years, especially recovery from setbacks, which are critical points of decline. But the idea of a natural limit suggests that productive aging, successful aging, and related concepts may be a kind of delusion. In Moody's phrase, promotion of such concepts might be "like being social director on a lifeboat."

The second direction, in fact a demographic revolution, is that economic development, technology, and individual behaviors can dramatically improve the odds of reaching the natural limit and maintaining functioning as one gets older. The practical conclusion is that more people are living longer, with greater functioning. In all likelihood, this trend will continue. Already the United States has over 33 million people over age 65 and more than 70 percent of these are basically fit and functioning. At retirement, the typical person in 1996 could look forward to 17 years of life expectancy, perhaps 12 of these active (U.S. Bureau of the Census, 1996). Moreover, it is altogether likely that the average age of dependency and death will continue to rise. This is a huge blessing and opportunity for individuals, a striking success for technology and economic development, and an enormous resource for the society and economy. The extent of this demographic change strongly suggests that we are going to have to do something differently, and on this there appears to be widespread agreement.

Overall, the conceptual and practical tension between these two great biological facts—a fixed limit to the human life span, but people living longer, healthier lives—underlies much of the debate surrounding productive aging. Typically a given scholar will be operating from one of these positions or the other.

Social Construction: Old versus Happen to Be Old

Somewhat related to the biological tension discussed above is a conceptual tension in the social construction of being old, and on this distinction rests a great many of the debates in gerontology. As we discuss in the next chapter, the two basic conceptual choices in productive aging are (1) productivity for old people, or (2) productivity for people who happen to be old. Emanating from these two different social constructions is the theoretical choice of (1) life stages, institutionalized roles, and marked changes or (2) no clear life stages, continuity across chronological age, and gradualism. Much of the discussion and theorizing among scholars in this volume seems to assume the latter: aging as a lifelong process, or aging on a continuum of life. Moreover, they would agree with Bytheway (1997) that to think otherwise would be to start from a position that reinforces fundamental prejudices about the elderly. This perspective is sometimes called "deinstitutionalization of the life course," and it presents us with questions that will be important to answer: To what extent is productive aging part of the movement trying to break down the distinction of aging as a separate period of later life? If so, what are the implications? What are the likely benefits to this viewpoint, and the likely costs? What are the implications for theory development? For one, the primary emphasis is on capacity and functioning rather than chronological age.

Policy: "Retirement" versus Something Else?

Although policy is not much discussed in this volume, we cannot help but bring up one major point: retirement as a separate period in later life was a creation of the industrial era, to provide relief from physical work and also to remove older people from the labor market to make room for others (Achenbaum, this volume). We should not forget that public policy has actively and strongly shaped the choices, expectations, and behaviors of the older population. A strong influence on decisions to "retire" is the Social Security retirement system, which is in fiscal terms the largest single public policy in the nation. It is well to bear in mind that this policy structure, so embedded in industrial production, will not necessarily fit the information era (Sherraden, 1997). There may be little reason to take retirement as we know it today as a "given" over the long term. Indeed, it seems likely that retirement, like all aspects of labor markets, will adapt to new systems of economic production (see Schulz's chapter). In some situations, older workers with skills will be in high demand. A likely adaptation is a blurring of the boundary between work and retirement that has characterized industrial era social policy. We are already seeing this in numerous forms of "phased retirement."

Toward Theory in Productive Aging

Our job in this chapter is to point toward theoretical pathways that might carry this new thinking into programs of scientific research, and eventually into new policies and programs. First, we point to the excellent work in the major chapters in this volume, especially the comprehensive conceptual model presented by Bass and Caro, the review of sociological theory by Taylor and Bengtson, the observations on economic theory by Schulz, and insights by Birren. With this work as a foundation, we can perhaps be of some help by specifying the territory for productive aging as an applied concept. As indicated above, the notion of productive aging suggests that (1) older people should, if they choose, be engaged in some way(s) that are beneficial to others; and (2) the society, economy, and polity should seek to increase the opportunities for this to happen. This is normative theory that implies a policy and/or program agenda.

Regarding theoretical structure, there are two fundamental options. The first is to examine productive aging as a dependent variable, with complex causation. This theoretical structure asks the general question: What leads to productive aging? The second is to examine productive aging as an independent variable, with multiple outcomes, both positive and negative. This theoretical structure asks the question: What are the effects of productive aging?

Numerous theoretical formulations are possible within each of these two choices. Many different theories can be used to understand a phenomenon, and each can be helpful; but not all theories are of equal usefulness in a particular situation. The field of productive aging would benefit, at this stage of development, from judicious specification of theories of both of these basic types. The scholars in this volume are among those best positioned to offer these specifications. Also, as the chapter by Taylor and Bengtson suggests, not all theories are of equal usefulness in a particular situation and there is a need to make some theoretical choices. In other words, it is time to place some intellectual bets. The bets are almost sure to be less than perfect, but that is how knowledge moves ahead. The essence of good theorizing for knowledge building is to specify and pursue with empirical evidence a theory that is most likely to be productive, and then discard, revise, or accept the theory as warranted by the evidence.

Much of the theory in productive aging is likely to draw on economic models or analogies. As especially the chapters by Schulz, Birren, and Bass and Caro make clear, the basic notions of supply and demand provide the fundamental micro-theory context. This implies a functioning "market" for productive roles on one hand and individuals to assume these roles on the other, operating much like a labor market.

A theoretical gem is found in Birren's chapter. Birren is a psychologist but he sometimes crosses boundaries, particularly into matters that are essentially economic. He offers an economic concept that is useful in macro theory building, the idea of "flows." He identifies the critical flows as time, information, and energy. Of these, he says, information may be the most important in an information age economy and society. Building on the concept of flows, Birren asks about "sources" and "sinks," that is, where the flows are generated and where they are absorbed. This conceptualization holds considerable potential in both theory building and policy analysis. One can think of a variety of ratios of sources to sinks. What would these ratios mean for different types of flows? What ratio level would be considered "productive"? Also, the idea of flows leads us to the related economic concept of "stocks," that is, storehouses of resources for future flows. This can in turn be related to capacities and functioning, a conceptualization that Nobel laureate economist Amartya Sen (1993) suggests for defining welfare or well-being at the individual and household levels.

Toward Specification:
A Model of Productivity in Later Life

The chapters in this volume have given us very excellent work in laying out the territory. The next theoretical steps will be in specification of these theories. We can turn to the considerable wisdom of sociologist Robert Merton's (1957) call for theories "of the middle range," by which he meant theories that are not so grand as to have no operational implications and not so narrow as to have no relevance beyond specific circumstances. Theories of the middle range would incorporate especially the institutional constructs indicated above, which can have clear operationalizations and applied implications, but are at the same time flexible in responding to many different circumstances. Also, for applied purposes, simplicity matters. We are in need of middle range theories that (1) have only a few operational constructs and (2) identify key relationships. The point of good theory is not to represent a complex reality, but to capture a fundamental dynamic that is highly explanatory—and in the applied social sciences, has large implications for action. To put this another way, we are in need "strategies for ignoring information," which is what a good theory does.* This is perhaps best articulated in Milton Friedman's classic *Essays in Positive Economics* (1953), in which he argues for the greatest simplicity possible.

The challenge in the applied social sciences is not to find out what is true, but rather to find out what is both true and useful. The second half of this standard—useful—has a number of dimensions that can be stated as follows: theory in the applied social sciences should have implications for action (policy, program, treatment, or intervention) that are (1) simple and clear, easily communicable, (2) highly explanatory (i.e., have meaningful effects), (3) readily transferable to application, (4) ethical, (5) subject to multiple tests in the real world, (6) politically within the realm of possibility, (7) affordable, and (8) doable by an average person or organization.†

Thus, we seek a middle range theory of productive aging that is mindful of the above guidelines and can be used to frame and generate questions for research that are oriented toward policy and practice. To reiterate, this is decidedly not a theory that seeks to encompass or explain everything about productive aging. With this general direction in mind, we can begin to identify categories and constructs for an emerging theory. We offer a beginning list below:

Sociodemographics (individual priors or givens): gender, race, age, socioeconomic status, education, and residence

Public policy (sets the macro stage for productive action): programs, regulations, taxation

Individual capacity (supply: possible targets for individual intervention): physical functioning, cognitive functioning, economic resources, time, knowledge and skills, social support, transportation

Institutional capacity (demand: possible targets for public policy and programs): number, types, and quality of roles, and linkages to roles

---

*We thank Jim Birren for this phrase.

†This list of desirable attributes of theory in the applied social sciences has been developed by Sherraden in teaching doctoral students how to think about theory in applied research. It is important to note that the theoretical demands are high, especially the last standard, which says that the implied action must be "doable by an average person or organization." Unfortunately, the implied action of many of our theories fails to meet this basic standard, yet without it little can happen beyond showcase events or demonstration programs.

Productive behaviors (resources applied to different types of productive activity): market activity, nonmarket activity with economic value, formal social or civic activity, informal social assistance

Productivity outcomes (measured by effects of behavior): assessed at different levels: individual, family, society

From these building blocks a variety of theories and models can be constructed. We offer our view of how a useful model might be constructed (Figure 12.1). This model draws from the work of the scholars contributing to this volume. As in the "aging and society paradigm" (Riley, Foner, & Riley, 1999), we emphasize the interplay between individual lives and social structures to explain productive behavior in later life. Regarding theoretical specification, this model (1) points to constructs that are measurable; (2) indicates logical relationships (i.e., it tells a sensible story about individuals, social structure, and productive behavior); and (3) is oriented toward action in the sense that most of the categories are subject to intervention and change.

It may be helpful to clarify and discuss a few points related to this model.

Sociodemographics are separated from individual capacities. As Svanborg and others have pointed out, we should be thinking about improving individual capacities, so it makes sense to distinguish the background characteristics from current capacities. Exogenous factors affecting individual capacity include sociodemographic characteristics such as gender, race, cultural background, age, education, and residence.

Individual capacity, like institutional capacity, has an effect on the appraisal that the individual makes about engagement in productive activities. Among numerous factors, an older adult's physical and cognitive functioning, social support, income and assets, as well as acquired knowledge and skills affect her or his productive behavior. Thus, the model seeks to sort out intracohort variability and creates the possibility of identifying different types of older adults vis-à-vis productive activity (Dannefer & Uhlenberg, 1999).

Note that this model does not include individual appraisal and decision making, not because these do not occur—obviously they do—but because the authors are making the judgment that decision making is unlikely to be highly explanatory in the model and opportunities for systematic intervention are limited. An alternative approach would be to include

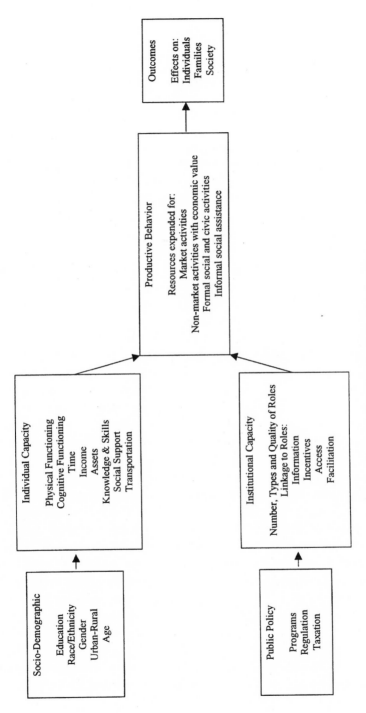

Figure 12.1 Productivity in later life

appraisal and decision making and look perhaps to social marketing strategies for intervention. Recent social marketing successes in reducing drunk driving and handgun violence indicate that this might be fruitful.

The macro environment is represented here only by public policy. This is not to say that many other macro factors—economic, political, social, and cultural—are not important. Indeed, the life course can be seen as a set of publicly shared meanings and expectations for the course of human lives. However, these age norms are gradually formalized in a matrix of policies and practices (Dannefer & Uhlenberg, 1999). The purpose of theorizing in our case is to construct theory that might, if substantiated, serve as a guide to action, and public policy provides a better handle on application. As mentioned above, the political state, through its social policies, is today a powerful determinant of decisions to "retire." What if the state were to create a different kind of policy? What would be the public policy for "productivity through the life course"? What would be the programs, regulations, and tax laws that defined this policy? And what institutional structures would these policies create? Especially, what would be the numbers and types of roles, and linkages to roles through information, incentives, access, and facilitation?

Institutional capacity refers to the ability of social institutions, like businesses, public and private agencies, churches, legal institutions, social/ civic clubs, and families to offer (or not offer), create (or not create), and promote (or not promote) productive roles for older adults. In these ways, institutions bring productive roles into a market in which individuals, with varying capacities, may connect with these roles. Institutions vary in the number and types of roles that they create, and they differ in the manner and extent to which they enable individuals to link to those roles. Linkage to roles is affected by the amount of information made available about the role, the accessibility of the role, incentives provided for engagement, and the degree to which the institution facilitates sustained involvement in the role. Each dimension can produce negative to positive effects on an individual's assessment of the role and on the productive behavior itself. Institutions can provide more or less information to individuals and the public about opportunities, benefits, and costs of a particular role. Incentives could include the use of stipends, wage compensation and benefits, and the development of social networks. Institutions can also create disincentives for participation, for example, the income test of Social Security reduces benefits to those who have earned incomes over a certain level, and this policy reduces employment effort by the elderly (Friedberg, 1999). Similarly, institutions can provide varying levels of access to productive roles by, for example, embedding the role within a program with eligibility guidelines, offering the role within a broad or limited geographic area, or making the physical environment in which the role is performed accessible to all qualified individuals. Finally, institutions may facilitate individual engagement in roles through such factors as transportation, training programs, the availability of good supervision, attitudes of co-workers in the organization, or supportive services.

Institutional capacity is important because it may explain a large part of the variance in productive behaviors, as suggested in the work of Bass and Caro. This is also the fundamental viewpoint in the structural lag theory (Riley, Kahn, & Foner, 1994), which suggests that institutions usually lag social reality. If one agrees with this analysis (it is hard not to) there are two basic ways to proceed. One is to do little because structural lag is a kind of historical inevitability. The other is perhaps more optimistic. Riley also points out that institutions are to some extent created and changed by people, which means that policy and program innovations are possible. As applied social scientists we choose to take this latter approach, although we remain mindful of the challenges. We turn our attention to a middle-range context of theorizing, to policy and program innovations and how these come about. The chapter by Freedman in this volume on structural lead sets the tone for this direction, although more academic work is required on how institutions are purposefully created and changed (Sherraden, 1997).

Freedman also reminds us that not all institutions that engage older adults are of equal impact. Some hold greater promise for individuals, families, communities, and society. To date, scholarship on productive aging has made little effort to set standards or distinguish among various types of productive activities and institutions. It seems likely that this will begin to change, and theory may begin to explain characteristics of more productive institutions and causal factors in their creation and successful operation. For example, Freedman (this volume) begins to document attributes of institutions that may be most attractive to elders; he points to the name, critical mass or presence, flexibility, leadership possibilities, opportunity to learn, and opportunity to work on a team.

The category of institutional capacity also suggests variation in how policy is implemented and in the capacities of local programs. As William Frey (1999) cogently pointed out, the circumstances of the elderly vary markedly in different localities, and productive aging strategies, along with all other policies and services for the elderly, should take local variations into account. In other words, one cannot assume that macro policy is actually "doing something" in a given location, and this is one reason why theory of the middle range that looks at institutions is preferable for applied purposes.

Although not specified as a category or construct, individual choice is central to the model. This reflects both the positivistic view of engagement of supply and demand in a market-like function, and the normative view that choice matters above all else in considering strategies for productive aging. This reflects the principle of human agency and self-regulation, that is, people plan and make choices among options that become the building blocks of their evolving life course. Contrary to an age grading viewpoint, peoples of the same age do not march in concert across major events of the life course; rather they vary in pace and sequencing (Elder, 1995). This is due in large part to the fact that they make different choices. In this model, institutionalized roles and individuals are brought together in a market in which individuals choose to engage or not to engage.

We have not modeled choice as a construct because, in our judgment, it may not be a fruitful approach for applied purposes. This is somewhat akin to neoclassical economic models, wherein market participants are assumed to have perfect information, act in unrestricted markets, and by definition make the "right" choices. To say the least, these assumptions are not a perfect fit with reality. Indeed, some social gerontologists have warned against unjustified faith in market functions and the role of choice. In the study of productive behavior, choice may be a problem to be analyzed, not a matter to be assumed. Dannefer and Uhlenberg (1999, p. 309) warn against "unwarranted affirmation of choice as an unproblematized determinant of the life course." This may be especially relevant in the study of marginalized or oppressed populations, who may face more restricted opportunities and may differently understand and differently value "productive behavior" (see chapters by Jackson, Estes and Mahakian, and Bass and Caro in this volume; also Herzog & Morgan, 1992; and Holstein 1992).

As this discussion illustrates, the essential dynamic in the social sciences is the tension between social structure and individual action. In the present model, this tension results in some type and level of productive behavior. This behavior should be defined, and as discussed in the following chapter, we define productivity as "any behavior, whether paid or unpaid, that creates a good or service." At minimum, this will require identifying arenas of action that constitute productive behavior and the resources that are expended in those arenas. The areas we suggest are: market activities, nonmarket activities with economic value, formal social and civic engagement, and informal social assistance. The ability to engage in these behaviors requires slack resources, or capacity that exceeds that needed to perform sufficient levels of self-care or household maintenance. These areas of productive behavior may be conceptually distinct, but in research will be challenging to isolate. Within each area, it will be necessary to measure resources expended, principally time and money. Inquiry must also be open to concurrent involvement in multiple forms of productive behavior by a particular individual.

Absent from the above definition of productive behavior are informal social relations that have no social product. Also, this definition excludes activities that benefit solely the actor, such as self-care; activities that are required to live independently, such as household work; and activities for self-improvement, such as education, physical exercise, or spiritual reflection. This is certainly not to say that these activities are not socially valued. It is generally agreed, for example, that the ability to live independently, to whatever extent one is able, is desirable and worthy of societal support. However, we are concerned that including such areas in a definition of productive aging, as some scholars have done, may lead to a diffusion of the concept and ultimately limit its utility.

Although we have emphasized the institutional context of productive behavior, not all such behavior occurs through defined roles within formal institutions. For example, an older adult may elect to provide informal volunteer assistance to a neighbor. The choice to perform this service will take into account the individual's capacity, and possibly the impact of public policy (e.g., a tax deduction for expenses) without going through a formal institution.

Productivity outcomes are the effects of productive behavior. These may include a wide range of effects on the individual, family, and society, both positive and negative. As Jim Birren notes in this volume, it will be necessary to look beyond the market value of an activity (e.g., the wage value of the individual's time, the market cost of the good or service) and determine the net value of that engagement, which includes the potential consequences of the activity or good produced for the producer, consumers, and spillover costs and/or benefits to the family, community, and society. The chapters by Bengston and Taylor, Jackson, and others look at outcomes at several levels. We think that some of the most important

effects are likely to be social, in community building and positive intergenerational relations. A significant challenge will be in how to measure
these.

Turning to analysis, Birren's thinking on sources and sinks points toward
a benefit-cost framework for analysis. This is an "ideal" policy analytic
framework, but possible only when all expended resources (productive
behaviors) and all effects (productivity outcomes) can be measured in dollar
terms with some degree of confidence. More often this will not be possible, in which case a less universal assessment, such a cost-effectiveness
analysis, may be appropriate. A key issue for integrity of analysis will be
that the effects that are selected for measurement are derived from theoretical statements and not piled up arbitrarily.

As a final point, this model is weak in historical terms. It does not have
a way to analyze variability across cohorts (Sampson & Laub, 1993; Riley,
Foner, & Riley, 1999). Human lives carry the imprint of their particular
social worlds, and times of rapid change can bring personal disruption
and incoherence of one kind or another. Social scientists are interested in
explaining how dynamic worlds change people and how people select and
construct their environments. Historical changes do not occur uniformly
across communities, regions, and societies, and a focus on the individual
may ignore social change (Elder, 1995; Riley, 1996). In productive aging,
we are reminded of this most profoundly by Achenbaum (1995, and in
this volume), when he points out that, prior to this century, productive
aging has been the norm. Out of necessity, older adults have had to be
productive until they could no longer work. This major historical fact by
itself repositions our understanding of this issue. We sacrifice this and
other historical insights in the model above because our purpose is applied and more immediate. This may serve as a sober reminder that every
theoretical construction has certain benefits and certain shortcomings.

Conclusion

A wise person once said that a good theory provides a "dazzling glimpse
of the obvious." The field of productive aging is ready for a few more
such dazzling glimpses. In our view, this is today the most important challenge in knowledge building in productive aging. A field initiated by advocacy and empiricism will gradually mature into a more scholarly endeavor with specified theories and programs of systematic inquiry. It seems
likely that some of the dazzling glimpses in the future will emerge from

the work of the accomplished authors represented in this volume. Based on the important groundwork they have laid, others will follow. As both reality and understanding of aging continue to change rapidly, scholars from diverse disciplines will join in this discussion, offering new and valuable conceptualizations that today we are not able to see.

REFERENCES

Achenbaum, W. A. (1995). *Crossing frontiers*. New York: Cambridge University Press.

Bass, S. (Ed.). (1995). *Older and active: How Americans over 55 are contributing to society*. New Haven: Yale University Press.

Bass, S. A., & Caro, F. G. (1996). Theoretical perspectives in productive aging. In W. Crown (Ed.), *Handbook on employment of the elderly* (pp. 265–275). Westport, CT: Greenwood.

Bytheway, B. (1997). Talking about age: The theoretical basis of social gerontology. In A. Jamieson, S. Harper, & C. Victor (Eds.), *Critical approaches to ageing and later life*. Buckingham, England: Open University.

Dannefer, D., & Uhlenberg, P. (1999). Paths of the life course: A typology. In V. L. Bengtson & K. W. Schaie (Eds.), *Handbook of theories of aging* (pp. 306–326). New York: Springer.

Elder, G. (1995). The life course paradigm: Social change and individual development. In P. Moen, G. H. Elder Jr., & K. Luscher (Eds.), *Examining lives in context: Perspectives on the ecology of human development* (pp. 101–139). Washington, DC: American Psychological Association.

Erikson, E. H. (1950). *Childhood and society*. New York: Norton.

Estes, C. (1991). The new political economy of aging: Introduction and critique. In M. Minkler & C. L. Estes (Eds.), *Critical perspective on aging: The political and moral economy of growing old* (pp. 19–36). Amityville, NY: Baywood.

Frey, W. H. (1999). *Beyond Social Security: The local aspects of an aging America*. Washington, DC: Brookings Institution.

Friedberg, L. (1999). *Social Security earnings test reduces work by the elderly* (NBER Working Paper 7200). Cambridge, MA: National Bureau of Economic Research.

Friedman, M. (1953). *Essays in positive economics*. Chicago: University of Chicago Press.

Herzog, A. R., & Morgan, J. N. (1992). Age and gender differences in the value of productive activities. *Research on Aging, 14* (2), 169–198.

Holstein, M. (1992). Productive aging: A feminist critique. *Journal of Aging and Social Policy, 4* (3–4), 17–33.

Jackson, J. S., Antonucci, T. C., & Gibson, R. C. (1990). Cultural, racial, and ethnic minority influences on aging. In J. E. Birren & W. Schaie (Eds.), *Handbook of the psychology of aging* (3rd ed., pp. 103–123). New York: Academic.

Kuhn, T. (1970). *The structure of scientific revolutions* (2nd ed.). Chicago: University of Chicago Press.

Lewin, K. (1951). *Field theory in social science: Selected theoretical papers.* D. Cartwright (Ed.). New York: Harpers.

Merton, R. (1957). *Social theory and social structure* (rev. ed.). London: The Free Press.

Peter D. Hart Research Associates. (1999). *The changing face of retirement: Older Americans, civic engagement, and the longevity revolution.* Washington, DC: Author.

Riley, M. W. (1996). Discussion: What does it all mean? *The Gerontologist, 36* (2), 256–258.

Riley, M. W., Foner, A., & Riley, J. W., Jr. (1999). The aging and society paradigm. In V. L. Bengtson & K. W. Schaie (Eds.), *Handbook of theories of aging* (pp. 327–343). New York: Springer.

Riley, M. W., Kahn, R. L., & Foner, A. (1994). *Age and structural lag: Society's failure to provide meaningful opportunities in work, family, and leisure.* New York: Wiley.

Sampson, R. J., & Laub, J. H. (1993). *Crime in the making: Pathways and turning points through life.* Cambridge, MA: Harvard University Press.

Schulz, J. (1995). *The economics of aging* (6th ed.). Dover, MA: Auburn House.

Sen, A. (1993). Capability and well-being. In M. Nussbaum & A. Sen (Eds.), *The quality of life* (pp. 30–53). Oxford: Clarendon.

Sherraden, M. (1997). Conclusion: Social Security in the twenty-first century. In J. Midgley & M. Sherraden (Eds.), *Alternatives to Social Security: An international inquiry.* Westport, CT: Auburn House.

Thyer, B. (1999). The role of theory in research on social work practice, keynote address, *Proceedings of the eleventh national symposium on doctoral research in social work* (pp. 1–25). Columbus: Ohio State University, College of Social Work.

U.S. Bureau of the Census. (1996). *65+ in the United States* (Current Population Reports, Special Studies, P-23-90). Washington, DC: U.S. Government Printing Office.

13

ADVANCING RESEARCH ON PRODUCTIVITY IN LATER LIFE

Nancy Morrow-Howell, Ph.D., James Hinterlong, M.S.W.,
Michael Sherraden, Ph.D., and Philip Rozario, M.S.W.

In this chapter, we seek to assess the current knowledge base on productive aging and recommend research questions to advance understanding of the phenomenon of productivity in later life and to inform the
development of programs and policies that influence this productivity.
This research agenda seeks to advance accurate perspectives about the
potential of older adults and to foster the development of social institutions that are appropriate to this potential.

Definitional and Value Statements

Given the definitional controversies in this volume, it may be helpful to
articulate our definition at the outset. Many definitions are offered in the
literature and used in research (see the first chapter of this volume for
reviews of definitions); and this book reflects the wide range of activities
and pursuits that are included under the various definitions of productive
aging. As Bass and Caro point out in their chapter, it would be helpful to
define productive aging in a "narrow, analytic sense" if we are to facilitate
comparison and replication and build a stronger knowledge base.

Following a careful reading of the gerontologists in this volume, we
prefer to define the concept of *productivity in later life* rather than the
concept of *productive aging*. The term *productive aging* is useful in bring-

ing attention to this topic, raising value issues, and advancing an advocacy agenda, but it may not be the best concept on which to base a research agenda. On reflection, this term may be at the root of some of the controversies around this topic. The term *productive aging* may imply that there is "unproductive aging." The term has caused some scholars to worry that we may come to view the highest attainment of late life as productivity. When we use the term *productive aging*, we may unwittingly participate in a rivalry among ideologies of late life. These ideologies include "successful aging" as offered by Rowe and Kahn (1998), "robust aging" as offered by Vailliant and Vailliant (1990), and "conscious aging" suggested by Moody in this volume. Perhaps the concept of "productivity in later life" minimizes some of these differences. The term suggests that productivity is among many possible pursuits of later life, including leisure and spirituality. There is less suggestion that productivity is the highest attainment of late life. Instead, productivity is one of many types of goals, all of which have value and can be promoted. The phrase *productivity in later life* has a more empirical tone that leads to research questions, rather than a value tone that leads to debate about the meaning of late life. The phrase also begins to move the discussion toward age-irrelevancy because age is but one factor in explaining productivity (one could also study productivity in middle age). Finally, the concept of productivity in later life in effect removes productive aging from the ideological competition. In obviating the demand for an all-encompassing concept, applied knowledge may develop more quickly.

Similar to other scholars, we define productivity in later life as activities that produce goods and services, whether paid or not. These activities include volunteering for an organization, engaging in civic affairs, providing assistance to relatives or friends of any age (caregiving to dependent relatives, grandparenting, assistance to adult children), and working in the labor force. We view these activities as making economic and social contributions to other people and to society. This definition does not include activities that are directed primarily to the self. We view self-care and self-development as important activities, and we believe that older adults should have access to education and other human capital building resources; but unlike Bass and Caro, we separate capacity-building from actual performance of productive activities, although both are important and should be addressed in a research agenda on productivity in later life. We separate these concepts because capacity-building involves the consumption of resources, and a person could engage in capacity-building activities and never engage in productive behaviors that result in economic or social contributions.

It is important that we distinguish between meaningful or valuable activities and productive activities. Many meaningful or valuable activities in which older adults engage are not productive in the sense we define above; these include artistic, introspective, relational, and spiritual activities. This does not mean that these activities should not be encouraged, but only that they are a different set of activities from those included in our definition of what constitutes productivity. To be sure, many other activities have important meaning and are essential elements of successful living.

Scholars should articulate the set of assumptions or values that underlie development of knowledge. This articulation is especially important, given the concerns expressed in the literature about the danger of the concept of productive aging. In this volume, Estes and Mahakian as well as Moody (citing Holstein, 1992), summarize these concerns. They warn that the promotion of productive aging could lead to the expectation that all older adults, no matter how frail, might be judged on their ability to be "productive" in an economic sense, for example, on their ability to hold a job or provide a certain number of volunteer hours. There is a fear that older adults who do not meet some arbitrary expectation about productivity would be viewed as unproductive and therefore of less value and undeserving. There is a fear that women and minorities would be further marginalized in late life when they continue to face discrimination in access to or support for engagement in productive activities, especially given their increased likelihood of having physical disabilities. Estes and Mahakian summarize these concerns powerfully: "the aged may find themselves dogged by market judgements to the end of life, and in ways that become troubling new sources of stigma and social control."

As scholars of productivity in later life, we do not want to contribute to the realization of these fears in the development of new programs and policies that punish elders who are not productive, by whatever definition. We start with this articulation of underlying values: policies and programs that seek to maximize the participation of older adults in productive roles should enhance engagement, not lead to exploitation. Thus, these programs and policies should seek to provide opportunities to older adults to engage in activities that they view as positive and valuable, that they choose to do, not that they are obliged to do.

However, this vision should also be applied to current circumstances.

In review, current practices in the employment, volunteer, and caregiving sectors may be oppressive to older adults in their lack of opportunity or lack of support and reward. Older adults are today oppressed in the predominant view of them as unproductive, as a sink rather than a source in the words of James Birren. As O'Reilly and Caro (1994) conclude, one should be able to choose to be productive throughout a life. Currently, older adults are in effect coerced into leisure activities by lack of opportunity for continued productive engagement. As Sicker (1994) notes, there is abundant opportunity for leisure in later life. The development of the productive aging concept should, at the heart, be about creating abundant opportunity and choices for productive engagement in later life.

Scholars should articulate to the extent possible underlying assumptions or values and then be vigilant about how these values are expressed in research endeavors. Values can be expressed through the questions that are developed, the samples that are chosen, the measurements that are used, the analyses that are chosen, and the interpretations that are made.

Current Knowledge on Productive Activities in Later Life

Extent of Involvement

Using definitions similar to the one we suggest, current research describes the extent to which older people are engaged in productive activities. In general, researchers have approached the question of extent of involvement by operationalizing various activities included as "productive" and measuring the level of each activity in hours per week. As reviewed in the first chapter of this volume, sampling strategies and sample sizes have varied, but several studies of large, random samples of older adults show that more than a quarter of the elderly population work, more than a quarter volunteer, more than a quarter provide assistance to a disabled person, and 40 percent help children and grandchildren (Caro & Bass, 1992). Analysis of this involvement demonstrates that engagement in one sector is largely independent of engagement in another; that is, the correlation between work hours and volunteer hours and between volunteering and caregiving is low (Caro & Bass, 1992).

Several authors point out that gerontologists began this documentation of productive engagement in late life to contradict the stereotypes of old age and to reverse the social devaluation of old age that Achenbaum (in Chapter 2 of this volume) suggests started at the turn of the twentieth century. Researchers have succeeded in accumulating this evidence. As Bass (1995) puts it, we can lay the misconception about the lack of involvement in productive roles to rest. Data demonstrate that neither the stereotype that elders are frail and dependent nor the stereotype that they are affluent retirees seeking leisure is correct. Although we have accumulated descriptive information about productivity in later life, this information has not been widely consumed nor transformed into common knowledge. It does not seem to have greatly influenced beliefs and attitudes about late life in the general population. The greedy geezer or dependent elder images are still more prominent in our society than the older adult making valuable contributions to families and communities. For example, surveys indicate that employers still hold negative perceptions of older workers, despite evidence of the positive impacts of older workers (Barth, 1997; Friedland, 1997). For gerontology advocates, a high priority for work in this area is the dissemination and utilization of accurate information on contributions of older adults.

Potential for Increased Involvement

Several studies have queried older adults about their desire to be more involved in employment and volunteer roles. Findings suggest that there is potential for increased involvement. Previous work shows that there is untapped potential of older adults to be involved in productive activities. For example, an estimated 12 percent of people over the age of 55 years are in good or excellent health and are not engaged in any work, volunteer, or caregiving activities; 20 percent of those in good or excellent health are engaged in these activities fewer than five hours a week (Caro & Bass, 1995a). A survey by The Commonwealth Fund (1993) documents that one in seven older adults who is not currently working is willing and able but cannot find a job; furthermore, more than half of all workers 50 to 64 years of age would continue working if retraining or transition opportunities were available and pensions were age-neutral. A survey sponsored by the Administration on Aging found that 37.4 percent of the older population are or may be willing to serve if asked (Marriot Seniors Volunteerism Study, 1991). The Commonwealth Fund Study found that 15 percent of people over the age of 55 who are not volunteering are willing to do so (Caro & Bass, 1995b). As pointed out by Caro and Bass (1992), for every two persons who are volunteering, another older person has reported being willing and able to volunteer.

However, research also raises some uncertainties about increasing involvement. Although survey researchers have documented that more people say that they want to engage in work and volunteer roles, it is not clear that they would do so if given the opportunity. This question is raised by studies of factors associated with *who is* involved in these activities versus factors associated with *who wants to be* more involved. For example, older adults who volunteer are more educated than nonvolunteers. Older adults who are willing to volunteer but not currently volunteering are less educated than those who are volunteering, although more educated than those not interested in volunteering. Given that those interested but not currently volunteering are "between" current volunteers and those not interested in regards to education (and the same holds for the variable religiosity), it could be that these persons are more similar to volunteers than nonvolunteers and are likely to be recruitable. On the other hand, they may be more similar to nonvolunteers and responding positively to questions regarding interest in volunteering out of social desirability.

Knowledge in this area might be advanced by a more specific understanding of what people want during later life (as suggested by Schulz in Chapter 7) and particularly what people want in terms of level and type of productive involvement in later life. The extent to which older adults increase their participation and the extent to which future generations plan on productive engagement in later life depend in part on preferences, which are shaped among other things by past experiences with productive engagement. Survey research indicates that older adults want "well-deserved leisure" and they want "to continue to be productive" (Rowe & Kahn, 1998). A survey conducted by Peter D. Hart Research Associates (1999) suggests that 50 percent of people between the ages of 50 and 75 say that volunteering/community service is an important part of their retirement plans; 12 percent reported being interested only in leisure activities.

Further quantitative and qualitative studies may be useful in clarifying such questions as how much leisure do older adults find optimal? How much productive engagement? What balance of the two in later life? What balance of the two in younger adulthood? Several scholars have pointed out that raising the Social Security pension age from 65 to 67 signals a change in expectation about older workers in this society (Friedland, 1997; Quinn, 1997), but what attitudes and expectations about employment and leisure are held by older people, by younger people, by employers? Riley and Riley (1994) have offered a vision of an age-integrated society where education, work, and leisure are allocated more equally across the life span. How do people envision this allocation? How do these visions vary by subpopulations within our society? Also, Freedman points out in Chapter 11 of this volume that all productivity is not created equal—some forms may hold greater promise to the individual, family, community, and society. Research could address the relative merits of various types of productive activity, from the perspective of older adults and younger adults.

These questions are particularly important to minority elders, whose life experiences in regards to work, caregiving, and volunteering differ from those of white elders. Allen and Chin-Say (1990) point out that the meaning of leisure and retirement may be different due to the domination of paid and nonpaid work over leisure throughout their lives. Further, definitions of retirement may differ and self-identification as a retired person may differ among ethnic groups (Gibson & Burns, 1991; Zsemblik & Singer, 1990). The documentation of minority elders' preferences, expectations, concerns, and experiences regarding productive engagement in later life is an important area of research.

Through survey research, we know that many older adults say that they want to be more engaged. We should now move to testing if they will become more engaged in the face of various opportunities and incentives to do so. What types of programs and policies are the most effective in engaging older adults? When testing the effect of a program or policy on tapping the unused potential of the older population, several outcomes may indicate success: the number of previously inactive older adults who initiate involvement, an increased level of involvement, a longer period of sustained involvement, increased satisfaction of those who are engaged, or increased benefit to the individual, family, or community. Rowe and Kahn (1998) propose that we keep a national count of social contributions through unpaid productive activities, akin to the GDP; they suggest that this counting effort will lead to increased attention to programs and policies that support productive engagement in later life.

Factors Associated with Engagement

The extent to which our society can maximize productive behaviors by any of its citizens relies on the explanation of productive behaviors. Who engages in productive behaviors and why? Most studies have been specific to particular types of productive behavior. For example, people who work more in later life are more likely to be in better health, have fewer disabilities, have more education, and be self-employed (Gibson & Burns, 1991; Harlow, Swindell, & Turner, 1991). Older people who volunteer are more likely to be younger, to be more educated, to have better health, to have more economic resources, to be married, and to be more active religiously than those who do not volunteer (Chambre, 1993; Okun, 1994; Fischer & Schaffer, 1993). People who are caregivers are older, female, wives or daughters, and unemployed (Brody, 1990; Dwyer & Coward, 1991; Stone, Cafferata, & Sangl, 1987).

One of most important and consistent findings from this work is that age is a factor in engagement in the workforce, but less salient in volunteering and caregiving. Studies by Caro and Bass (1992) and Herzog et al. (1989) show that age-related decrease in total productive hours exists but this decrease in primarily a function of decreased hours of paid work and childcare; there are no major age differences in volunteer, housework, and home maintenance hours. Herzog and Morgan (1992) suggest that retirement from paid work is at least as much a function of age-based societal norms and policies as inherent limitations of any aging organism and that reduction in involvement does not generalize from employment to other productive activities. Chambre (1993) suggests that the link between volunteerism and age is further weakening, due to demographic and cultural changes. From these previous works, we can comfortably conclude that chronological age is only one of many factors associated with productive engagement; moreover, it is a weak factor. Previous work clearly points toward the study of institutional and organizational factors, rather than individual factors, in understanding productive engagement.

Unfortunately, there has not been any study of the multifaceted explanations of productivity that would allow us to draw conclusions about the relative contribution of various factors, including physical health, individual preferences and attitudes, learned behaviors, culture and social norms, and institutional structures. Although the conceptual model presented by Bass and Caro in Chapter 3 depicts the multiple levels of factors associated with engagement in productive activities, only parts of this model have been tested. It may not be possible to test the relative influence of these various multilevel factors (and Taylor and Bengtson in Chapter 6 warn against confusing micro and macro levels of analysis). However, this model should encourage researchers to explore the full set of possible explanatory factors.

In the research to date, there has been more focus on individual characteristics than on social structures. For example, Rowe and Kahn (1998) write about "what it takes to be productive," and they list health, function, participation in social relations, education, and self-efficacy. They do not list "opportunity" or "facilitative institutional structures." When challenged by Riley and Riley (1998) on the lack of attention to social structures in their thinking about successful aging, Rowe and Kahn (1998) point to intradisciplinary work and methodological challenges as limiting factors in their work. Glass et al. (1995) documented individual factors associated with changes in productivity in a three-year longitudinal study. They found that being hospitalized and having a stroke were risk factors for decline in productive engagement. Married elders were at significantly lower risk for decline in productivity than nonmarried, and black elders increased levels of productivity more than whites over the observation period. These authors point out that they do not have the data to consider the role of the larger institutional context or the environmental determinants of activity. Of course, it is easier to measure individuals than institutions; and this tendency confirms Estes and Mahakian's fear (Chapter 9) that we will make the individual responsible for productivity and that social/environmental factors will continue to be underresearched.

Previous research has solicited from elders the barriers they experience in productive engagement, and this work suggests that individual factors (e.g., health and family obligations) are more often cited than organizational or structural characteristics (e.g., transportation, nature of the assignment, and expenses) (Glickman & Caro, 1992). It appears that when queried about barriers to engagement, people are more likely to think of personal reasons than be attuned to characteristics of the organization or nature of the assignment. It may be that these personal barriers are the most powerful; but this approach to studying barriers to productive engagement invites findings that focus on the individuals. We propose that researchers ask different questions that focus on structural factors that enhance or impede engagement. We suggest a focus on structural factors because they are likely to be important; that is, if our society seeks to maximize the potential of its older citizens, then an increase in productive engagement is most likely to be achieved through manipulating policy and institutional factors. Additionally, by focusing on organizational structures, researchers will be actualizing the values about productivity articulated above and avoiding a focus on individuals.

There is a good deal of discussion in the literature about institutional policies and practices that limit employment of older workers—lack of training and retraining programs; inflexible work schedules; pension plans that discourage employment beyond a certain age; restrictive job certification procedures; weak enforcement of age discrimination laws; and lack of transitional or bridge job opportunities (Barth, McNaught, & Rizzi, 1993; O'Reilly & Caro, 1994). There is less discussion on organizational structures and volunteerism, but several concerns have been identified: the lack of attention that organizations pay to the specific concerns of older volunteers; the undemanding or unfulfilling nature of volunteer tasks; and the lack of training and supervision (Gerson, 1997; Glickman & Caro, 1992; Morris & Caro, 1996). In regards to caregiving, there are institutional structures that impact caregivers' ability and willingness to engage or continue in caregiver roles: the availability and affordability of formal services to assist with the caregiving tasks; tax credits and other financial incentives to offset costs; laws affecting job security (Family and Medical Leave Act); and company policies that affect elder care (Gonyea, 1997; Hooyman & Gonyea, 1995).

Through research, we should increase our understanding of the impact of these arrangements on the level of engagement and the cost-effectiveness of these arrangements. In the area of employment, we must demonstrate and evaluate the impact of job sharing, bridge employment, job retraining, "niche" employment, and benefit options on older workers and their employers. As O'Reilly and Caro (1994) point out, there have been only limited efforts by employers to design and demonstrate these strategies and very little research regarding their effectiveness. Rowe and Kahn (1998) suggest the introduction of the four-hour work module to increase flexibility in work arrangements to the potential benefit of younger and older workers alike. Bass, Quinn, and Burkhauser (1995) suggest that new policies provide part-time employees with pro-rated benefits and reduce private health care costs for employers employing older workers. We must increase efforts to understand how the characteristics of volunteer assignments affect involvement; the extent to which constructive working relationships between workers and volunteers can be achieved if volunteers assume more challenging roles; and the impact on different types of compensation or reimbursement on recruitment, commitment, and satisfaction (Morris & Caro, 1996). The issues regarding the nature of volunteer assignments are especially salient given the increasing educational levels of older volunteers and the likelihood that unskilled and clerical tasks will not be fulfilling (Chambre, 1993). In the area of caregiving, we should increase efforts to understand the impact of public policies, like tax credits or "cash and counseling" programs, on caregiving involvement. Gonyea (1997) warns that companies must now be family-friendly to be politically correct, but that policies that support elder care may not represent substantive organizational change.

Research on caregiving as a productive activity in later life may lead to greater resolution of a tension that seems to exist in our society: caregiving as productive activity versus caregiving as a threat to productivity. Caregiving, although included in most all definitions of productive aging, may be the least valued of the enumerated activities. Researchers focus on its negative consequences and evaluate services designed to prevent burnout. Caregivers are given respite to pursue other activities; and caregivers sacrifice current and future financial resources to undertake the responsibility. These perspectives have not encouraged the promotion of caregiving as a valued role (Doty & Miller, 1993). Yet, due to demographic changes ahead, caregivers will become scarcer and therefore more valuable to dependent elders, families, and society (U.S. Bureau of the Census, 1992). Programs and policies can be created or extended to encourage and reward caregivers for engaging in this productive role (Doty & Miller, 1993).

Finally, O'Reilly and Caro (1994) pose a most interesting question related to maximizing involvement of those switching between types of activities, for example, from working to volunteering or from working to caregiving: What institutional arrangements facilitate transition from one productive activity to another? Findings in the volunteer literature highlight the importance of this question. In one study, 33 percent of older adults who were not currently volunteering were volunteers in the past, and reasons for stopping volunteering included assignment completed, moved to new area, and organization closed down (Glickman & Caro, 1992). Chambre (1993) suggests that volunteer opportunities should be responsive to seasonal migration patterns of retirees, who may be willing to continue volunteer involvement in various locations. Innovations in ensuring continuity among volunteer experiences may retain these older adults as experienced volunteers. Along these lines, we should increase understanding about facilitating transitions in the workplace as older workers move from full-time work to part-time work or less demanding work before full-time retirement. This is a growing trend among older workers (Quinn, 1997) and a common practice in Japan (Bass, 1994). We should further explore workers' and employers' expectations and desires regarding this transition within the employment sector. We also need to test institutional structures that give caregivers a choice to move between work and caregiving, or do both simultaneously with less negative consequences.

Valuation of Productive Activity

Research on the costs and benefits of various policies and programs that affect productive engagement depends in part on estimating the value of activities. Scholarly work on the valuation of productive activities has begun but there is much to do. This work is challenging, and Estes and Mahakian (Chapter 9) state that the task of valuing nonmarket efforts in this society where the market is king is formidable. When activities fall outside of the market economy, they have been invisible, socially and economically; and scholars have discussed the biases inherent in counting only paid work as productive (Herzog et al., 1989; Arno, Levine, & Memmott, 1999). It is clear that this traditional approach has severely underestimated the productive contributions of all ages, but that women more than men, and older adults more than younger adults have been disadvantaged (Rowe & Kahn, 1998). As part of the research agenda on productivity in later life, we should develop better techniques to estimate the value of the full range of productive activities. These valuation techniques will allow cost-benefit and cost-effectiveness analyses of programs and policies seeking to maximize productive engagement. Additionally, the development and use of better valuation methods may increase understanding about the full value of certain activities that to date have been underestimated, such as caregiving or civic engagement.

Current research often uses cost-to-purchase (wage rate) or opportunity cost as the measurement strategy to assess the value of volunteering, caregiving, and household maintenance activities. For example, a recent study uses a cost-to-purchase approach to conclude that caregivers provided $196 billion of service to this country in 1997 (Arno, Levine, & Memmott, 1999). Coleman (1995) uses the cost-to-purchase approach to estimate that current volunteer and caregiving activities of older adults are worth $102 billion. He argues that this substantial figure demonstrates the critical contributions that older adults make, outside the marketplace, to businesses, charitable organizations, and families. Further, by estimating that another $33 billion can be added by those older adults who report being willing and able to work or volunteer, he argues for increased investment in attracting older adults to these activities.

To date, studies regarding the value of late-life productivity resemble descriptive studies of amount of time devoted to work, volunteer, and caregiving activities in that they both seek to document extent of involvement and to impress readers with the contribution that is currently being made by older adults. Perhaps valuation studies advance this argument further by attaching a monetary value. They provide a more compelling challenge to the view of older adults as nonproductive and as a burden, and they are extremely useful in convincing the public or Congress to take the productive contribution of older adults seriously. However, the data remain largely descriptive, and future research should use valuation techniques for more analytic purposes. Researchers should address questions about the costs and benefits associated with programs and policies that affect caregiving, work, and volunteering; questions about how the value of activities affect older adults' participation rates; and questions about the effect of productive activities on the lives of individuals, families, and communities.

Analytic studies require sound estimation techniques; however, there are problems with these traditional approaches of valuing nonmarket activities of older adults. First of all, the cost-to-purchase and opportunity cost approaches are less applicable to productive activities in late life because opportunity costs are different for retired people and cost-to-purchase methodologies do not include other costs incurred or benefits reaped by the exchange. These monetary values fail to capture the emotional, cultural, and societal values expressed through informal caregiving (Arno, Levine, & Memmott, 1999) or volunteerism. For example, Herzog and Morgan (1992) point out that the wage rate for child care is low, yet there is widespread agreement that rearing the next generation successfully is extraordinarily valuable.

Further, these scholars demonstrate that different age and gender patterns in productivity result from different estimation techniques, and they present a "benefit approach" technique where the value of an activity is not specified in monetary terms. Rather, the beneficiaries of the activity use a Likert-type rating scale to fix the value of the action. Unlike monetary approaches, the benefit approach is applicable to all types of behavior and highlights the social benefit of activities. Using this approach, Herzog and Morgan (1992) demonstrated that child care is more valuable than its wage-rate value suggests. Rowe and Kahn (1998) also document that people rate unpaid work as highly as paid work in terms of benefit to themselves and higher in regard to benefit to others. Clearly, valuation approaches that capture social benefit in addition to monetary benefit are necessary, especially for cost-effectiveness studies.

Despite the groundbreaking work of costing productive activities in later life by Herzog and Morgan (1992) and Coleman (1995), greater consensus is needed on the best way to value the nonmarket activities that are included in most definitions of productive aging. It is essential that we utilize valuation strategies that mix economic and noneconomic estimation methods if we are to accurately represent the importance of all forms of productive activity. Furthermore, these estimation techniques must take into account the trade-offs that are made when older adults choose one activity over another (both within types of productive activities and across various types of activities). And not every effect is positive. Hidden costs should be assessed, such as the costs caregivers incur in health or mental health declines. Ultimately, solid valuation techniques must be available for researchers seeking to document the returns to the individual, family, and society on investments made in developing the productive potential of people in late life.

Capacity-Building for Productivity in Later Life

As Svanborg discusses in Chapter 4 of this volume, the functional capacity of the older population increased greatly in the last half of the twentieth century, and this increased capacity has been a major impetus behind the productive aging movement. As Freedman (Chapter 11) puts it, older adults represent a "vast reservoir of capacity." Despite the potential windfall of volunteers, workers, and caregivers to our society, we are only beginning to discuss how to develop this capacity for productive engagement. O'Reilly and Caro (1994) posed the question: "How can we strengthen skills and knowledge for productivity within each sector?" These authors point out that work-related training for older adults is limited and that educational institutions have not given high priority to strengthening the capacity of our older population.

Research has clearly demonstrated that physical and cognitive capacity of the current cohort of older adults can be enhanced and that older adults can learn and be trained for productive roles. Most of this research has been directed toward capacity-building among older adults for employment roles, and there is ample evidence that older adults can learn new skills required in the changing workplace (Rowe & Kahn, 1998; Sterns &

Sterns, 1995). Less attention has been paid to capacity-building for volunteering and caregiving.

Health, education, and experience are critical to productive capacity and both are harder to increase after lifelong deprivation. Further, continuity theory suggests that productive engagement in later life may stem from earlier opportunities and experiences, especially regarding volunteerism. In Chapter 10, Jackson argues that a life course perspective is important for understanding the involvement of older minority elders in social and economic networks. Thus, we propose that a research agenda on productivity in later life should focus on capacity-building across the life span. Knowledge regarding the most effective timing of capacity-development efforts is required. For example, it may be fruitful to focus capacity-building for volunteering in the middle years, when volunteerism is at its height and when patterns for the future are being established. It may be fruitful to focus capacity-building for providing care to grandchildren and disabled elders when these issues initially become salient in the person's life experience.

We suggest that the most fruitful research approach to capacity-building may focus on institutional capacity in contrast to individual capacity. There is a large body of institutional theory that asserts that societal institutions shape and give meaning to individual behavior (Beverly & Sherraden, 1999; Neale, 1987). Many important questions remain unanswered regarding the development of institutional capacity for productive engagement of older adults.

Morris and Caro (1996) challenged us to expand the capacity of community service organizations to assign more challenging responsibilities to older volunteers. In doing so, we must explore the extent to which older people respond to opportunities to make more significant contributions as volunteers and the circumstances under which community services can be restructured so that some responsibilities are shifted from paid personnel to volunteers. We should aim for greater understanding about the impacts of supervision, the match between participant's interest and his or her assignment, and the staff's relation to the volunteers. We should know the extent to which volunteers in meaningful roles threaten or displace paid workers (Chambre, 1987; Danzig & Szanton, 1987; Fischer & Schaffer, 1993).

The role of public policy in expanding involvement in productive roles is demonstrated by the Foster Grandparents and Senior Companion programs, where the government provides ongoing infrastructure to stimulate, support, and sustain service efforts. Freedman (1994) suggests that the government's niche may be in supporting high-commitment, stipended volunteer work aimed at community development. These national service programs raise many important questions that apply to both publicly supported programs for low-income elders and privately supported programs for a broader range of elders. How can access to these programs be increased?

Currently, many of these programs offer small compensations to offset transportation cost, to supplement income, and to provide minimum wages for community services rendered. Numerous questions should be raised about the impact of these incentives: How can we expand stipended programs beyond poor elders? How can we provide incentives to attract elders from all socioeconomic backgrounds? What are pros and cons of alternative forms of compensation, such as tax credits, service credits, education credits, and long-term care credits (Peter D. Hart Research Associates, 1999)? What is the cost-effectiveness of various strategies?

As for caregiving, we should increase our understanding of the capacity of programs and policies to make caregiving roles more attractive, less burdensome (Applebaum, 1997). On a larger scale, we should continue to test ideas about such matters as giving caregivers tax credits, allowing caregivers to accrue Social Security benefits during caregiving periods, and allowing care recipients receiving public subsidies to use that money to pay relatives for caregiving services. We should focus research on the capacity of legal, financial, and governmental institutions to support caregiving involvement as opposed to focusing on individual capacity of the caregiver.

A research agenda on increasing institutional capacity for productivity in later life could focus on constructs such as number of productive roles, types and nature of roles, and linkages to roles, including information about, access to, incentives for, and facilitation of roles. As discussed in the previous chapter, institutions can create roles, increase the number of roles, improve the quality of roles, change the nature of roles, or provide more or less information about the availability of roles. Institutional arrangements can increase access to roles. Incentives can influence individuals' appraisals about the value of the role in their lives. Facilitation, including training, support, and elimination of ongoing barriers, may lead to sustained involvement and more positive outcomes. These concepts provide researchers with ways of measuring institutional characteristics and forwarding a research agenda on institutional capacity in regards to late-life productivity. It will be important in this line of inquiry to keep issues of gender, race, and class inequities vis-à-vis institutional capacity in the forefront.

The Impact of Productive Engagement in Later Life

To some extent, there is an assumption in the productive aging literature that productive engagement, in and of itself, is a good thing. This assumption may stem from gerontology's roots in activity theory. Bass and Caro's model (Chapter 3) presents participation rates as the dependent variable in the conceptual framework. Evidence suggests that participation is a positive end in itself; and certainly, productivity rates may be the outcome of interest in evaluations of policies and programs designed to increase engagement. We suggest that researchers should test the effects of productive involvement on the individual, the family, the community, and society. In such studies, participation is an intermediate outcome that determines ultimate outcomes of a broader nature.

Considerable evidence demonstrates the positive impact of productive engagement on the individual. A long tradition in health and mental health research associates engagement in meaningful roles and social involvement with positive outcomes (as examples, see Berkman & Syme, 1979; Billings & Moos, 1982; Mendes de Leon et al., 1999; Moen, 1998). Some studies look specifically at the positive benefit of productive engagement in later life. For example, Herzog, House, and Morgan (1991) find that older people whose work patterns reflect their personal preferences report higher levels of physical and psychological well-being than people whose involvement in work is not under their control due to involuntary retirement or other factors. Moen, Dempster-McClain, and Williams (1992) studied women over time and document that participating in volunteer work and belonging to an organization are positively related to various measures of health. Musick, Herzog, and House (1999) documented in a prospective study that older adults who volunteer have lower mortality hazard than nonvolunteers. Freedman (1994) reviewed the evidence of the psychological and social benefits associated with participation in national service programs, including Senior Companions and Foster Grandparents. Although evaluation methods vary, some wait-list control studies show positive effects of participation on mental health functioning and life satisfaction.

Overall, there is enough evidence from related studies of health, mental health, and life satisfaction to conclude that engagement in productive roles is beneficial to the participant's well-being. However, we should pursue a more refined research agenda that considers differential impacts of this engagement on subpopulations (minority elders, chronically ill elders, etc.); differential impacts of various types of productive engagement on the participant; and differential impacts of various institutional structures. Musick, Herzog, and House (1999) demonstrate the importance of specification of conditions leading to positive outcomes by documenting that volunteers are not affected equally by their participation. This research reveals a curvilinear relationship between level of involvement and mortality, with moderate involvement offering the most benefit. Although their findings are not conclusive, their work suggests that volunteering has the most protective effect on those older adults with lower levels of informal social interaction. Similarly, Rushing, Ritter, and Burton (1992) report that for whites, being employed is a protective factor for mortality, whereas blacks, whether employed or unemployed, are at greater risk for poorer health. These studies demonstrate that future research on benefits of productive engagement to the individual must move toward specification of these relationships within the context of the individual's life and the context of certain organizational structures.

Similarly, research on outcomes of caregiving shows the need to specify the conditions of the involvement on consequences for the caregiver. Given evidence that there are positive and negative outcomes associated with caregiving, we should seek to better understand what conditions of engagement maximize positive outcomes for the caregiver. There is abundant evidence, from almost 20 years of research, that caregiving for a dependent relative can negatively impact a person's physical health, mental health, and financial status (Cantor, 1983; George & Gwyther, 1986; Doty & Miller, 1993; Wilcox & King, 1999). Therefore, some individuals may benefit from respite from one type of productive engagement (e.g., caregiving) to engage in another that carries different benefits and costs for that person (e.g., employment). This example of exchanging productive engagement in caregiving for engagement in employment highlights questions about transitions between sectors of productive engagement and about policies and organizational structures that provide choice to individuals for productive involvement, depending on individual preferences, cultural preferences, and family circumstances. Gender and race issues are of importance in this line of inquiry because movement between these types of productivity is more frequent for women and minority elders, and financial costs are associated with going in and out of the employment sector. It would be helpful to demonstrate policies and programs that reduce the cost of choosing caregiving over other types of productive engagement.

Some studies of productive engagement focus on benefits to service recipients. For example, evaluations of intergenerational tutoring programs document academic gains and behavioral improvements of the children (Hamon & Koch, 1993; Dellman-Jenkins, Lambert, & Fruit, 1991). Caregiving research documents the benefits to care recipients, in terms of reduction of unmet needs and life satisfaction (Kane & Kane, 1987). We suggest a research agenda that focuses on benefits beyond individuals— benefits to communities and society. In productive aging discussions, there are aspirations about the potential role of older volunteers in alleviating the country's pressing domestic problems, bolstering our nation's flagging sense of community, and increasing intergenerationalism (Freedman, 1994). The potential of older adults to increase community through civic engagement has been noted by Putnam (1994). However, these potential societal impacts may be overstated, and it is not clear if these impacts can be estimated, simulated, or measured directly.

Cost-benefit and cost-effectiveness analyses of programs and policies that maximize engagement should assess benefits at multiple levels. Trade-offs to increased productive behavior should be considered at each of these levels as well, as there may be risks and potential downsides of increased participation.

Theoretical Considerations in Developing a Research Agenda

Scholars have expressed the concern that productive aging research is developing without the use of guiding theoretical frameworks. In fact, work in this area reflects Bengtson and Schaie's (1999) observation that gerontology is data rich and theory poor. There is a wealth of survey data about work, volunteer, and caregiving activities; but fewer efforts use theory to explain processes and outcomes of productive involvement. In this chapter, we suggest a number of important research questions, and we urge scholars to adopt specific theoretical perspectives when they shape questions and interpret findings. As Bengtson and Schaie predict, there will be an "avalanche" of data about later-life phenomena, and the use of theory is critical to the cumulative development of knowledge regarding productive aging.

Many theoretical perspectives will prove useful to productive aging researchers. In Chapter 3 of this volume, Bass and Caro's model highlights the complexity of factors that affect productive engagement as well as points to the need for multidisciplinary nature of the research. Various theoretical perspectives can be used to explore specific relationships. As Taylor and Bengtson suggest in Chapter 6, different theories will be more useful for different levels of analyses. For example, social exchange theory may be helpful in studying individual motivation and participation level; and political economy perspectives may be helpful in focusing on public policies that affect the assignment of roles and responsibilities and how these relationships vary according to factors like race and gender. The life course perspective and role theory have influenced research in this area, and these frameworks will continue to be influential. Critical gerontology perspectives may influence the development of concrete experiments that create new roles for older adults, and as Moody (Chapter 8) hopes, widen the sense of possibility for later life.

From our perspective, the aging and society paradigm (Riley, Foner, & Riley, 1999) offers promise in forwarding a research agenda that focuses on social structures that facilitate late-life productivity. This paradigm considers the interplay between individual lives and social structures, helping us further explore and explain how individual lives and social structure evolve and effect each other as each changes to accommodate the phenomena of an aging society. The model offered in the previous chapter highlights the dynamic relationship between individuals and social structures in regards to late-life productivity. Institutional capacity and individual capacity together lead to productive behavior, and outcomes from this engagement in turn change individuals and institutions.

Conclusion

Overall, we have a good deal of descriptive information about levels of productive engagement of older adults, about the potential for increased involvement, and about individual factors related to engagement. Researchers should move from the descriptive to the analytic and evaluative. Regarding the analytic, we suggest the use of well-specified theory to explore factors associated with productive engagement, with a focus on social and organizational structures. Regarding the evaluative, researchers should test the actualization of productive potential through the demonstration of programs. Whenever possible, cost-effectiveness analyses that capture the full value of nonmarket activities should accompany demonstration programs.

We are concerned that the focus of research has been on the individual (which results in part from our person-focused research methodologies), fueling worries that productive aging will lead to a devaluation and further marginalization of "unproductive" elders. In our view, productivity in later life is more about social institutions, policies, and programs than about individuals. As stated by O'Reilly and Caro (1994): "A clear and direct pathway to improving productivity for older people lies in strengthening institutional supports for them." Thus, we suggest that further research should emphasize social institutions more than individuals. We propose a focus on institutional variables such as number, type and nature of roles, and linkages to these roles (information, access, incentive, and facilitation). As a general policy principle, we suggest that the ultimate limiting factors for productivity should be individual capacity and interest, not institutional capacity.

For the long run, it may be useful to focus on factors early in life that affect late-life productivity, indeed productivity across the life span, particularly health and education. With this focus on capacity-building at the individual level, research agendas on productivity in later life and successful aging overlap, which is consistent with a perception that productivity may be one aspect of successful aging. In fact, the unique importance of productive activity in the larger context of successful aging should be explored, building on Rowe and Kahn's (1998) proposition that there are three main components of successful aging: low probability of disease, high mental and physical functioning, and active engagement in life.

Since Robert Butler and his colleagues introduced the term *productive aging* almost 20 years ago, scholarship on the topic has come quite a long way. Beginning with an advocacy agenda, researchers collected data to demonstrate the contributions of older adults to society and to challenge the negative images of aging that prevailed. As academic and public discussions increasingly focused on the costs of population aging, productive aging proponents pointed to a potential windfall of human resources. Although productive capacity of older adults is limited to some extent by age-related decline, productive aging scholars argued that this is not the entire picture. They discussed outdated social policies, organizational structures, and employment practices that restrict the opportunities for older adults to remain productive.

As questions arose about the process and outcomes of various forms of productivity in later life, the advocacy agenda shifted to a research agenda. A body of literature began to take shape, although its boundaries are still diffuse. As in most fields of inquiry, this study has proceeded without the advantages of commonly accepted definitions and guiding theoretical frameworks. This volume has devoted attention to these definitional and theoretical issues as well as to research questions that deserve attention. Hopefully, these discussions will help galvanize and coalesce scholarship on productive aging, with the promise of generating a solid knowledge base for policy and program developments related to the productive engagement of older adults.

References

Allen, K., & Chin-Say, V. (1990). A lifetime of work: The context and meanings of leisure for aging black women. *The Gerontologist, 30,* 734–742.

Applebaum, B. (1997). The emergence of community-based long term care. *The Public Policy and Aging Report, 8,* 3–5.

Arno, P., Levine, C., & Memmott, M. (1999). The economic value of informal caregiving. *Health Affairs, 18,* 182–188.

Barth, M. (1997, July 25). Older workers: Perception and reality, U.S. Senate Special Committee on Aging Forum.

Barth, M., McNaught, W., & Rizzi, P. (1993). Corporations and the aging workforce. In P. Mirvis (Ed.), *Building a competitive workforce* (pp. 156–200). New York: John Wiley & Sons.

Bass, S. (1994). *Productive aging and the role of older people in Japan.* New York: The Japan Society and the International Leadership Center on Longevity and Society.

Bass, S. (Ed.). (1995). *Older and active: How Americans over 55 are contributing to society.* New Haven: Yale University Press.

Bass, S., Caro, F., & Chen, Y.-P. (Eds.). (1993). *Achieving a productive aging society.* Westport, CT: Auburn House.

Bass, S., Quinn, J. F., & Burkhauser, R. V. (1995). Toward pro-work policies and programs for older Americans. In S. Bass (Ed.), *Older and active: How Americans over 55 are contributing to society* (pp. 263–294). New Haven: Yale University Press.

Bengtson, V. L., & Schaie, K. W. (Eds.). (1999). *Handbook of theories of aging.* New York: Springer.

Berkman, L., & Syme, S. (1979). Social network, host resistance and mortality. *American Journal of Epidemiology, 109,* 186–204.

Beverly, S. G., & Sherraden, M. (1999). Institutional determinants of saving: Implications for low-income households and public policy. *Journal of Socio-Economics, 28* (4).

Billings, A. G., & Moos, R. H. (1982). Social support and functioning among community and clinical groups: A panel model. *Journal of Behavioral Medicine, 5* (3), 295–311.

Brody, E. (1990). *Women in the middle.* New York: Springer.

Cantor, M. H. (1983). Strain among caregivers: A study of experience in the United States. *The Gerontologist, 23,* 597–604.

Caro, F., & Bass, S. (1992). *Patterns of productivity among older Americans.* Boston: Gerontology Institute, University of Massachusetts Boston.

Caro, F., & Bass, S. (1995a). Dimensions of productive engagement. In S. Bass (Ed.), *Older and active: How Americans over 55 are contributing to society* (pp. 204–216). New Haven: Yale University Press.

Caro, F., & Bass, S. (1995b). Increasing volunteering among older people. In S. Bass (Ed.), *Older and active: How Americans over 55 are contributing to society* (pp. 71–96). New Haven: Yale University Press.

Chambre, S. M. (1987). *Good deeds in old age. Volunteering by the new leisure class.* Lexington, MA: Lexington Books.

Chambre, S. M. (1993). Volunteerism by elders: Past trends and future prospects. *The Gerontologist, 33* (2), 221–228.

Coleman, K. (1995). The value of productive aging of older Americans. In S. Bass (Ed.), *Older and active: How Americans over 55 are contributing to society* (pp. 169–203). New Haven: Yale University Press.

Danzig, R., & Szanton, P. (1987). *National service: What would it mean?* Lexington, MA: Lexington Books.

Dellman-Jenkins, M., Lambert, D., & Fruit, D. (1991). Fostering preschoolers' prosocial behaviors toward the elderly: The effect of an intergenerational program. *Educational Gerontology, 17,* 21–32.

Doty, P., & Miller, B. (1993). Caregiving and productive aging. In S. A. Bass, F. G. Caro, & Y.-P. Chen (Eds.), *Achieving a productive aging society.* Westport, CT: Auburn House.

Dwyer, J. W., & Coward, R. T. (1991). A multivariate comparison of the involvement of adult sons versus daughters in the care of impaired parents. *Journal of Gerontology: Social Sciences, 46,* S259–S269.

Fischer, L. R., & Schaffer, K. B. (1993). *Older volunteers: Enlisting the talent.* Newbury Park, CA: Sage.

Freedman, M. (1994). *Seniors in national and community service: A report prepared for the Commonwealth Fund's Americans Over 55 at Work Program.* Philadelphia: Public/Private Ventures.

Friedland, R. (1997). Lesson from the past and opportunities for the future: The labor market for older workers. *The Public Policy and Aging Report, 8,* 9–19.

Gallagher, D., Rose, J., Rivera, P., Lovett, S., & Thompson, L. W. (1989). Prevalence of depression in family caregivers. *The Gerontologist, 29,* 449–456.

George, L., & Gwyther, L. (1986). Caregiver well-being: A multidimensional examination of family caregivers of demented adults. *The Gerontologist, 26* (3).

Gerson, D. (1997, April 28). Do do gooders do as much good: Most volunteers aren't solving core problems. *U.S. News & World Report, 122* (16), 26–33.

Gibson, R. C., & Burns, C. J. (1991). The health, labor force, and retirement experiences of aging minorities. *Generations, 15,* 31–35.

Glass, T., Seeman, T., Herzog, A. R., Kahn, R., & Berkman, L. (1995). Change in productive activity in late adulthood: MacArthur Studies of Successful Aging. *Journals of Gerontology, 50B* (2), S65–S76.

Glickman, L., & Caro, F. (1992). *Improving the recruitment and retention of older volunteers.* College Park, MD: National Eldercare Institute on Employment and Volunteerism.

Gonyea, J. (1997). The real meaning of balancing work and family. *The Public Policy and Aging Report, 8,* 1–8.

Hamon, R., & Koch, D. (1993). The elder mentor relationship: An experiential learning tool. *Educational Gerontology, 19,* 147–159.

Harlow, K. S., Swindell, D., & Turner, M. J. (1991). *Productivity in late life: Does contribution continue?* (Agedata: Special Issues report #16). South Bend, IN: Heartland Center on Aging, Disability and Long Term Care.

Herzog, A. R., & House, J. S. (1991). Productive activities and aging well. *Generations, 15* (1), 49–54.

Herzog, A. R., House, J., & Morgan, J. N. (1991). Relation of work and retirement to health and well-being. *Psychology and Aging, 6* (2).

Herzog, A. R., Kahn, R. L., Morgan, J. N., Jackson, J. S., & Antonucci, T. C. (1989). Age differences in productive activities. *Journal of Gerontology: Social Sciences, 44,* S129–S138.

Herzog, A. R., & Morgan, J. N. (1992). Age and gender differences in the value of productive activities. *Research on Aging, 14* (2), 169–198.

Holstein, M. (1992). Productive aging: A feminist critique. *Journal of Aging and Social Policy, 4* (3–4), 17–33.

Hooyman, N. R., & Gonyea, J. (1995). *Feminist perspectives on family care: Politics for gender justice.* Thousand Oaks, CA: Sage.

Kane, R., & Kane, R. (1987). *Long term care.* New York: Springer.

Kaplan, G. A., Strawbridge, W. J., Camacho, T., & Cohen, R. D. (1993). Factors associated with change in physical functioning in the elderly: A six-year prospective study. *Journal of Aging and Health, 5* (1), 140–153.

Marriott Seniors Volunteerism Study. (1991). Commissioned by Marriott Senior Living Services and United States Administration on Aging. Washington, DC: Marriott Senior Living Services.

McIntosh, B. R., & Danigelis, N. L. (1995). Race, gender, and the relevance of productive activity for elders' affect. *Journal of Gerontology: Social Sciences, 50B,* S229–S239.

Mendes de Leon, C. F., Glass, T. A., Beckett, L. A., Seeman, T. E., Evans, D. A., & Berkman, L. F. (1999). Social networks and disability transitions across eight intervals of yearly data in the New Haven EPESE. *Journal of Gerontology: Social Sciences, 54B* (3), S162–S172.

Moen, P. (1998). Women's roles and health: A life-course perspective. In K. Orth-Gomer, M. Chesney, and N. Wenger (Eds.), *Women, stress, and heart disease* (pp. 111–132). Mahwah, NJ: Erlbaum.

Moen, P., Dempster-McClain, D., & Williams, R. (1992). Successful aging: A life-course perspective on women's multiple roles and health. *American Journal of Sociology, 97* (6), 1612–1638.

Morris, R., & Caro, F. (1996). Productive retirement: Stimulating greater volunteer efforts to meet national needs. *The Journal of Volunteer Administration, 14* (2), 5–13.

Musick, M., Herzog, R., & House, J. (1999). Volunteering and mortality among older adults: Findings from a national sample. *Journal of Gerontology: Social Sciences, 54B,* S173–S180.

Neale, W. (1987). Institutions. *Journal of Economic Issues, 3,* 1177–1206.

Okun, M. (1994). The relation between motives for organizational volunteering and frequency of volunteering by the elderly. *Journal of Applied Gerontology, 13,* 115–126.

O'Reilly, P., & Caro, F. (1994). Productive aging: An overview of the literature. *Journal of Aging and Social Policy, 6,* 39–71.

Peter D. Hart Research Associates. (1999). *The changing face of retirement: Older Americans, civic engagement, and the longevity revolution.* Washington, DC: Author.

Putnam, R. (1994). Bowling alone: America's declining social capital. *Journal of Democracy, 6* (1), 65.

Quinn, J. (1997). Retirement trends and patterns in the 1990's. *The Public Policy and Aging Report, 8,* 10–14.

Riley, M. W., Foner, A., & Riley, J. W., Jr. (1999). The aging and society paradigm. In V. L. Bengtson & K. W. Schaie (Eds.), *Handbook of theories of aging* (pp. 327–343). New York: Springer.

Riley, M. W., & Riley, J. W., Jr. (1994). Age integration and the lives of older people. *The Gerontologist, 34* (1), 110–115.

Rowe, J., & Kahn, R. (1998). *Successful aging.* New York: Pantheon.

Rushing, B., Ritter, C., & Burton, R. P. D. (1992). Race differences in the effects of multiple roles on health: Longitudinal evidence from a national sample of older men. *Journal of Health and Social Behavior, 33* (2), 126–139.

Russo, J., Vitaliano, P. P., Brewer, D. D., Katon, W., & Becker, J. (1995). Psychiatric disorders in spouse caregivers of care recipients with Alzheimer's disease and matched controls: A diathesis-stress model of psychopathology. *Journal of Abnormal Psychology, 104,* 197–204.

Schulz, R., Visintainer, P., & Williamson, G. M. (1990). Psychiatric and physical morbidity effects of caregiving. *Journal of Gerontology: Psychological Sciences, 45,* P18–P191.

Seeman, T. E., Berkman, L. F., Charpentier, P. A., Blazer, D. G., Albert, M. S., & Tinetti, M. E. (1995). Behavioral and psychosocial predictors of physical performance: MacArthur Studies of Successful Aging. *Journal of Gerontology: Medical Sciences, 50A* (4), M177–M184.

Sicker, M. (1994). The paradox of productive aging. *Ageing International, 21* (2), 12–14.

Sterns, H., & Sterns, A. (1995). Health and employment capability of older Americans. In S. Bass (Ed.), *Older and active: How Americans over 55 are contributing to society* (pp. 10–34). New Haven: Yale University Press.

Stone, R., Cafferata, G. L., & Sangl, J. (1987). Caregivers of the frail elderly: A national profile. *The Gerontologist, 27,* 616–626.

Strawbridge, W. J., Cohen, R. D., Shema, S. J., & Kaplan, G. A. (1996). Successful aging: Predictors and associated activities. *American Journal of Epidemiology, 144,* 135–141.

The Commonwealth Fund. (1993). *The untapped resource: The final report of the Americans Over 55 at Work Program.* New York: Author.

U.S. Bureau of the Census. (1992). Current Population Reports, P25-1092, *Population projections of the U.S. by age, sex, race, and Hispanic origin: 1992–2050.* Washington, DC: U.S. Government Printing Office.

Valliant, G. E., & Vailliant, C. O. (1990). Natural history of male psychological health: A 45-year study of predictors of successful aging. *American Journal of Psychiatry, 147,* 31–37.

Wilcox, S., & King, B. (1999). Sleep complaints in older women who are family caregivers. *Journal of Gerontology, 54B,* P189–P198.

Zsemblik, B. A., & Singer, A. (1990). The problem of defining retirement among minorities: The Mexican Americans. *The Gerontologist, 30* (6), 749–757.

INDEX

AARP, ix, 115, 253, 268
Achenbaum, W. Andrew, xi, 6, 19–34, 282, 288
Achieving a Productive Aging Society (Bass, Caro, and Chen), 7
ACL. *See* Americans' Changing Lives Study
activities, productive: *versus* busyness, 11–12, 146, 181, 245; and life portfolio, xii, 107, 262; tables of, 230–34; value of, 108, 214–15, 227–28, 281, 296–98. *See also* caregiving; education; employment; volunteer work
activity theory, 6, 121, 128–29, 163, 181, 215, 301
ADA, 51–52, 68
Adams, John, 23
Adams, John Quincy, 23
advocacy: and ageism, 5–7, 181, 191; agenda for, ix–x, 185, 286, 305–6; for productive aging, 4–5, 38, 184, 191, 260, 289
African Americans, 26, 227. *See also* race
Age and Achievement (Lehman), 31
Age Discrimination in Employment Act (1967), vii, 33, 68
ageism, 2, 20, 26, 122, 183; and advocacy, 5–7, 181, 191; and

discrimination, vii, 10, 33, 44, 50–51, 68, 164, 182; and human rights, viii, 197, 210; institutionalized, 9, 53–54
age stratification, 133–35, 138, 163–64, 182–83, 215, 262, 290
aging: and apocalyptic demography, 175, 181; and assisted suicide, 179; of baby boomers, vii, ix, 58, 149–53, 176, 179, 188, 248, 252, 256; biomedical perspective on, xii, 6, 8–9, 14, 81–97, 200–201, 261, 270; conscious, xiii, 137, 176, 186–87, 192, 263, 286; costs of, 19, 37, 131, 149–53, 163, 281; and disease, viii, 50, 81–87, 124, 305; and economic status, 12, 14, 31, 121–22, 146, 228; and elements of transcendence, 166, 186, 286–87; exogenous factors of, xii, xv, 81, 85–88, 91–96, 198–200, 261, 276; genetics of, viii, 50, 81, 86–87, 114, 180; inequalities in, 124, 128, 184, 206, 209–10; life course perspective on, 133, 138, 187–91, 215, 290–91, 299, 304; longitudinal studies on, xiv, 14–15, 86–87, 228, 293; negative images of, 4–6, 25–27, 32–33, 54, 160, 166, 288–89; of population, 82, 157, 175, 188, 215, 248; positive images of, 34, 103–4, 117, 120, 122, 127, 176, 192;